T0331732

A Concise History of Veterinary Medicine

From Ayurvedic texts to botanical medicines to genomics, ideas and expertise about veterinary healing have circulated between cultures through travel, trade, and conflict. In this broad-ranging and accessible study spanning 400 years of history, Susan D. Jones and Peter A. Koolmees present the first global history of veterinary medicine and animal healing. Drawing on inter-disciplinary and multidisciplinary perspectives, this book addresses how attitudes toward animals, disease causation theories, wars, problems of food insecurity, and the professionalization and spread of European veterinary education have shaped new domains for animal healing, such as preventive medicine in intensive animal agriculture and the need for veterinarians specializing in zoo animals, wildlife, and pets. It concludes by considering the politicization of animal protection, changes in the global veterinary workforce, and concerns about disease and climate change. As mediators between humans and animals, veterinarians and other animal healers have both shaped and been shaped by the social, cultural, and economic roles of animals over time.

SUSAN D. JONES is a Distinguished McKnight University Professor at the University of Minnesota and a trained veterinarian and historian. Along with her co-author, Peter A. Koolmees, she served as co-president of the World Association for the History of Veterinary Medicine, 2008–2014.

EMERITUS PROFESSOR PETER A. KOOLMEES is a member of the Descartes Centre for the History and Philosophy of the Sciences and the Humanities of Utrecht University and a trained BSc and historian. He served as president in 2000–2004, and co-president in 2008–2014, of the World Association for the History of Veterinary Medicine.

New Approaches to the History of Science and Medicine

This dynamic new series publishes concise but authoritative surveys on the key themes and problems in the history of science and medicine. Books in the series are written by established scholars at a level and length accessible to students and general readers, introducing and engaging major questions of historical analysis and debate.

Other Books in the Series

A Concise History of Veterinary Medicine

Susan D. Jones
University of Minnesota

Peter A. Koolmees
Utrecht University

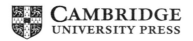
CAMBRIDGE
UNIVERSITY PRESS

CAMBRIDGE
UNIVERSITY PRESS

University Printing House, Cambridge CB2 8BS, United Kingdom

One Liberty Plaza, 20th Floor, New York, NY 10006, USA

477 Williamstown Road, Port Melbourne, VIC 3207, Australia

314–321, 3rd Floor, Plot 3, Splendor Forum, Jasola District Centre, New Delhi – 110025, India

103 Penang Road, #05–06/07, Visioncrest Commercial, Singapore 238467

Cambridge University Press is part of the University of Cambridge.

It furthers the University's mission by disseminating knowledge in the pursuit of education, learning, and research at the highest international levels of excellence.

www.cambridge.org
Information on this title: www.cambridge.org/9781108420631
DOI: 10.1017/9781108354929

© Susan D. Jones and Peter A. Koolmees 2022

First published 2022

A catalogue record for this publication is available from the British Library.

ISBN 978-1-108-42063-1 Hardback
ISBN 978-1-108-43070-8 Paperback

Contents

Illustrations

Tables

Note on Translations

Translations from the following languages, into English, were completed by the authors: Dutch, German, Afrikaans, French, Spanish, Italian, and Russian. We thank the late Ivan Katič for translations from the Danish; Ilkka Alitalo for Finnish; Roar Gudding for Norwegian; R. Tamay Başağaç Gül for Turkish; Myung-Sun Chun for Korean; Junya Yasuda and Marcia Yonemoto for Japanese; Shawn Foster for Chinese; and Bíbor Bán'fi-Klekner for Hungarian. All errors are the responsibility of the authors alone.

Preface

In 2010, as members of the World Association for the History of Veterinary Medicine, we were fortunate to hold our annual congress in the delightful Mediterranean port of Antalya, Turkey. Over potent glasses of *raki*, our hosts immediately got down to business. Turkish law required all veterinary students to take a course in veterinary history. Where, our hosts asked, could they find a general textbook on the history of veterinary medicine to use in their courses? The book needed to be concise, written in English, with an international scope. We exchanged glances. No such book existed. We began then to think about writing this book. Our goal is to provide a broad framework, informed by global and world history, for the past 500 years of animal healing and veterinary medicine's development.

There is so much excellent research about the history of veterinary medicine and animal healing available. Unfortunately, we could not include all important events and research in a "concise" book. Instead, this book will trace broader themes that can (and should) be filled in with the exciting stories, discoveries, and episodes of each proud national tradition. As a global history, we have also sought to highlight the less well-known voices and stories, and to consider "veterinary medicine" as a broad set of animal care practices. Some of these stories are appearing in English for the first time, and they represent the authors' twenty-plus years of collaborating with scholars from around the world.

The daunting task of writing a global history of modern veterinary medicine could not be successfully completed without the work of many scholars. From Spain to South Korea and Kenya to Brazil, many people are interested in the history of animals and veterinary medicine. It is impossible for us to thank every person who has contributed to this book, but we have some special debts we would like to acknowledge. Our colleagues in the World Association for the History of Veterinary Medicine have generously shared their own research with us, and we especially thank: Ilkka Alitalo, Tamay Başağaç Gül, Martin Brumme, Myung-Sun Chun, Ferruh Dinçer, John Fisher, Joaquín Sánchez de Lollano, Miguel Marquez, Johann Schäffer, and Abigail Woods. We remember scholars no longer with us whose work informs veterinary history, especially: Jean Blancou, Miguel Cordero del Campillo, Angela von den Driesch, Robert Dunlop, Denes Karasszon, Ivan Katič, William McNeill, Wilhelm Rieck, Leon Saunders, Calvin Schwabe, and Fred Smithcors. This book stands on their shoulders.

We thank our editor, Lucy Rhymer, and the staff at Cambridge University Press; and our employers, the Universities of Minnesota and Utrecht. Universiteit Utrecht's Descartes Center for the History and Philosophy of the Sciences and Humanities and its Director, Bert Theunissen, generously funded a writing semester together in Utrecht in 2018. Finally, history cannot be done without the substantial help of librarians, archivists, and museum curators. Of many, we specially mention Trenton Boyd, Christophe Degueurce, the late Ivan Katić, the late Guus Mathijsen, and Susanne Whitaker.

We are completing this book during two important historical events: the COVID-19 pandemic, caused by a coronavirus originating in wild bats and possibly spread by animals and raw food at open-air markets; and renewed concerns about worldwide socioeconomic inequality due to racism, discrimination, lack of education, wars, and colonialism, including the dangers of disease exposure and violence. These events have necessarily influenced how we address some of the issues in this book, specifically: the history of zoonotic diseases; the interactions between human populations and wildlife in the environment; the development of agricultural practices such as raising livestock in close confinement; and the roles of veterinarians in "One Health" and other approaches that help an increasing global population of humans live with disease risks.

COVID-19 has shown how pandemics can still cause serious disruptions of modern life despite advanced scientific knowledge and technological progress. At its basis is a reminder that people cannot simply control nature. Socioeconomic inequality still plays a role in the development of veterinary medicine in terms of possessing and exploiting food and other animals and enabling veterinary care for these animals. Therefore, we have sought to make this book inclusive of cultures, beliefs, and practices from around the world. Political ideology, religion, wars, and socioeconomic inequality, including ideas and practices on serfdom and slavery as well as social-Darwinist and other concepts of racism and discrimination, also influenced the history of human–animal relationships, and thus the development of veterinary medicine. Within these contexts we shall also address human and animal suffering from wars, epizootic and zoonotic pandemics, disturbed production, and supply of foods of animal origin, as well as the inclusion or exclusion of people from the veterinary profession based on gender, ethnicity, and other factors.

We have much work to do. Let us all, as informed citizens and dedicated professionals, pledge to use our abilities to make the world a better place for people, animals, and their environments.

Introduction
Human–Animal Relationships and the Need for Veterinary Medicine

The word "veterinary" can be traced back in time to the Latin *veterinum*, which meant "beast of burden." Of course, "veterinary" has come to include many types of animals, not only beasts of burden, and the history of animal healers and veterinarians is a rich one. This book is a synthesis of broad themes, not a catalogue of every important event or individual in veterinary history; indeed, that would be impossible in a concise history. Yet there are so many fascinating stories we want to tell from all around the world. In India, sacred animals (especially cattle) warranted special feeding and care; what happened when the British colonizers arrived (1800s), with their habit of eating beef? In eighteenth-century Spain, horses were more valuable than men on the battlefield; while in France, Charles Vial de St. Bel, first director of the London veterinary school, died in agony of glanders (a horse disease). The model of veterinary education still used today developed amidst the violence of the French and American revolutions (late 1700s), and veterinarians found themselves at the forefront of wars and imperial invasions for the next 150 years. Human–animal relationships and the need for animal healers have reflected the impacts of environmental changes, cultural encounters, food production, international trade, economic developments, and imperialism and colonialism. By focusing on the uses of animals for food, transport, the military, and companionship, we situate our history of veterinary medicine over the past 500 years within these broader perspectives while highlighting some of the stories and experiences that make this history so interesting.

"Veterinary medicine" can be defined as the diagnosis and treatment of animal health problems in the context of human–animal relationships. Therefore, we use a broad definition of "veterinary medicine" to include many types of animal healing throughout history. In each place and time, a veterinary marketplace existed that could include formally educated veterinarians, botanical healers, castrators, disease specialists, and many other types of animal healers (including the animal's owner). Today's veterinarians work in the spotlight of local and global social concerns. Whether an urban "pet vet,"

1

a manager of huge cattle populations on feedlots, a wildlife conservationist, medical researcher, or the last resort for a farmer with a sick animal, veterinarians mediate between the interests of animals and their owners, animal producers, consumers, and government authorities. It is a complex task, requiring more than just technical skills and knowledge. Like other animal healers through the centuries, today's veterinarians must understand the sociocultural and economic pressures driving (or limiting) their activities. For them, history is a guide that deepens their understanding of veterinary medicine today. We organize the chapters of this book around different problems and how people have responded to them over time: keeping animals alive and well in (sometimes) dangerous places and situations; communicating with individuals in multiple cultures; and working within political, economic, and social opportunities and constraints. Our goals are twofold: to frame veterinary history in the larger social and cultural context of global and world history, and to help students think critically about their profession and the broad scope of the sciences that inform it, from anatomy to epidemiology.

History also offers windows into how animals themselves have functioned as important actors in human history, and how their roles have affected the development of veterinary healing and medicine through time. Animals have shaped the human-built environment around the world: animals' needs determined the geographical spread of agricultural societies and structured cities while their labor powered industrialization, human migrations, and wars. Animal behaviors, as well as human interactions with them, have both guided and limited their healers' work. Therefore, every chapter will include attention to animals' behaviors, social lives, ecology, and environments as well as human sociocultural contexts. We also integrate the ever-changing philosophical thinking about human–animal relationships and how this impacted the treatment of animals. This contributes to our "new veterinary history" approach, which reflects relatively recent changes in the scholarship. The history of veterinary medicine is based on texts from antiquity onward, and scholars around the world specialize in translating and analyzing these classic texts. Over the past twenty-five years, professionally trained social historians have joined veterinary writers. They have built on and revised existing veterinary history, adding critical analysis to translations and narratives, broadening the focus beyond a handful of professional veterinarians and well-known scientists, and adopting new sources and methods from anthropology, environmental history, and global history. One milestone in global history, the beginning of the exchange between the Old and New Worlds, sets our choice of time period to begin around 1500. Although the scope of this book dictates narrowing the time period to the past 500 years, we next outline some of the major themes in earlier human–animal healing that inform this book.

Early Animal Healing

Domestication

The story of veterinary medicine begins with the age-old human problem: food. For thousands of years, humans fed themselves by hunting wild animals and gathering plants. Domesticating plants and animals yielded more food than the foraging way of life, resulting in denser human populations in permanent agricultural settlements. Domestication may be defined as selectively taming, feeding, and breeding animals in captivity, thereby modifying them from their wild ancestors for the benefit of humans. (Experts believe domestication started in the Middle East around 10,000 BCE.) On prehistoric farms, domesticated animals replaced wild animals as the main source of animal protein. Milking sheep, goats, bovines, or camels kept for several years produced much more food than when they were hunted and eaten as meat. Livestock also provided manure for fertilizer, contributing to higher crop yields.

Animals' superior muscle power created bigger fields and revolutionized agriculture. With the invention of the yoke, collar, hame, and harness, the power of oxen and horses could be applied to ploughing more soil for growing crops. The breast-strap or breast-collar, invented in China in the period 481–221 BCE, became known throughout Central Asia by the seventh century and was introduced to Europe by the eighth century. This preceded the horse collar, which is a part of a horse harness that is used to distribute the load around a horse's neck and shoulders when pulling a wagon or plough. A yoke is a wooden beam normally used between a pair of oxen or other animals to enable them to pull together on a load when working in pairs, as oxen usually do. There are several types of yokes used in different cultures, and for different types of oxen, horses, mules, donkeys, and water buffalo. When the horse was harnessed in the collar, the horse could apply 50 percent more power to a task than could an ox within the same time period, due to the horse's greater speed. For this reason, oxen were largely replaced by horses, a technological change that produced more food, boosted economies, and reduced reliance on subsistence farming. All these technologies not only increased the efficiency of agriculture (to feed rapidly growing human populations) but also increased the importance and value of the animals using them.

Domestication shaped the development of human societies in other ways. Taming horses, donkeys, and camels made it possible to transport people and heavy goods overland for long distances. Next to transport, horses became crucial in warfare, and their essential military role lasted into the twentieth century. First, horses were ridden bareback; later, they were yoked to wagons and battle chariots, which changed warfare in the Near East, the Mediterranean, and China dramatically. For instance, the Hyksos with their horse-drawn chariots conquered Egypt in 1674 BCE. Similarly, Attila the Hun invaded the Roman Empire with his horsemen. In South Asia, elephants were crucial beasts of war due to their strength, size, and ability to endure harsh conditions and attacks. Next to large mammals, small animals such as chickens, ducks, geese, guinea fowls, other birds, and insects (honeybees) were domesticated because of their usefulness for human societies. Some wolves co-evolved with humans, becoming dogs that worked as hunting companions and guards or supplied food or companionship. Cats began to live near human settlements to hunt mice and rats eating grain. Domestication meant increasing human control over nature, enabling the growth of ever-larger human populations.

Veterinary medicine is as old as the process of domesticating and utilizing these animals. Provision of veterinary care seems obvious because these animals were so valuable to agrarian societies. To secure and sustain food production, prehistoric farmers and shepherds worked to keep their horses, camels, elephants, sheep, goats, bovines, and pigs healthy. Traces of veterinary activities can be found in prehistory. For example, in 2018 paleo-pathologists found evidence for trepanation in a cow's skull from the Neolithic period found in France. Castration of bulls, healed broken legs in cattle, dog breeding, and crossbreeding horses and donkeys have also been well documented in the literature. Such ancient veterinary activities were performed by experts, probably mainly farmers and shepherds themselves. Disease in humans as well as in animals was probably considered the result of magical forces, a supernatural intervention, or a divine castigation. Thus, treatment of humans and animals was based on a combination of ritual healing and medical or surgical therapies that corresponded to theories about disease causation

Traces of Veterinary Medicine in Antiquity: Keeping Animals Healthy

We define these early veterinary activities broadly as keeping animals healthy (the formal veterinary profession only developed much later, as we discuss in Chapter 3). Archaeological and written sources, including bones, statuettes, murals, mosaics, and reliefs, show that animal diseases were a major problem for ancient societies. In 2015, archaeologists analyzed bones of cattle from the Middle East dating to 8,000 years ago and found the bones to be infected with bovine tuberculosis. The oldest written account of an animal disease is about rabies (caused by infected domesticated dogs). This infectious (zoonotic) disease, which is lethal for humans if not treated, was already feared in antiquity. One part of the legal code of Eshnunna, from ancient Mesopotamia (Tell Asmar in present-day Iraq) dated in the twentieth century BCE, states that the owner of a rabid dog had to pay a fine if his dog bit a human and caused death because the owner did not control his dog. Controlling diseases in animals used for food, transport, and agriculture was essential to the success of domestication, and human intervention in animal health is as old as domestication.

History helps us to interpret the activities of past peoples; histories show the continuity of change over time and the fact that past events could have created very different outcomes. For example, domestication progressed most rapidly in particular regions due to a combination of environmental and social developments. The existence of several domesticable species in the environment was crucial, but so was the development of social patterns that encouraged people to seek more efficient food production. Fast-forwarding several millennia, we see that we are shaped by the past but that nothing has been *inevitable*. Wars, famines, natural disasters: all these events affected different societies in different ways.

We must also remember these lessons of history when we explore veterinary history. Animal healing has a long history, but, of course, we can recover only a small part of it because many texts and other sources have not survived. A popular theme within veterinary history has been the search for the oldest known veterinarian in the ancient Middle East; however, from our point of view, this is a futile undertaking because animal healing was so obviously widespread by this time. We may never obtain the full picture of ancient animal healing. What we can do is to situate the surviving historical sources within the social activities and cultural beliefs of the time. We can gain some insight into how people and animals lived so long ago, and that insight has great value today. This new model of veterinary history focuses not just on "finding the first," but on understanding "the most": the histories of how the common people and their animals lived.

This new model of veterinary history also incorporates a global history approach, because most Western-based veterinary historians' works have not included information from unfamiliar cultures, especially those in Asia and Africa. But to explore early veterinary activities, we must investigate places such as ancient India, where Vedic tradition says that both human and animal medicine arose from observing how animals and birds healed themselves. Veterinary activities were part of the ancient *Ayurveda*, or science of life. During the Vedic period (c. 1500–500 BCE), cattle played important roles as sacred animals and prized possessions, and early animal hospitals and sanctuaries were dedicated to cattle. Early treatises also focused on the Asian elephant (prized in warfare and for transportation), but healing practices were well developed for many species. At this time, veterinary activities were financed by the state, and the emperor Ashoka the Great sponsored the early Ayurvedic veterinary hospitals (still visible in edicts engraved on pillars and rocks). Ashoka's motivation was reportedly spiritual: the practice of *dharma* linked human and animal welfare. Thus, these ancient institutionalized veterinary activities arose in a sacred society where early veterinary and medical practice was connected to sacred rituals and spiritual beliefs. Ayurvedic theories on physiology and health and disease spread from India into China via Buddhist texts and were successively linked to indigenous perceptions of human and animal bodies within a religious context.

Medical and veterinary practices in the ancient Arab and Mediterranean worlds were likewise related to religious rituals at first. Priest-physicians working in healing temples created theories of health and disease that guided their activities in human and animal healing. Although religion and rituals continued to play a role in medical treatments, a secular medicine based on natural theories of health and disease also emerged. Regular horse-doctors (ἱππιατρός or hippiatros) in ancient Greece appeared as early as 130 BCE, with one treatise naming "Metrodoros" as a hippiatros. The most renowned early Greek horse-doctor was probably Apsyrtos from Bithynia (c. 280–337 CE), who served in the cavalry of Constantine the Great and whose writings were praised for centuries. Apsyrtos outlined a coherent system of belief about animal diseases and based treatments on his theories. For example, he observed the contagious nature of anthrax, farcy, and glanders and as a result recommended isolation for sick animals.

During the Roman Empire, professional animal healers, responsible mainly for the health of equines, were known as *veterinarius* and *mulomedicus*. The Roman scholar Publius Vegetius Renatus (c. 385 CE) used the term "veterinarian" in his writings; Arabic scholars translated this to "*bitar*" or "*baytār*," meaning a surgeon of animals (especially horses). And this observation demonstrates another theme important in this book: both animals and medical knowledge about them traveled between very different cultures, often due to the activities of trading (economics) or conquest (war). This was certainly the case in Iberia (medieval Spain and Portugal), which Muslim armies invaded to establish the Islamic Al-Andalus region (711–1492), thereby bringing people, animals, and the learned traditions of Northern Africa and the Middle East into contact with Europe. The word for professional animal healers in medieval Iberia, *albeitar,* was derived from "*baytār*," and this was only the Western appendage of a much larger intellectual empire that extended into central Asia. The early development of veterinary specialization accelerated during the ancient period, when large groups of animals were used in agriculture, in armies, and in supplying the needs of enlarging human settlements.

Veterinary Activities in the Middle Ages: Translation and Exchange

Past historians of Europe characterized the centuries between c. 500 and 1000 CE as the Dark Ages, characterized by warfare, famine, and a decline in intellectual developments (including those associated with medicine and healing). Today we understand that the centers of intellectual development did not disappear; they shifted East and were thriving there by the time of the Iberian invasion in 711. Constantinople, the capital of the Byzantine Empire, was a center of scientific knowledge (further described in Chapter 1) during this time. Later, the Islamic Golden Age (786–1258) included probably the greatest assemblage of scholars from around the world, based on the House of Wisdom (established 825), the great library of Baghdad. Veterinary knowledge was also significantly advanced by the scholars of the Mamluk Sultanate based in Cairo, Egypt (1250–1517).

Islamic human and veterinary medicine, based on the sacred idea that humans and animals were interrelated, became the most advanced model worldwide for centuries. Influential veterinary contributions were made by Ibn Akhī Ḥizām, commander and stable master to caliph Al-Mu 'tadid (who reigned from 892–902). He wrote *Kitāb al-Furūsiyya wa 'l-Bayṭara* (*Book of horsemanship and hippiatry*). Later, Ahmad ibn al-Hasan included horse, cattle, sheep, and camel medicine in his *Kitāb al-Baiṭara* (c. 1209). A very important medieval source for spreading veterinary knowledge was the tenth-century *Hippiatrica*. This Byzantine compilation by an unknown editor was based on Greek and Roman texts on horse medicine from late antiquity, among others from Xenophon, Pelagonius, and Apsyrtos. The *Hippiatrica* was often copied and referred to for centuries. It contains no overall medical theory or etiology, but instead emphasizes practical treatment of injuries, lameness, colic, cough, glanders, and parasites.

Animal and human health were closely related at this time. Around the world, most people lived in small shelters, houses, or stables with horses, cows, goats, or sheep. Such animals carried diseases that could infect humans, either directly or through the bites of external parasites such as fleas. In hindsight, it can be concluded that these circumstances were ideal for spreading zoonotic diseases. Wars also spread diseases. An important example from this time period was the eight crusades during which Europeans invaded the Arabic and Mediterranean regions. With them came diseases adapted to Western European human and animal populations. The invaders themselves suffered from poor food and water, lack of personal hygiene, and stress, which must have weakened resistance among high concentrations of people in a new and strange environment. Such favorable circumstances for the transmission of infectious diseases took their toll on the crusading armies. Dysentery, cholera, typhoid fever, leprosy, and bubonic plague ran rampant in the armies and occupied regions. The thousands of animals on both sides suffered from similar conditions, circulating diseases such as glanders among high concentrations of animals with weakened resistance. Military horse-doctors were skilled in wound treatment but often remained practically powerless against such infectious animal diseases.

Animals' key military roles meant that knowledge about animal healing was often sponsored by expanding regimes and quickly translated. During the eleventh through the thirteenth centuries, Islamic medical and veterinary knowledge spread northward into Europe from the Mediterranean. The Islamic works were translated back into Latin, and from there into Italian, Spanish, French, German, English – thus circulating both Islamic and ancient veterinary knowledge. A few important works appeared from Christian Europe also. Giordano Ruffo's *De medicina equorum* was apparently not derived from older Byzantine or Arabic sources but is mainly based on his own observations and experience. It was quickly translated into European languages and remained a standard veterinary text for centuries. The same happened with *Marescalcia* from the veterinarian Laurentius Rusius, who worked in Rome in the period 1320–1370, and *El libro de menescalcia et de albeyteria* written by Juan Alvarez de Salamiellas between 1340 and 1360.

In Europe, the Middle East, and Asia, veterinary knowledge continued to circulate with human invasions and migrations. The Mongols, by enfolding other cultures' knowledge and technologies into their vast empire, had helped collapse the geographic and intellectual distances between the ancient civilizations of China, Persia, Arabia, and the West. After the conquest of Constantinople in 1453 by the Ottoman Turks and the consequent fall of the Byzantine Empire, many scholars fled to Italy where they contributed to the Renaissance (c. 1350–1600), a golden age in European cultural history. With a new focus on humans as individual and unique beings (humanism), the Renaissance also included changes in understanding animals and the animal body. This was reflected in art and in a new critical approach to anatomy (see Chapter 1). People, animals, ideas, and the everyday practices of animal husbandry traveled and encountered each other.

These circulations of veterinary knowledge and practice intensified when people from the Eastern and Western Hemispheres (the Old World and New World) contacted each other around 1500. Not only knowledge but also animals, microorganisms, and parasites themselves traveled and altered the disease ecologies of both animal and human populations. These transformations may have intensified the need for animal owners to act as healers or to consult professional healers (we take up this topic in Chapter 2). The central question for anyone concerned with practical veterinary health (and scholarly treatise-writers) was, How and why did animals get sick?

Theories of Disease and Types of Healing

Although animal healing also addresses injuries and other problems, we will focus on disease for a moment. Disease has been central to the history of human–animal relationships, and people have understood the causes and processes of disease in different ways at different times. The way we understand many diseases today, using sciences such as bacteriology and virology, is quite recent: only 80 to 150 years old. And our knowledge is constantly changing, even at a basic scientific level (think of prions, only discovered in the 1990s). As we will see in this book, an understanding of diseases did *not* begin with bacteriology in the late 1800s. Many disease causation theories, and the diagnostic and treatment techniques arising from them, dated back thousands of years to animal domestication. By 1500, healers of animals and humans had several logical and well-established theories of disease from which to choose; and they selected treatments based on their ideas of disease causation and experiences. Some persist in one form or another today. While this pre-modern period arguably yielded mixed results, animal healers, then and now, used the tools that were available according to the beliefs of the time – just as we do today.

Although no organizational scheme is perfect, we can place animal healing methods into five categories of systems: (1) *self-healing*, or methods of instinctual healing on the part of the animal; (2) *mystical* (religious, spiritual, or magical); (3) *empirical* (therapy based on educated guess); (4) *ethnoveterinary medicine* (traditional methods used by laypeople and professionals); and (5) *contemporary veterinary medicine* ("modern" Western professional veterinary medicine that has developed during the past two centuries, based on sciences such as bacteriology. Except for self-healing, *all these healing systems were based on theories and observations of how the animal's body worked and what caused the animal's illness or injury.* In other words, they all made sense in their own time and place. This point bears repeating, because we often assume that the only rational healing methods for animals are those of the present time. But obviously, knowledge and technologies change quickly. Today, people around the world consider veterinary medicine and many other animal healing methods to be effective and rational. We do not want future generations to judge us negatively for what we do not yet know (we have not yet discovered a cure for cancer, for example). In the same way, we cannot judge people of the past who believed firmly in their chosen theories and methods of healing animals (regardless of whether we now find those methods to be effective).

The first animal healing system is *self-healing*, or instinctive healing on the part of the animal. The most well-known method is the instinct of injured or sick animals to hide and rest. Animals are also observed to eat certain plants or substances to self-medicate (such as self-induced vomiting in domesticated dogs with gastroenteritis). Biologists and evolutionary anthropologists have discovered several examples of these behaviors in wild animals. Mountain gorillas eat clay to absorb and neutralize ingested toxins; Ethiopian baboons eat the leaves of a plant that helps them expel parasitic flatworms. Capuchin monkeys collect and rub themselves with millipedes, whose bodies contain benzoquinone insecticides that reduce heavy external parasite infestations. Elephants in western Kenya travel to the caves of Mount Elgon and eat the soft, salt-laden clay found there, which helps them to digest toxins in the plants they eat. Despite these activities, animals still get sick, fall prey to parasites, and die; but researchers believe that some instinctive animal behaviors have evolved to address illnesses and injuries. Of course, this is a human interpretation of certain animal behaviors that may or may not be true, and therein lies the mystery (since we cannot communicate directly with the animals). But researchers assert that animals' behaviors are "self-medicating" when the specific medicinal plants (and other things) they use are not normally part of their diet; provide no nutritional benefit; are not used by all animals in the group; and are usually used during certain seasons or life stages (for example, pregnancy). Self-treatment, in other words, is the most likely explanation. "Zoopharmacognosy" is the academic field that links observations of eating behaviors with the theory that animals have evolved ways to heal themselves to survive. The development of this interesting field is beyond the scope of this book, so we turn now to the other healing systems.

These types of healing are conducted by humans, on animals. *Mystical medicine*, *empirical medicine*, and *ethnoveterinary medicine* are the oldest approaches in the human repertoire. Some of these methods continue to be important around the world today in various cultures. *Mystical* healing methods, usually a combination of rituals and petitions to a deity or higher power(s), correspond directly to a culture's major spiritual and religious beliefs about how animals' bodies function, what causes illness in them, and how they are expected to respond to magical procedures or prayers. In the first two chapters of this book, mystical and sacred healing traditions will be an important context for our discussion of animal healing circa 1500–1700. However, such healing methods are still important today, especially in sacred-based cultures and societies around the world. In *empirical* healing systems, practitioners select therapies based on observation, experience, and trying several likely treatments. While empirical systems did not exclude theories of health and disease, they placed emphasis on clinical experience and what we would call trial and error. In the modern era, empiricism has been derided as unscientific; however, contemporary veterinary medicine obviously still includes reliance on experience, observation, and clinical response to treatment.

Likewise, *ethnoveterinary medicine* encompasses the uses of treatments learned or identified by laypeople, the folk medicine that has been woven into today's veterinary treatments. (And as we will see in Chapter 3, natural history and medical botany were key components of the first veterinary schools in France in the 1700s.) Most animal healing conducted in the non-Western world is still done by laypeople and professionals using traditional methods. *Contemporary veterinary medicine* refers to the version of school-based, Western veterinary medicine that has been practiced professionally since the late 1700s (Chapters 4–7). This system of animal healing has incorporated many components from the other systems, yet like any "new" system it has commonly disavowed them to distinguish itself. With many successes and many continuing challenges, the practice of contemporary veterinary medicine today is enriched by understanding how practitioners of the past have envisioned and taken action to restore health in their

How to Use This Book

We have organized the book around themes: social/cultural and scientific. This book may be read chapter by chapter or *in toto*, either integrated into scientific courses (such as anatomy) or as a textbook for a veterinary history course. The book is built around eight learning objectives. A table of these learning objectives and the chapters that focus on them is found in Appendix B. Appendix C provides suggestions of which chapters to assign within standard veterinary courses, such as anatomy, physiology, pathology, surgery, food hygiene, and ethics/deontology. Appendix A lists early veterinary schools, and the dates founded, for many nations. Veterinary professors can therefore easily insert history into existing courses in the veterinary curriculum. In this concise history of veterinary medicine, we do not attempt to include all important topics in the history of animal healing. Instead, we frame the history of animal healing and veterinary medicine using a global and world history approach, and we include activities at the end of each chapter that encourage readers to explore the veterinary history of their own region and nation. Every chapter considers how animal healing interacted with tensions between the economic, military, and emotional (religious) value, status, and uses of domesticated animals. Who were the animal healers? What was their social status? How were they trained? What skills and knowledge did they have? How did people explain or theorize animal health problems in each place and time period?

In Chapter 1, we highlight traditions of animal healing around the globe, from South American, to Islamic and Ottoman, to Ayurvedic and Chinese. We broadly analyze early veterinary activities, including professionalization, and link them to the more well-known histories of military animal healers and the development of veterinary anatomy since 1500. In Chapter 2, we describe the impact of large-scale animal epidemics and pandemics enabled by the ecological exchanges of animals, parasites, and pathogens. Developments in international trade, colonialism, and conquest frame Chapter 2 and set up the military and economic needs that shaped the professionalization of modern veterinary medicine in Europe, which we explore in Chapter 3. Some questions of importance in these chapters include the following: Which medical concepts, popular beliefs, and therapies were used in animal health care? How were animal diseases circulating around the world due to exploration, colonialism, war, and trade? What was the impact of these diseases on human health and well-being, and on the projects of colonialism and state formation? In terms of the modern veterinary curriculum, Chapter 2 highlights the development of physiology and new disease causation models; Chapter 3 details the growth of veterinary surgery. Chapter 3 also asks, How did the Western veterinary professionalization process of the eighteenth and nineteenth centuries proceed? How was the circulation of veterinary knowledge organized, particularly with reference to the challenges of animal disease outbreaks that had accompanied war, trade, and colonialism? How did the modern veterinary school develop, and why did this model spread around the world?

The dramatic political as well as scientific developments of the nineteenth and twentieth centuries frame Chapters 4–6: the rise of germ theories, the world wars, problems of food insecurity, and the various manifestations of modernity implied by new regimes of animal production. How did new domains for animal healing arise (such as preventive medicine in intensive animal agriculture and the need for veterinarians specializing in "exotic" zoo animals and pets)? How did veterinary public health grow during this time, especially as circulations of scientific knowledge (and animal diseases) increased in scope? What roles did laboratory research, germ theories, and comparative medicine play? Chapter 7, the final chapter of the book, considers how veterinary medicine has continued to change in the early twenty-first century, with the dramatic worldwide increase in companion animal practice, the availability of new medical and digital technologies, and the politicization of animal welfare and animal rights.

The Epilogue concludes the book by discussing veterinary medicine circa 2021 and the traditional concerns and new realities it faces. These new realities include the need to ensure food animal and herd health in a world increasingly affected by emerging diseases and climate change – while most European and North American veterinarians specialize in individual treatment of companion animals (pets). With technological developments, such as the ability to genetically modify and clone organisms, we have unprecedented levels of control over animals' biology. How are veterinarians navigating these dramatic changes and potential ethical concerns? These questions and many others ensure that the future of veterinary medicine will be as dynamic as its past has been. As mediators between humans and animals, veterinarians and other animal healers have both shaped and been shaped by the social, cultural, and economic roles of animals over time.

1   Animal Healing in Sacred Societies, 1500–1700

Introduction

In this chapter, we focus on what historians in the West call the early modern time period, approximately 1400–1700, although we also provide necessary historical background from earlier times and several cultures. Along with using animals for food, transport, and cultural status, many societies incorporated animals into their sacred traditions and developed elaborate systems of knowledge about animals (including animal healing). In the early modern period, animals' ability to contribute to societies depended on animals' bodies being healthy and fulfilling the specific needs of cultures. Regimes of animal healing developed within these world-ordering cosmologies to provide for specific material requirements of complex societies.

Animals in Medieval and Early Modern Sacred Societies

"In the year 1492, Columbus sailed the ocean blue." This children's rhyme describes one of the early encounters between the Eastern Hemisphere (Old World) and the Western Hemisphere (New World), a major milestone in history. The vast and wealthy empire of the Inca (12 million people) predominated in the Western Hemisphere and Incan encounters with Europeans during the sixteenth century would forever alter both civilizations. But the centers of power and activity in the Eastern Hemisphere were also changing at this time, as the old empire created by Mongol conquests dissolved and new centers of power arose in the West. On the African continent, the Congo and Songhai kingdoms included some of the world's most experienced animal pastoralists; in the North, Africans encountered the Ottomans, and in the east, Chinese explorers. With the Old World's centers of power shifting to the Moghul empire in South Asia, the Ottoman empire in the middle east, and the Spanish and Portuguese in Western Europe, an already interconnected world became more expansive and extensive from the turn of the sixteenth century onward.

This world was the beneficiary of knowledge from ancient civilizations and the medieval Islamic scholars, who had preserved, translated, and revised texts about animal healing from around the world. The most important corpus of medieval animal healing knowledge was collected in the Bayt al-Hikma, the Abbasid caliphate's great Baghdad library, and the Islamic influence spread this knowledge widely. In addition to circulations of knowledge, printing technologies and print culture spread westward from China and became increasingly important. (This development allows historians today to use many types of sources, including archaeological, oral history, manuscripts, and printed documents, for the period 1500–1700.) Finally, the Iberian-instigated connections between the animals and civilizations of South, Central, and North America in the West with those of Eurasia and Africa dramatically influenced the animal-cultures of all peoples. By 1700, the Iberian empire was joined by two other rising world powers: the Manchus' Qing, successors of the Ming Dynasty in China in 1644, and the Russian empire, under its leader Peter I (who became Tsar in 1682).

Animals were central to all these events: equines and elephants for war, transport, and power; cattle and other food-producing animals; and many types of animals as markers of social hierarchies and cultural beliefs. Vast empires could not be created and sustained without healthy animals. In this chapter, we explore animal healing based on how different societies understood animals' bodies and how this reflected the sacred and practical values attached to different domesticated and wild animals from the end of the fifteenth through the eighteenth centuries. We begin with theories of health and disease and the positions of animals in the cultural beliefs of different historical societies. We consider various species and their uses, and we highlight the development of knowledge about animal anatomy during this time. All these developments occurred within a time of strong theological and cosmological influences on beliefs about animals and how to keep them healthy.

Early Theories of Animal Health and Disease

What caused an animal to be healthy or sick? The answer depended not just on pathogens, but was influenced also by time, place, and the roles different animals played. Overall, diseases in humans and animals in early modern times were often considered to be caused by magical forces, supernatural interventions, or divine punishments for sinful behavior. The old idea of disease as a divine punishment still appears today (for example, with outbreaks of HIV/AIDS, Ebola, avian influenza, and foot and mouth disease).

The Americas

When Europeans crossed the Atlantic Ocean and encountered the vast empire of the Inca (1438–1533), they immediately noticed the different species of animals and their importance in sacred rituals (as well as for food and fiber). The Incan people kept large numbers of domesticated guinea pigs, alpacas, and llamas for meat and wool (llamas could also be used as pack animals). Incans also kept llamas as sacred animals that could be ritually sacrificed to the gods, and skilled artisans created solid gold llama-shaped idols. The *Ayllu*, or local kinship community, held llama herds in common. Given the llama's sacred status, its health is likely to have been understood within the cosmological framework of the *Chakana* (three universes) in which all living creatures' bodies held vital energy and consciousness. We know of very few sources (none in English) mentioning animal husbandry and animal healing in the empire of the Inca, but practitioners of this specialized role probably existed in such an advanced agricultural society. Due to the tremendous practical and sacred value of llamas, it is likely that healers used well-articulated theories and practices to heal these animals.

Further north in Central America, the Aztec empire (an alliance of three societies) was also distinguished by a carefully ordered pantheistic society that included dogs and turkeys as domesticated animals. Aztec citizens hunted wild game (peccaries, antelope, and birds), although the main foods were vegetables, grains, and fruits supplemented by fish; they also consumed specially bred dogs. Animals played important roles in Aztec beliefs: animals mediated with and represented the deities, and artists created numerous animal sculptures and images. Aztec-era medicine, especially knowledge of medicinal plants, was highly developed and a wide variety of treatments were available for specific diseases. (Many of these formulations are still available today.) Medicine was a holistic practice that included rituals to invoke spiritual healing as well as material therapies (such as bloodletting) that corresponded to theories of disease causation. Wounds were sutured; broken bones could be set with external plasters or as necessary, inserting a stick as an intramedullary pin. As one poem described the healer's role: they should examine the patient, address the symptoms, and experiment with prevention and treatment, within a holistic framework of theory and practice. As with the Incan empire, we know very little about animal healers in the Aztec era; but such healers surely existed within this society's advanced development and medical knowledge.

East Asia

On the other side of the world, in Chinese medicine (also a basis for Japanese, Korean, and other Asian healing regimes), generally an animal's body was healthy when it was in balance. This balance, in both human and animal bodies, reflected the harmonic balance of all Nature and the entire cosmos. This was a system based on rational principles of knowledge rather than sacred beliefs, but it nonetheless relied on a coherent cosmological framework.

Ancient Chinese philosophy is beautifully complex, and we can give only the most superficial description here as it pertains to animal health. Bodies were influenced by the five material elements of fire, water, earth, metal, and wood and the six abstract concepts of *yin, yang*, wind, rain, darkness, and brightness. The functional relationship between organ systems corresponded to elements, which in turn related to the seasons. Bodies also demonstrated these forces in different layers, from the most superficial to the deepest, with the *qi* (vital energy or life force) flowing throughout.

Bodies changed, and disease resulted, with six stages of *qi* transformation described and connected in a diagnostic system by Zhang Zhongjing in his *Shanghan lun* (second century). The causative forces included combinations of wind (*feng*), heat (*re*), damp (*shi*), fire (*huo*), dryness (*zao*), and cold (*han*), which could affect the normal opening and closing cycles of the body's functions. Disturbances to the balance of these forces' normal cycles could originate internally or externally. Important sources of external disturbance were the *zhangqi*, toxic or poisonous gases and vapors, originating from specific environments (especially hot and damp places with large amounts of rotting vegetation). Breathing the air in these places endangered the health of animals and humans alike, and many medical authorities and laypeople believed that *zhangqi* caused epidemics. (This conclusion made sense: many people or animals became sick at the same time because they breathed the same poisonous air.)

In the *Shanghan lun*, Zhang based the complex system of medical diagnostics and therapeutics on the practitioner's ability to detect these changes by examining signs such as the pulses. Treatments, keyed to signs and diagnosis, included herbs, special diets, manipulation, and moxibustion (burning bits of the herb *Artemesia* at points on the skin to affect the body's interior), as well as external interventions such as cautery, cutting, and a type of bone-setting. This system has been the basis of traditional Chinese medicine for centuries, although of course it was changed and used in different ways over time. These changes often incorporated vernacular (indigenous or local) knowledge since the vast regions of East Asia encompassed multiple types of climate and various cultures. Circulations and transfers of animal healing knowledge proceeded most smoothly when incorporating vernacular ideas and practices.

Print culture also ensured the centuries-long popularity and influence of the most important Chinese texts written during the sixteenth to eighteenth centuries. The most important compendium of herbal *materia medica* was Li Shih-Zhen's *Ben Cao Gang Mu*, which described over 11,000 herbal formulas. The wide popularity of Yu Ben-Yuan and Yu Ben-Heng's 1608 treatise on horses, *Yuan Heng Liao Ma Ji*, along with the same authors' books on cattle and camels, established the Yu brothers as the fathers of early modern professional Chinese animal healing. The ruling Ming Dynasty greatly expanded foreign trade, and these books were available outside China and translated into European languages by the early 1600s.

The treatments described in these treatises corresponded to the underlying theory of imbalance in the body. For example, moxibustion brought blood and *qi* flow and heat to a specific area of the body that was overly cold (*han*), damp (*shi*), or suffering from blocked energy flow. In human medicine, moxibustion has also been used for chronic conditions and to help turn breech babies. Its function of redirecting heat to combat cold was synchronized with knowledge of the energy pathways in the body. Printed texts based on Chinese ideas about health and disease often included anatomical diagrams of the important points on the animal's body for the detection of pulse and energy and for the corresponding focus of treatment modalities (Fig. 1.1).

These treatment regimens based on theories of imbalance often got combined with local folk remedies. Sources on professional animal healing often dealt with military horses, for instance, the collection on care for such horses provided by hostlers (innkeepers' professional stable men): *Si mu an ji ji* written by Li Shi in the ninth century. From China, such hippiatric texts were transferred to Korea and Japan where further combinations with local

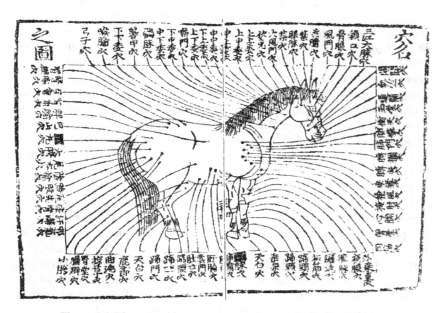

Figure 1.1 Diagram with acupuncture points on the body of the horse.
Source: Ma Niu I Fang (China, 1399 CE); reproduced in Lu Gwei-Djen & Joseph Needham, *Celestial Lancets. A History and Rationale of Acupuncture and Moxa* (Cambridge: Cambridge University Press, 1980) 238.

knowledge systems were incorporated. This is shown in illustrated scrolls on equine medicine from Japan, for instance, one from 1267 that was given to Tadayasu, a veterinarian responsible for cavalry horses. In Korea, horse-doctors (*Maui*) were active from the tenth century onward. The oldest Korean compilation on equine medicine, *Sin pyeon jip seong ma ui bang*, contains remedies for thirty-four horse diseases. It was written in 1399 by Confucian scholars who integrated knowledge from Chinese hippiatric sources and Korean folk remedies. These early animal treatment systems worked for the local people because they successfully combined vernacular (folk) ways of understanding equine diseases (and their treatment) with the more scholarly theories.

South Asia

Important influences on Chinese medicine were the older Ayurvedic medical principles, which continue as the basis for traditional medicine in India and other nations today. Ayurveda, literally "life knowledge system" or "science of life," is also based on a rational belief system in accordance with ancient Indian cosmologies dating back at least to 1000 BCE. Ayurvedic knowledge was recorded in old Sanskrit texts, the *vedas*. Anatomy, or *Śarira Sthana*, is important in Ayurvedic knowledge. Ayurvedic principles guided the treatment of elephants and horses, valued as pack and war animals, as well as other animals and humans in South and Southeast Asia. Cows (water buffaloes and zebu) were especially valued for milk and milk products, and references to cows are plentiful in the *vedas*. Boiled cows' milk, buttermilk, and *ghee* (clear butter fat) were (and are) important components of vedic Indians' diet. Cows were also highly regarded as symbols of blessing and sacred life under Buddhism, the formal religion based on the *vedas* that arose around 500 BCE. For Buddhists, cows provide five sacred products: *ghee*, milk, curds, urine, and dung (the latter used for fertilizer). The Buddhist prohibition against harming or killing any living creature applied especially to cows.

  These sacred cows were cared for and healed according to the sophisticated Ayurvedic system of medical knowledge. Ayurvedic medicine (again, far more complex than we can describe here) is based on five elements that interact with the body's vital energy, the *prana* (analogous to the *qi* in Chinese medicine): earth, water, wind, fire, and ether. Together these elements contributed to one of three *doshas* or humoral-metabolic body types (including the mind and consciousness): the *vâyu* (dry and cold; movement and elimination or catabolism; or wind), *kapha* (water and earth; tissue structures and anabolic processes; or phlegm) and *pitta* (water and fire; chemical processes or metabolism; or bile). Assessing these *doshas* formed the basis of a rich and intricate medical system that included problem-based diagnosis and treatment.

An individual animal's normally healthy constitution always included a combination of the three *doshas* in a unique individual balance. Disease resulted when external (breathing bad air; eating improperly) or internal forces (often a decreased digestive energy) caused imbalances in the body. Diagnosis was based on the pulses, the condition of the tongue, and careful physical examination (including bodily excretions, such as urine). The treatments, consisting mainly of dietary changes and herbal medications, depended on the diagnosis and corresponded to the missing elements. Treatment aimed to re-balance the *doshas* by reducing excesses and remedying deficiencies. If the animal's constitution, the nature of the disease, and the season/climate all belonged to the same *dosha*, then the case was considered almost impossible to cure. Thus, early Ayurvedism was a theory-based "ethnoveterinary" practice. Although it underwent many changes over time, Ayurvedism continues as an important veterinary healing system today

Some of the world's oldest institutions of animal healing were located in India where elephants, horses, and cattle were very valuable to the state. Few veterinarians outside South Asia or Africa will ever treat an elephant today, unless in a zoo or circus; but elephants were important in military campaigns and as beasts of burden from ancient times through the sixteenth to the eighteenth centuries. Some elephants were also kept as sacred animals or sent as valuable gifts between rulers and emperors. (A famous example was the Asian elephant Abul-Abbas, gifted by Harun al-Rashid, the fifth Caliph, to Charlemagne in 802. This elephant traveled from India to Baghdad to Aachen, and its keepers managed to keep it alive and healthy.) With key roles as both sacred and working animals, elephants have been the subjects of animal healers' attention, and many South Asian Ayurvedic animal healing treatises are devoted to them. The *Shalihotra Samhita*, dating to the third century BCE, is an early treatise on horse and elephant medicine. The author Shalihotra is praised as the founder of veterinary medicine in the Indian tradition. This treatise, which covers equine and elephant anatomy, physiology, surgery, and how diseases of these animals could be prevented and cured, was translated from Sanskrit into Persian, Arabic, Tibetan, and, much later, English.

In the modern period, Ayurvedic principles guided the diagnosis and treatment of cattle along with elephants and horses, according to the *Sivatattvaratnâkara*, the printed Indian eighteenth-century encyclopedia of knowledge. Particular attention was devoted to surgical methods, proper diets, and external manipulations such as inducing sweating or administering enemas to balance the animal's three *doshas*. More invasive or dramatic treatments, such as cauterization, were reserved as last resorts in particularly difficult cases of sickness or injury. Overall, animal healers derived their diagnoses and corresponding treatments from their judgment of how vigorous or well balanced the animal's *doshas* were. Since the *Sivatattvaratnâkara* included three chapters on animal medicine – one each for cattle, horses, and elephants – we can conclude that these valuable animals were the most important patients for South Asian animal healers in the eighteenth century. Cows, as the givers of milk, were also givers of life; and protecting cows meant ensuring life and health for all people.

Mediterranean Region and Arabic World (Near East)

As in Asia, extensive knowledge about animal medicine supported the crucial roles of camels, goats, sheep, horses, and other animals essential for food, transport, and military use in the ancient Arabic world. In the desert and semi-desert regions, the nomadic *badawī* (Bedouins) lived as herders and possessed a great deal of knowledge about animal care and medicine. (Bedouin peoples live today in many nations, including Israel, Palestine, Syria, and Saudi Arabia.) Animal medicine (like human medicine) in these tribal cultures was mostly empirical and included spiritual rituals and botanical knowledge, learned through apprenticeship. Camels, thought of as the "gift from God," supplied milk, food, fiber, and transport for goods and people because these animals could survive the harsh desert conditions. For the *badawī*, keeping animals alive and well ensured survival. Experts in animal medicine (such as the famed Al-as ibn Wa'il) would have been important members of the community. It is notable that, in the pre-Islamic period, famed animal healers included women such as Ibn al-Qosh. Recovering the history of Bedouin animal healing practices is important: like other nomadic peoples, the Bedouin had a great deal of practical experience with animals and theirs was the most important livestock-based society in the vast desert regions. Although few written texts survive, historians can consult the rich oral tradition of these peoples today.

In other ancient cultures in this region, texts focused mainly on animals valuable for their theological, cultural, or practical roles in societies. The most important animals were equines and, secondarily, bovines and camels. Historians have argued over who was the oldest known "veterinarian" in the ancient Middle East. Some historians believe that a relief on the so-called *Ur-Lugal-edina* cylinder seal from Sumeria, circa 2020 BCE, shows an animal healer with instruments used in obstetrics. Lexical texts from this period also mention doctors of oxen and doctors of donkeys. Other historians have pointed to the Egyptian Sekhmet priest Aha-Nakht, who treated oxen. We do not know much about the practices of these healers. By the 1750s BCE, the legal Code of Hammurabi established the separate practices of human and animal medicine and the fees that could be charged by professional animal healers. Rarely, extant sources mention professional animal healers: a cattle-doctor named Abil-ilisu is mentioned in a court record from Babylonia (circa 1739 BCE) and the term "cattle-doctor" (*a.zu gu.hi.a*) continued to be used in Babylonian records and laws. Therefore, the sources that survive today support the idea that an officially recognized class of animal healing practitioners existed in these ancient societies.

Although regular horse-doctors in ancient Greece existed earlier, the first testimony of the Greek word for horse-doctor, ἱππιατρός (hippiatros), appeared within a long treatise written around 130 BCE. This document described the work of Metrodoros the hippiatros. Metrodoros was a native of Lamia in Thessaly, a region well known for horse-breeding. The most renowned ancient Greek horse-doctor was probably Apsyrtos from Bithynia (c. 280–337 CE), who served in the cavalry of Constantine the Great and whose writings were praised for centuries. He observed the contagious nature of anthrax, farcy, and glanders and recommended isolation for ill animals. However, the oldest surviving Mediterranean animal healing texts did not originate in Greece, but in Egypt (Fig. 1.2). The association of cats with ancient Egyptian goddesses and sacred rituals is well known. The papyrus of *El-Lâhūn* (c. 1850 BCE) reveals that animal medicine and surgery were practiced by professional healers in ancient Egypt. The papyrus contained instructions on how to diagnose and treat diseased bovines, dogs, ducks, and fish. The first evidence for literature on hippiatry (horsemanship) appeared in cuneiform tablets from the fourteenth century BCE found during excavations at Ras Shamra-Ugarit in Syria.x

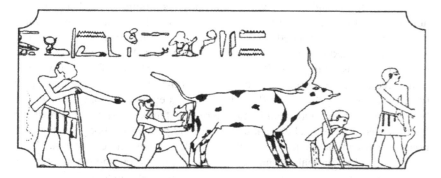

Figure 1.2 Egyptian tomb relief depicting veterinary care during delivery. Remarkably, the cow is in a standing position. It also shows a division between hands-on work by an operator while an experienced herdsman instructs. The accompanying text says: "Herdsman, catch gently" (Egypt, Old Kingdom, 1990–1970 BCE).
Source: A.M. Blackman, *The Rock Tombs of Meir*. Vol 1 (London: Cambridge University Press, 1914) Table X, detail; text p. 33.

Medical and veterinary practices in the ancient Near East were based on magic, rituals, religious beliefs, and practical knowledge of healing. Initially, physicians were also priests working in healing temples. It was the ancient Greeks who extended sacred healing knowledge into the basis of what is generally known as the Western medical tradition. Less well known is that their theories also applied to animals. Although religion and rituals continued to play a role in medical treatments, a secular medicine based on natural theories of health and disease emerged. Hippocrates (c. 460–370 BCE) who lived on the island of Cos, is often praised as the father of Western secular medicine, which was documented in the Hippocratic *Corpus*. However, Hippocrates' actual contribution to this *Corpus* is unclear: it is a collection of about 60 works composed by various unknown authors throughout two centuries. These treatises included various aspects of medicine which were later integrated into one framework, Hippocratic medicine.

Hippocratic medicine combined a holistic approach and naturalism. As in medical traditions from other parts of the world, ancient Greek doctors carefully observed the whole patient to obtain information about his health status. Naturalism dictated that the body was able to heal itself, with the role of the healer to "do no harm" and help the body to restore its own health. Western, Arabic, and Persian theories of health and disease had some similarities to those of Asia during the early modern period (although these theories were framed within very different cultural contexts). An important external cause of disease was *miasma* (toxic or bad air); the climate and seasons also influenced the state of an animal's body. Health was maintained by vital forces and balances of fluids and energy within the body according to the theory of the humors. The four humors of Greek medicine – blood, yellow bile, black bile, and phlegm – corresponded to the overall Hippocratic system of elements, temperaments, and seasons (similar to the structure of Ayurvedic and Chinese medical systems) (Fig. 1.3). The four elements – earth, air, fire, and water – influenced and corresponded to the behavior of the four humors: the black bile (dry, cold; earth); yellow bile (hot, dry; fire); phlegm (wet, cold; water); and blood (hot, wet; air). Different combinations, or temperaments, accounted for the observed differences between the organs and parts of the body (such as the bones). We cannot do justice to this complex system here, but overall, it defined a healthy animal as one whose body contained combinations of these humors, in correspondence with its external environment, functioning in a kind of equilibrium.

Disease and some injuries appeared or failed to heal when these humors were out of balance, reducing the animal's vital energy or life force. Therapeutic choices (for both humans and animals) proceeded from the healer's diagnosis of which humors were in excess (*materia peccans*) or deficient in the body. For example, it was widely believed that horses

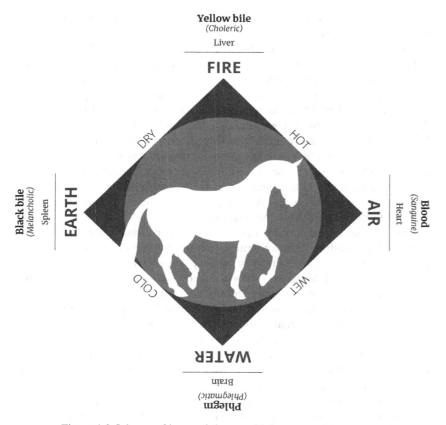

Figure 1.3 Scheme of humoral theory with humors and temperaments, elements, and qualities.
Courtesy: Lisanne van der Voort, Faculty of Veterinary Medicine, Utrecht University.

contained too much blood in springtime by which the animals became over-heated (feverish). Bloodletting of horses after wintertime remained a regular treatment until well into the nineteenth century. As with Ayurvedic medicine, healers applied enemas, induced vomiting (purging), or held hot cups on the skin to draw out toxic or surplus bodily fluids. Other treatments to reestablish balance included changing diets, massage, warm or cold baths, and exercise. Animal healers worked within a nosology (or classification) of diseases based on these internal and external forces, and treatment procedures were designed to restore the body's balances.

Another Greek scholar, Aristotle (c. 384–322 BCE), is considered one of the greatest philosophers and scientists of the ancient Western world. He laid the basis for biology by classifying about 500 different animal species. Once again, his contributions to animal health and disease are less well known. Aristotle named several animal diseases with their symptoms but mentioned only bloodletting as treatment. He described breeding of horses, donkeys, and mules, as well as the castration of bulls and boar and how these animals grow fatter. Aristotelian and Hippocratic texts were augmented later by the work of the influential Greek/Roman physician Claudius Galen (130–210 CE). Although humors were key elements for the careful observation of patients, Galen provided some anatomical knowledge to support the humoral theory. He dissected pigs (which he viewed as most similar to humans) to obtain a deeper insight into the function of the various organs. For example, he noted that urine was produced in the kidney and not in the urinary bladder. Next to vomit, sweat, urine, and feces, pus was an important expression of *materia peccans* that had to be removed from the diseased body

Treatises on animal healing from Greek authors were cited, copied, and translated into Latin by Roman writers after the conquest of Greece. This was the case with the treatise on horsemanship (*hippiatrica*) by Xenophon (c. 430–354 BCE), philosopher, historian, and soldier from Athens. Classic Roman works from late antiquity entirely devoted to veterinary medicine are *Ars veterinaria* by Pelagonius and *Mulomedicinae* by Vegetius. In the Roman Empire, professional animal healers, responsible mainly for the health of equines (horses, donkeys, mules, hinnies), were first known as *medicus equarius* (horse-doctor) and *veterinarius*, and later (fourth century) as *mulomedicus* (mule-doctor). (Often these terms were later incorrectly translated into "farrier.") The word *veterinarius* (caretaker of *bestia veterina*: equines, according to Latinist James Adams), appeared in Columella's treatise on Roman agriculture, written around 60 CE. Agricultural production was mainly based on slavery. It is not clear whether the (low) status of the *veterinarius*, who also belonged to this group of agricultural workers, was free or servile; however, it is possible that many were slaves.

The ancient Greek and Roman economies heavily depended on livestock and crop production. Animals were indispensable because they provided for transport, food, animal traction, and warfare. But equally important was the cultural role of animals in menageries and for entertainment in the circus, including horse chariot racing in amphitheaters. Animal healers were needed to support all these activities. Ancient Roman mosaics and reliefs provide evidence for veterinary care, including racehorses wearing leg bandages. The most common representations of instruments include variations of the nose-twitch, the hipposandal (*soleae ferreae*), and instruments for cauterizing, trimming hooves, and castration. Besides horse races, fights between gladiators and wild animals were also part of public entertainment. Over the centuries of the Roman empire, thousands of exotic animals were captured to supply the more than seventy amphitheaters. (Ecologists have argued that this practice caused permanent declines in wildlife populations, particularly in Africa.) As for practical veterinary medicine, the boundary between the work of herdsmen, owners, interested laymen, stable masters, breeders, other healers, and the professional *hippiatros, veterinarius,* and *mulomedicus* was small.

A final cultural role for animals and animal healers was the widespread aristocratic sport of hunting. Animal assistants in the hunt included horses, dogs, and hunting birds such as falcons and raptors. These practices ranged widely across Eurasia and persisted for centuries (even into the twenty-first century in some places), thus providing a thread of continuity for the *longue durée* history of human–animal relationships. Elite hunting was common in early Mesopotamia, China, and India; and it persisted into the modern era in Iran, Northern India, and the Middle East. Its practices instigated innovations in animal breeding, care, and healing. For example, the manuscript "On Hunting" presented in 1247 to al-Mansur (the Hafsid Sultan of North Africa) also detailed the proper treatment of the sultan's saluki hunting dogs. The dogs were carefully bred, fed special diets, and given expert care for diseases and injuries. Historians can often find information about animal healing practices in documents and other sources describing the use of animals in cultural activities.

The Islamic Scholarly Tradition

After the fall of Rome in the fifth century CE, Constantinople, the capital of the Byzantine empire, became an important center of scientific knowledge – and a return to the importance of theological knowledge. A shift occurred from the Latin West to the East where Jewish, Islamic, and Christian authors added to the existing medical and veterinary writings. For example, Maimonides (1135–1204) worked as a rabbi, philosopher, and physician in Spain, Morocco, and Egypt and wrote texts that included veterinary treatments. With the rise and expansion of the Islamic empire around the Mediterranean, Greek, Latin, and Indian sources were translated into Arabic, Persian, and other Middle Eastern languages. Medieval Islamic scholars integrated Greek, Roman, Persian, and Ayurvedic concepts and adapted human and veterinary medicine based on new anatomical and physiological research (pulmonary circulation of blood, the eye as an optical instrument, physiology of the stomach), drugs (the use of papaver), and practices (mercuric chloride to disinfect wounds, cauterization of wounds to prevent infection and to stop bleeding). Islamic human and veterinary medicine became the most advanced worldwide for centuries. During the Middle Ages (fifth–fifteenth centuries), the most important collections were written by Islamic scholars in Mamluk Egypt, including Abū ʿAlī b. Abd Allāh b. al-Ḥusayn Ibn Sīnā (Avicenna,

980–1037) for human medicine; Ibn Rushd (Averroes, 1126–1198); and Muḥammad al-Bakhshī al-Ḥalabī (1246–1324) and Ibn al-Mundhir (writing c. 1339–1340) for veterinary medicine. These medical texts applied the theory of the humors to understanding human and animal diseases and linked treatment to anatomical knowledge.

Although the more scholarly authors had little hands-on experience with animals, their extensive reading and sophisticated analytical abilities meant that their texts were highly influential. Al-Bakhshī al-Ḥalabī, for example, was primarily a poet, calligrapher, and important generator of documents for the governor of Damascus and other Mamluk leaders. He wrote his treatise on horses because his high-ranking patrons were interested in horses for practical reasons (hunting and racing, for example) and for theological reasons (explained below). According to another scholar, every ruler needed a range of professional services to be provided by his staff, including veterinary medicine, falconry, chess, medicine, music, astrology, and agriculture. Veterinary treatises were essential to court life and to the ongoing success of every ruler in the fourteenth century.

For the more middling classes of hands-on veterinary practitioners, the most famous book on veterinary medicine, the *Kāshif* or *Al-Kitāb al-Nāsirī*, was written by Abū Bakr al-Bayṭār in the 1330s. "Al-Bayṭār" meant "veterinarian" or "horse-doctor." (Derived from this term, albeitar became the word for professional animal healers in medieval Spain.) Abū Bakr was the son of a highly ranked court veterinarian and a distinguished practitioner in his own right. While serving as chief veterinarian for the powerful sultan Nāsirī, Abū Bakr combined his family's practical knowledge with Greek, Byzantine, South Asian, Arabic, and Persian texts; he cited Vegetius, Aristotle, Hippocrates, and Galen as well as Persian and Indian experts. He also tested some of the treatments recommended by his predecessor authors, and his analysis could be quite critical. Of course, the state of knowledge had changed over seven centuries; but Abū Bakr was one of the few writers who could speak authoritatively about both the classical texts and the current practices of his time.

Abū Bakr's work allows us to envision how Islamic scholars analyzed, questioned, and revised classical texts, often adding new ideas and practices to the accumulated wisdom. The volumes of the *Kāshif* demonstrate that the basis for knowledge about animal health and disease was the theory of humors. Humoral imbalance (as well as external factors such as *miasma*) led to the manifestations of disease, as the ancients had believed. But the originality of the *Kāshif* lies with Abū Bakr's recommended treatments, particularly formulations of medicines, which reflected his experiences and his times. Historian Hosni Alkhateeb Shehada cites the example of *al-baqar* disease (Arabic: ox or cattle disease), which classical texts deemed incurable. He argues that Abū Bakr rejected this, instead recommending a complex medication made from several minerals and plants such as *kahrabā*, *ṭabāshīr*, seeds of the *rijlah* plant, and a decoction of the *lisān al-ḥamal* plant. Another treatment for *al-baqar* disease was based on the seeds of *ḥummāḍ*, *qaṭūnyā*, and *kathīrah*, mixed with the *lisān al-ḥamal* decoction. Modern ingredients, such as sugar, also appeared in Abū Bakr's medical recipes. To us today, Abū Bakr's recommendations look more humane overall than some of the treatments advocated by classical texts (bleeding and purging).

This brings us to a final point: most of these treatises and texts were meant to be used by practitioners, and surviving examples demonstrate just how innovative veterinary practitioners were (Fig. 1.4). As we mentioned earlier, the

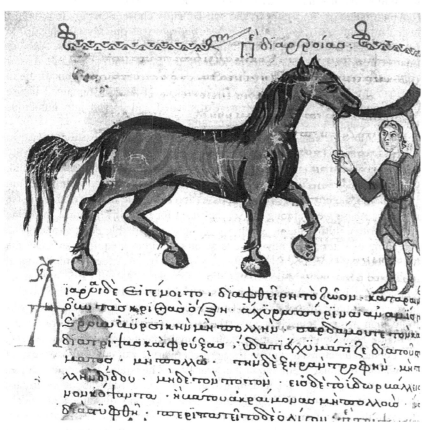

Figure 1.4 Treatment of a horse with diarrhea. A drug is administered with a horn.
Source: Fourteenth-century copy of *Corpus Hippiatricorum Graecorum*. Courtesy: Bibliothèque nationale de France, Paris, Ms Gr. 2244, folio 74v.

Islamic works were translated back into Latin, and from there into Italian, Spanish, French, German, and English, indicating how widely they spread around the West. Veterinary knowledge traveled from the Near East and Northern Africa through southern Italy, Spain, and Armenia. The court of Emperor Frederic II from Hohenstaufen (Barbarossa, 1198–1250) in Sicily became an important clearinghouse of knowledge about veterinary medicine from the Islamic and Latin traditions. For example, Jordanus Rufus (c. 1200–1256), Frederic II's *marescallus* (marshall or master of the cavalry), wrote *De medicina equorum*, a systematic work on equine medicine. In *De medicina equorum*, Rufus addressed the learned stable masters: he described the symptoms of illnesses; tried to determine a material or mechanistic cause (beyond magic or superstition); and subsequently chose a therapy that he had tested in practice himself. *De medicina equorum* was quickly translated into several European languages and remained a standard for centuries. Another treatise from Frederic II's court, written by the blacksmith and stable master Albrant, became the most widespread booklet on practical equine medicine in German during the Middle Ages. The therapies of Albrant remained in use until around 1900 because they were translated and copied into numerous books of recipes for equine medical treatment.

Circulations of veterinary knowledge between cultures also took place in Cilicia (part of modern Turkey), which circa 1200–1375 was a largely Armenian Christian enclave at the crossroads of the Mongol and Mamluk (Egyptian Islamic) empires. In 1258, Cilician forces under King Het'um I conquered Baghdad and obtained possession of Arabic manuscripts on horse medicine; these were among the sources used for the Cilician horse medicine books written during the next century. A quite remarkable book showing the spreading of veterinary knowledge is a compendium on equine medicine, the horse book sponsored by King Smbat, co-written by an Armenian multilingual monk and a Syrian horse-doctor in Cilicia between 1295 and 1298. Among its sources, the book mentions an Indian manuscript and two Arabian works; however, a study of these original references has shown that this book was more than a mere translation of earlier work. Rather, the Smbat-era equine medicine book synthesizes ideas from animal healing in the Indian, Arabic, and Persian literatures and provides a critical overview of contemporary expert knowledge on horse medicine in the Near East. The equine medicine treatises of thirteenth-century Cilicia demonstrate how knowledge about veterinary medicine was appropriated, translated, added to, and disseminated widely between the many learned cultures of the early modern period. This veterinary knowledge, in turn, contributed to the later corpus of works in European languages.

Among contemporary European treatises was the *Mulomedicina* from the Italian bishop Theodoricus Cerviensis (1205–1298), an influential equine medicine book in Latin. Cerviensis' book tells us the types of herbal-based medications used in the early modern period, for example, henbane as an anesthetic to calm horses before surgery. Later, mandrake and poppy were used for this purpose – precursors to the opioids still used in veterinary anesthesia today. The invention of printing (circa 1450) dramatically stimulated translations and compilations of writings on animal breeding and healing from antiquity onward. Older classical texts were re-published, such as *Artis veterinariae sive mulomedicinae* from Flavius Vegetius Renatus (Basel 1524); expanded editions were now possible. The most striking example is *La Gloria del Cavallo* (Venice 1566) written by Pasquale Caracciolo. This treatise of about a thousand pages with a comprehensive number of references mainly deals with horses and horsemanship. It also includes a chapter on cattle diseases. Another important encyclopedist was Conrad Gestner with his *Historia animalium* (Zürich 1551–1558) in which he described the natural history, breeding, and veterinary treatment of the horse. Eventually, the printing press would make animal healing books available to larger sectors of societies, at least, to literate animal owners.

To write treatises and books, however, authors needed patronage from sultans, kings, or religious institutions. Next to courts and monasteries, medical schools of universities increasingly became centers of veterinary knowledge with libraries containing veterinary manuscripts. For example, around 1080 the first medical school started in Salerno, Italy, while the first university in Europe was opened in 1188 in Bologna. Medical faculties formed the basis for university-trained physicians. Lectures were mainly based on Greco-Roman and Islamic texts and students did not get training with hands-on skills. This led to the occupational division between the educated *doctor medicinae*, who theorized and instructed; and the (lower-class) surgeon and apothecary, who obtained their knowledge by apprenticeship, performed the practical manual labor, and regulated their professions in medieval guilds. These and later European traditions of veterinary knowledge owed a great debt to the Islamic scholars who created this rich global corpus of veterinary knowledge. Blending the healing traditions of secular systems (such as the Greco-Roman) and sacred ideas, these early modern animal healers most often worked within sacred traditions and institutions.

New Ideas: Breaking from the Ancient Traditions

However, this dynamic transfer of veterinary knowledge almost came to a standstill during the devastating spread of bubonic plague (Black Death) during the fourteenth century. Originating in wild rodent colonies in eastern Central Asia and western China, bubonic plague spilled over into populations of hunters, farmers, and invading armies during the late 1200s into the mid-1300s. The disease then spread throughout Asia and to Europe along trade routes (plague infects not only rodents and humans, but also camels, cats, and other domesticated animals). Bubonic plague devastated parts of South and East Asia, killed around one-third of Europeans, spread to the continent of Africa, and continued to cause sporadic epidemics for 400 years. In local areas around the world, the plague outbreak changed agriculture and livestock production significantly. In some places, whole cultivated areas were abandoned. As crop-farming decreased, more meadows became available for livestock production. As human populations began to recover from the devastation, meat consumption increased in some areas, and higher livestock numbers demanded veterinary care. Existing veterinary knowledge did not disappear, and it continued to be recorded in treatises that survive today. In Europe, for example, farms belonging to feudal courts and monasteries were the centers of hunting, agriculture, and livestock production, where veterinary knowledge and practices were concentrated. At one monastery, Abbess Hildegard von Bingen's (1098–1179) *Causae et Curae*, for instance, included treatments for livestock diseases along with those for human diseases; these treatises were kept safely in the monastery's library and survived the centuries as one of the few written by a woman. As in the Islamic tradition, religious institutions were important centers for knowledge in the European tradition, both before and after the Black Death era.

Legal texts and trade rules represent another source of information about animal disease, especially among livestock for food and other products, in the fourteenth to sixteenth centuries. In Europe, for example, liver fluke parasites in sheep are mentioned in late medieval trade rules. A seller of sheep guaranteed that the buyer would be given a refund if the animals proved to have internal parasites or a liver sickness within six weeks of purchase. Along with writings on horses and livestock, works were also dedicated to care for dogs and birds used at courts for hunting. A famous example is the *Livre de chasse*, a medieval book on hunting, written in the late fourteenth century by the French count Gaston Phébus. One part of the work is about the nature and care of dogs. This classic was translated many times with editions available even today. Besides the skilled handlers caring for hunting dogs, great value was attached to falconers, who were responsible for the health of birds of prey. Falconry books with extended descriptions of bird diseases were already written in early medieval Persia. Arabic knowledge on falconry was then translated into Latin and used at European courts. The higher educated nobility and clergy used these treatises to instruct their servants on practical animal health care for centuries.

Recovery of agriculture, governance, and learning was slow; but after this dark period of bubonic plague, a new era emerged. In the West, the Renaissance (c. 1400–1600), a golden age in European cultural history, began when many scholars fled to Italy after the conquest of Constantinople in

1453 by the Ottoman Turks and the consequent fall of the Byzantine Empire. From Italy, Renaissance ideas spread across Europe and stimulated art, philosophy, and the sciences. This cultural context not only shaped the relationship between veterinary and human medicine but also potentially challenged the Christian doctrine that God had created humans to be separate from (and superior to) animals.

Ars nova: Anatomy in Europe

The Renaissance changed the ways animals and animal bodies were understood and represented, and this was reflected not only in art but also in a new critical approach to existing knowledge of anatomy. No longer was anatomical training conducted mainly from Galenic treatises; it was now based on active observation and dissection of animal (and occasionally human) bodies. By 1500, all of Europe's approximately seventy medical schools included anatomy lectures based on animals and, increasingly, dissection demonstrations. As part of comparative medicine, elite *doctores medicinae* studied animal anatomy and physiology, as well as animal diseases, for centuries. One early anatomy text (dating to the beginning of the twelfth century) dealt with the pig, the animal considered the closest to humans in terms of anatomy and physiology. This text was used as the anatomical instruction book for students in the medical school of Salerno. A major contribution was made by the universal genius Leonardo da Vinci (1452–1519), who as an artist studied the anatomy of various domesticated animals as well as humans. Following in the footsteps of earlier Islamic scholars working to correct the errors of Galenic anatomy, da Vinci made his superb drawings of human and animal anatomy based on his own observations during dissections. Based on a comparison of human and equine anatomy, he concluded that horses walk on their tiptoes. He also left a very detailed drawing of a gravid bovine uterus, placenta, and innervation of blood vessels.

The scientific basis for human anatomy was laid in 1543 by the Flemish physician Andries van Wesel (Andreas Vesalius, 1514–1564). Vesalius learned to dissect animal bodies during his study at the university of Paris, but he criticized the usual methods of instruction. Ignorant surgeon-dissectors, he wrote, did nothing more than cut up body parts to be examined by students according to the instructions of a physician-lecturer (who never touched the body) reading from a Galenic treatise. For a long time, dissecting human corpses was forbidden and criticized due to cultural and religious restrictions, but from the fourteenth century onward, anatomical demonstrations during lectures slowly became more common. Dissections even attracted the curious public to anatomical theaters, sometimes creating a carnival atmosphere or public spectacle. After dissecting several human corpses (often executed criminals), Vesalius concluded that Galen had probably never seen a human body on the inside, and had obtained his anatomical knowledge from dissecting pigs, dogs, and monkeys. For example, Galen had written that the human liver consisted of four or five lobes instead of two, as Vesalius observed. Based on his own observations on internal structures and functions of the body, and after comparing these with those of ancient Greek, Roman, and Islamic scholars (which was typical for science in the Renaissance) Vesalius wrote *De humani corporis fabrica* [*On the fabric of the human body*]. *De humani corporis fabrica* was a breakthrough: a new detailed and comprehensive anatomy of the human body, including a systematic Latin nomenclature of organs, bones, nerves, blood vessels, and muscles which we still use today. The magnificent drawings to illustrate Vesalius' text were probably made in the studio of the great Renaissance artist Titian. Linked with art and spectacle as well as science, anatomy became the leading scholarly discipline within European human and animal medicine in the sixteenth and seventeenth centuries. Mostly, veterinary anatomy focused on the horse because this was the most valuable animal (with some attention to bovines and other animals).

By 1600, art, science, and aesthetics merged in a fascinating style in printed veterinary anatomical texts. The most important text, a veterinary equivalent of Vesalius' anatomy, was *Dell'Anatomia et dell'Infirmita del Cavallo* (*On anatomy and disease of the horse*, 2 volumes, Bologna 1598) from the Bologna lawyer and senator Carlo Ruini (c. 1530–1598). Ruini was inspired by Vesalius, and although he did not attend the University of Bologna, he became one of the famous horse anatomists of the late sixteenth century. As a member of a rich family, Ruini owned and rode horses and thus had a great deal of experience with them. (He likely learned a great deal from the family stable-masters and other practitioners as well.) Ruini's treatise, the first one exclusively devoted to the anatomy of a species other than humans, appeared shortly after his death. The *Dell'Anatomia* set a new standard for high-quality anatomical illustrations, remaining unsurpassed for centuries. It contains detailed studies on osteology (bones), myology (muscles), splanchnology (viscera), the nervous system, and blood vessels – all captured in very accurately drafted and beautifully rendered woodcut images (Fig. 1.5). The identity of the artist who created these images remains a mystery, and some historians have speculated that he wished to remain anonymous due to the humble practicality and lowly artistic status of his subject, *veterinary* anatomy. Numerous editions of Ruini's book were published, and errors made in the first edition (even in the title) were corrected in the second edition of 1599. As scholars have argued for human anatomical treatises, Ruini's work represented the high value placed on the horse, both for its practical importance and the natural majesty of the equine body in the animal kingdom. His treatise's success in capturing this cultural, as well as practical, value was demonstrated by how widely *Dell'Anatomia* would be copied in the ensuing years.

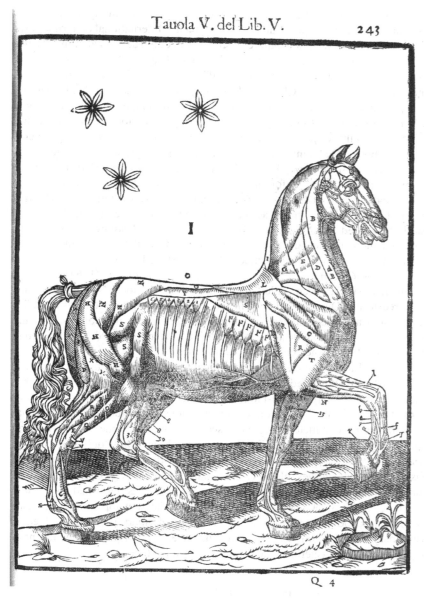

Tauola V. del Lib. V.   243

Q 4

Figure 1.5 Woodcut plate from Carlo Ruini, *Anatomia del cavallo, infermità, et suoi rimedii* (Venice: F. Prati, 1618) 243.
Courtesy: U.S. National Library of Medicine Historical Anatomies Collection.

The text, as well as the 49 beautiful woodcut images, regularly reappeared in later anatomical works without acknowledgment. (International copyright laws did not exist at that time.) Andrew Snape (London 1683), Valentin Trichter (Nuremberg 1715), Gaspar de Saunier (The Hague 1734), and François Garsault (The Hague 1741) all "borrowed" images from Ruini. Andrew Snape, the court horse-doctor of Charles II from England, even claimed that he was the first person to describe the anatomy of the horse, despite the fact that he copied 22 plates from Ruini (reversing the plates in an attempt to hide the plagiarism, which placed the viscera on opposite sides of the body and confused students using his book). De Saunier went even further, asserting that the 61 plates in his horse anatomy were drawn from his own observations when 51 of them were plagiarized from Ruini. Unfortunately, quality did not always improve after the new standard was set by Ruini. An example is Gervase Markham's *Maister-Piece* (London 1610), which has been criticized for its inaccuracies. One historian has declared that Markham's *Maister-Piece* harmed progress in veterinary medicine more than any other text. However, it did circulate widely, including to the British colonies in the Americas. An interesting fact is that the American version, *The Citizen and Countryman's Experienced Farrier* (1764), included treatments that European settlers had learned from the local Native Americans (referred to as "Discreet Indians" in the text). These were botanical remedies based on local plants that were unfamiliar to the European newcomers; thus, the *Experienced Farrier* reflected circulations of veterinary medical knowledge between natives and newcomers in North America.

The final European veterinary anatomical text we will highlight was written in English and illustrated by the London artist George Stubbs (1724–1806). Stubbs, who was largely self-taught, embodied the realist tradition in art and sought to connect the horse's underlying anatomical structures with its external appearance. He conducted his own dissections and, like some of his predecessors, sought to depict the equine body as noble and well designed. In *The Anatomy of the Horse* (1766), Stubbs depicted the skeleton, muscle layers, fascia, ligaments, nerves, blood vessels, glands, and cartilage of the horse from three positions (side, front, and back). Stubbs' book was published, as we will see in Chapter 3, at about the same time as the development of modern veterinary schools. Anatomical dissections for veterinary purposes revived in veterinary schools from the 1760s onward, and anatomy has remained a central subject within the veterinary curriculum ever since then.

Differentiating Animals and Humans

Our focus on anatomy, especially veterinary texts, raises an important cultural question: what do these books reveal about European beliefs regarding the relationship between humans and animals, circa 1600–1750? By studying human and animal bodies, many scholars found similarities. Since ancient times, curious dissectors had studied animals' bodies as proxies for human bodies. Some parts of animal bodies looked almost identical to those of humans, and the notion of "comparative anatomy" was based on homologous structures (such as the human forearm and the horse's front leg). Natural philosophers studying animals' bodies also linked their findings to observations about animals' ability to reason and communicate, like humans. However, there was a problem: in the European Christian sacred context of this time period, only *man* was created in the image of God, not animals. The observed anatomical similarities forced theological scholars to find another way to divide humans from animals, and they focused on debating whether animals had souls, as humans did. In this way, the developing sciences of anatomy (and embryology and physiology, as we will see) challenged the firm theological boundary between humans and animals by uncovering layers of material similarity between species' bodies and stimulating debates about how closely related animals were to humans.

Anatomy was not the only developing science to challenge the human–animal boundary: embryology and physiology added more knowledge about how human and animal bodies developed and functioned. Girolamo Fabrizio (Hieronymus Fabricius ab Aquapendente, 1537–1619) is often considered the father of embryology. He was professor of surgery and anatomy at the University of Padua, and based on dissecting horses, bovines, sheep, pigs, dogs, and mice, he wrote the first comprehensive study on comparative embryology: *De formato foetu* (1600). It contains a detailed description of the outer shapes of the various fetuses and the characteristics of the membranes. In addition, Fabricius studied the anatomy of the eye, ear, intestines, stomach, larynx, and esophagus. Three years later he published a treatise on valves within veins. (The small pulmonary circulation was already described by the Arab physician Ibn al-Nafis (1213–1288), the Spaniard Miguel Serveto (1511–1553), and the Italian Realdo Colombo (c. 1515–1559).)

The University of Padua became the center of comparative anatomy and physiology, led by Fabricius' brilliant student (and later competitor), Giulio Casseri (Julius Casserius, 1552–1616). Casseri, a physician, performed dissections for students on different animal species and human cadavers. Based on these, he authored three reference books on comparative anatomy and physiology. Both Fabricius and Casseri (who succeeded Fabricius as professor in 1604) were teachers of the British physician William Harvey (1578–1657). Harvey's observation of valves within veins triggered his theory and experiments on capillaries and the large blood circulation, which was published in 1628 (see Chapter 2). Further supporting similarities between humans and animals, Harvey also wrote that humans and other mammals originated from eggs and that the reproductive cycle was the same for all. These were milestones in the history of the modern sciences; and they were challenges to the Christian doctrine that God had created humans to be completely different from (and superior to) animals.

However, the anatomical and embryological scientific evidence was not strong enough to make animals "more human" for two major reasons: theological doctrine and religious rituals were more powerful than science at this time; and most people had no opportunity to study scholarly texts and thus continued relying on older, well-established beliefs and healing practices. Although many anatomy texts (including Ruini's) included sections on treating injuries and diseases, these findings did not greatly affect disease causation theories or change contemporary healing practices (in part because Ruini's therapeutics were quite traditional). Methods of surgery could have benefited from greater knowledge of internal anatomy; however, seldom did surgeons attempt to work on the internal organs because neither antisepsis nor anesthesia were yet available. Animal healers continued to rely on correcting an imbalance of humors with bleeding or purging; fighting inflammation in horses' legs with blistering and cauterizing; and administering medicines made from plants and simple chemical compounds. They learned these skills through apprenticeship with a more experienced practitioner (this was also true of most physicians for humans). In the medical marketplace in most of Europe, a strict hierarchy existed: a few educated scholars at the top, then the physicians for upper-class and wealthy people; followed by more humble physicians; and then, at the lower levels, surgeons and apothecaries and veterinarians. The social distinction between physicians and surgeons was preserved through the mid-1800s (and that between veterinarians and the various human medical practitioners even longer). Surgery, apothecary work, and veterinary medicine were considered (in most places) to be trades, not professions; and they all did the manual labor disdained by the more socially exalted physicians. The social differences between physicians and veterinarians reflected the differentiation between humans and animals in the Western Christian tradition: according to the Bible, God placed animals on the earth to serve man, and the value of animals lay in the resources and services they could supply to the growing numbers of humans populating the earth in the 1600s and 1700s.

Conclusions

From this very brief survey of several centuries, we can conclude that:

1. The domestication of elephants, horses, poultry, bovines, and other animals supplied animal bodies for food, transport, power, and cultural status. Also, many societies incorporated animals into their sacred traditions and developed elaborate systems of knowledge about animals (including animal

healing). All these uses made animals valuable economically and culturally within human societies.

2. Animal healers, like human medical practitioners, gained knowledge mainly through experience and apprenticeship. Some texts were written and kept in libraries (especially by Islamicate scholars), and a few writers in Europe began publishing printed texts about animal anatomy and medicine by the 1500s.

3. Globally, the most common theories of disease causation in humans and animals in early modern times were probably supernatural ones: magical forces, divine intervention, or punishment for sinful behavior. Within the same time, place, and culture, supernatural or sacred theories could be combined with natural ones; they were not mutually exclusive.

4. Natural (not supernatural) theories were important in Southeast and East Asia, and in ancient Greece and Rome. In the Greco-Roman tradition, they included the theory of the humors; the miasma theory; and contagion. Ayurvedic theories (India) incorporated the theory of humors into a universal cosmology of elements and seasons. Traditional Chinese medicine sought to balance and nurture the essential energy of the body, the *qi*.

5. Treatments corresponded logically to the theories. Depending on the tradition, sacred rituals could be combined with bodily treatments in attempts to cure patients. Treatments for the imbalance of humors included removing excess blood (bleeding) and bile (vomiting and purging); for nurturing the *qi*, these included acupuncture and guided movements or massage. Sacred rituals included invocations to the gods, prayer, blessings, and others.

6. Knowledge about animal healing circulated between different cultures. For example, Abū Bakr al-Bāytar wrote an important veterinary medical text in the 1330s that combined his family's practical veterinary knowledge with Greek, Byzantine, South Asian, Arabic, and Persian texts; he cited Vegetius, Aristotle, Hippocrates, and Galen as well as Persian and Indian experts. Islamicate scholars in the medieval and early modern periods were especially important to collecting, revising, and circulating veterinary knowledge.

7. In Europe during and after the Renaissance, the development of sciences such as anatomy and embryology had the potential to challenge the Christian doctrine that God had created humans to be separate from (and superior to) animals. Comparative anatomy demonstrated many similarities between the bodies of humans and other mammals, for example.

8. However, the anatomical and embryological scientific evidence was not strong enough to make animals "more human" for two major reasons: theological doctrine and religious rituals were more powerful than science at this time; and most people had no opportunity to study scholarly texts and thus continued relying on older, well-established beliefs and healing practices.

9. In the early modern period, animals' ability to contribute to societies depended on animals' bodies being healthy and fulfilling the particular needs of that culture. Regimes of animal healing developed within these world-ordering cosmologies to provide for specific material requirements of complex societies.

Many complex societies were built with large numbers of domesticated animals. However, keeping animals close to or inside people's houses effectively altered the environments of both. People and their domesticated animals shared microorganisms (which also co-evolved with them over time). A major problem with the closeness of human and domesticated animal populations was the spread and evolution of pathogens, and healers for both humans and animals faced the challenges of emergent diseases then (as we do now). Increasingly, human activities shaped the ecologies of health and disease around the world. When the peoples of the Western and Eastern Hemispheres encountered each other in the late 1400s, for example, the invading Europeans brought their domesticated animals, plants, and diseases with them. As we will see in the next chapter, these demographic and ecological transformations ushered in a new era for animal healing and veterinary medicine.

Question/Activity: Can you find examples of how healers in your region or nation contributed to knowledge about animal disease, from ancient times until 1700? What were the major theories about disease causation, and what were the major treatments used on sick animals?

2　Animal Healing in Trade and Conquest, 1700–1850s

Introduction

Globalization is not new. People and other animals, plants, and microbes traveled great distances from the time of ancient migrations to the Americas, and the Polynesians; through the early Chinese dynastic empires; to the invasions of the Crusades and the Mongols. Besides archaeological evidence, we have few sources for understanding how the transfers of ancient civilizations and ecologies affected the world inherited by later generations. Traces disappear and become naturalized, as if they had always been present; but this is an illusion. Our world has been continually re-made by peoples (and microorganisms, plants, and animals). What roles did animal healing play in early modern globalization, and how did global forces affect the development of veterinary medicine? We must necessarily limit our scope in this chapter to only two centuries (circa 1650–1850) and a few case studies. Overall, we show how the history of animal healing in this time period was mainly shaped by two important aspects of globalization: trade and conquest.

By the late 1600s, human activities had dramatically interconnected the world's continents, transforming environments as well as societies. By engaging in colonialism, opening trade routes, and geopolitical conflicts, humans knowingly and unknowingly transported animals, plants, microbes, and diseases across vast distances (this is known as ecological exchange). All these activities required healthy domestic animals for food, warfare, power, and transport. Keeping these animals alive and well in new environments or dangerous conditions was a major challenge. A more interconnected planet also meant new circulations of human and animal diseases. Responding to these challenges caused significant changes in animal healing and veterinary medicine.

This chapter analyzes three phenomena and their influences on the development of animal healing: ecological exchanges, imperialism, and animal epidemics; how people responded to animal epidemics; and the development of military veterinary surgery. Ecological imperialism, as defined by historian Alfred Crosby in the 1970s, is the theory that domesticated animals (and plants) were crucial to conquering newly discovered lands and newly encountered peoples. One example is Portuguese and Spanish adventurers bringing horses to the Americas, where horse-like animals had been extinct for millennia. Likewise, diseases traveled on ships and overland, infecting groups of people who had never encountered these microorganisms (as described by the historian William McNeill). A similar (but less well-studied) effect occurred with *animal* diseases, such as rinderpest and contagious pleuropneumonia in cattle. Finally, armies began appointing professional animal healers to keep cavalry and artillery horses healthy.

These problems were not new, but by 1700 new social institutions began to offer new solutions. These included the spread of book printing by which knowledge could be quickly disseminated to literate people; the establishment of universities; and the birth of modern scientific studies of animal bodies (such as physiology and pathology). These institutions developed within the frameworks of the European Enlightenment, the Qing Dynasty in East Asia, and other learned cultures. They built on the traditions and institutions that already existed from the ancient through early modern periods discussed in Chapter 1, but the scope was wider and pace of development relatively faster. Yet books, universities, and the developing sciences probably did not change the treatments used by animal healers very much. Treatments corresponded to centuries-old theories about animal bodies, and popular beliefs and practices were slow to change. But in this era of global interconnection, animal healing systems could incorporate knowledge from multiple cultures on multiple continents. Overall, the animal diseases and problems that mattered were those that threatened the society's cultural, commercial, political, and military interests – and these interests shaped early modern developments in animal healing and veterinary medicine.

Ecological Exchange: Natives, Newcomers, and Invaders

The Americas, Western Africa, and Europe

What happened when different cultures of animal healing and veterinary medicine encountered each other? Did these healing cultures communicate information to each other at first? (Few historians or anthropologists have analyzed these first encounters, and this is an exciting area for further veterinary history research.) In Chapter 1, we introduced the travels of European adventurers that brought the Western and Eastern Hemispheres into contact with each other. Christopher Columbus' second voyage in 1493 brought European species of domestic animals to the West Indies on the small ships that crossed the Atlantic. These animals not only survived but also multiplied well and served as the foundation stock for the Spanish colonies in Mexico. When animals escaped their owners, they established wild herds. (There is a

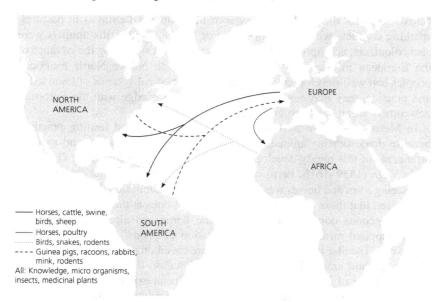

Figure 2.1 Map showing the New World, the Atlantic, and Western Africa with arrows indicating the exchanges of animals and knowledge.
Courtesy: Lisanne van de Voort, Faculty of Veterinary Medicine, Utrecht University.

famous example of most Central American rabbits descending from one pregnant female who escaped her cage.) This is ecologically interesting: sometimes species die in new places, and sometimes they succeed as invasive species. European domesticated animals (horses, cattle, dogs, chickens) proved themselves to be successful invaders in the Americas, adapting to new environments. With each voyage, more animals arrived: in 1520 European cattle were introduced in Florida (now part of the United States) by the voyage of Juan Ponce de León, and large animals (horses, cattle) came to the Virginia colonies about 1611. (Few larger livestock animals were brought into New England until 1620) (Fig. 2.1).

Domestic animals' needs shaped social and economic relations between the Native peoples of North America and the European colonizers. At first, European ideas about animals and land as property astonished North American Native peoples, many of whom had a holistic cosmology that considered animals and people to be closely related. European newcomers, whose lifeways were built around domesticated animals, in turn viewed Native beliefs and lifeways as "uncivilized," partly because they did not raise livestock. For their part, Native peoples recognized the Europeans' animals as both a resource and a threat. They often killed European animals that strayed onto

Native lands for the meat; and they sometimes attacked animals in pastures, sparking conflicts with the Europeans. For Native peoples, the animals were also colonizers, appropriating land and resources and signifying the advance of the European invaders. In this situation, although Native North American peoples had well-developed (often plant-based) medical systems of knowledge and practice, they may not have shared much knowledge with the European newcomers when they first encountered them.

In Mesoamerica, we have more evidence about animal healing practices because domesticating animals was more common in the urban and agricultural areas of this highly developed society. The *mestizo* chronicler Garcilaso de la Vega (1539–1616, Peru) observed that the Incan peoples' reactions to first seeing oxen and horses was astonishment and admiration; but they quickly recognized that these were *animals* – and useful ones at that. Incans had their own indigenous domesticated animals, the llama and alpaca, for example, which supplied meat, fiber, and transportation of goods. Medical treatments for animals (similar to those of humans) were based on spiritual beliefs, herbal knowledge and empiricism. For example, Garcilaso de la Vega described a great epidemic of *carache* (llama mange) and Incan experiments with several herbs trying to cure it. (Finally, only warm pig-fat rubbed on the skin helped.) He catalogued medicinal plants indigenous to what is now Peru, and he described how the Incans used them medicinally. In this way, de la Vega's treatises demonstrate a robust system of healing practices for humans and animals already present in Central America when Europeans arrived. From the early modern treatises such as de la Vega's that survive today, we surmise that the European invaders did get medical knowledge (especially useful plants) from Indigenous Central Americans.

In North America by 1630, domesticated animal numbers in the Virginia colonies exceeded 5,000, despite many animal deaths during Native American–European battles in 1622. This included mainly chickens, swine, and cattle but not yet many horses. Horses were less useful in Virginia because they required more care than cattle. Also, oxen were better suited to plowing new fields, which was very hard work for horses. There appears to have been some transfer of animal treatments from England, as there are references to an expert cow-doctor practicing in Virginia as early as 1625. We do not know what types of treatments were being used; however, the colonists probably brought the veterinary practices of their homelands with them. Several handbooks and treatises for the treatment of animals existed in vernacular languages (English, Spanish, Portuguese) at this time and we will briefly discuss them below.

The other major influences on this complex culture of animal healing were the people from the continent of Africa who were forcibly relocated or migrated to the Americas. By 1600, about 500,000 Africans lived in the

Americas. Historians have recovered evidence that Africans brought with them extensive knowledge about agriculture and animal husbandry. Western Africa (the homelands of many African Americans) was (and is) home to large animals such as antelope, gazelle, wildebeest, primates, hogs, giraffe, and wild dogs. Africans successfully domesticated guinea fowl and donkeys and bred groups of cattle and goats acclimated to the local conditions. Western Africans were also familiar with horses. The great Malian empire (1217–1255) had been united by the powerful leader Sunjata and his generals using horses purchased from North African traders. By 1500, when larger numbers of African people began to arrive in the Americas, African pastoralists brought their experience and knowledge about keeping cattle alive and well in difficult environmental conditions (high temperatures, for example). Because ticks and flies were a constant problem in sub-Saharan regions, Africans from certain regions had much more experience with insect-transmitted tropical diseases than Native Americans or Europeans did. Their knowledge was probably crucial to successful livestock-keeping, especially in the hot climates of the southern and equatorial Americas

In current studies of animal-keeping in Africa and surviving historical documents from early modern America, we find evidence of African knowledge about cattle disease that influenced early modern American animal healing. In Tanzania and Zimbabwe, pastoralists have demonstrated a vigorous understanding of ticks and tick-borne diseases and a complex system of *materia medica* based on local plants. Maasai cattle owners, for example, described eight different tick-borne diseases they said were caused by the bites of six tick species. They used hand-picking and application of kerosene-based skin treatments to clean ticks off the animals and burning and smoking to kill ticks in pastures. If the animal became sick, cattle owners applied botanical remedies based on plants such as *Aloe*, *Cissus*, and *Terminalia* (all with medicinal properties recognized by Western medicine today). In the midlands of Zimbabwe today, ingredients such as snail shell and more than twenty plant species, compounded into drenches and ointments, are used by livestock owners and animal healers to treat injuries and diseases (mainly common diseases such as diarrhea). Of course, we do not know if this accurately represents the state of knowledge in the sixteenth–eighteenth centuries; but it gives us some idea of the traditional types of animal healing still practiced by people in these regions of Africa.

Historical studies demonstrate the transmission of plants and medical knowledge from Africa to the Americas, as part of the ecological exchange across the Atlantic Ocean. Africans provided crucial expertise for growing rice, for example, and brought new plants such as okra (*Abelmoschus esculentus*) and watermelon (*Citrullus lanatus*). Kola nuts (an ingredient in the original "Coca-Cola") and the Ethiopian coffee plant (*Coffea arabica*) also originated in Africa and traveled to the Americas. Both kola and coffee were used as components of medicinal preparations and as stimulants. Africans also brought knowledge about inoculation (causing immunity in a healthy animal or person by introducing small amounts of infectious materials) to the Americas. Inoculation, long used in China to prevent smallpox, spread west through the Turkish empire via Circassia and into eastern and northern Africa. (Chinese naval expeditions reached eastern Africa even earlier, so it is possible that knowledge about inoculation arrived with them in the sixteenth century.) We are only beginning to uncover the rich history of medical knowledge circulations between East Asia, Africa, and the Americas. But domesticated animals were very valuable, and they traveled. Knowledge about keeping them healthy surely traveled with them, just as botanical knowledge, plants, and seeds journeyed from one continent to another.

Early printed treatises and books, which were widely available by 1600, targeted animal owners and lay healers as well as professionals. One of the early sources of veterinary knowledge is *El Libro de Albeitería*, written in 1575 in New Spain by Juan Suárez de Peralta (1541–1613). This equestrian was born as son of one of the conquistadores in the city México-Tenochtitlan. With this work, Suárez de Peralta imported the *albeitería* legacy from Spain into Central America. Written English texts traveled to the Americas in both handwritten and printed form, including recipes that described how to make medications. These texts tell us that Europeans learned from Native Americans and Africans, creating a New World veterinary tradition that braided together the knowledge people chose to share. For example, based on Gervase Markham's English book, American treatise *The Citizen's and Countryman's Experienced Farrier* was updated and edited by John Millis (a farrier) and George Jeffries (a gentleman farmer). In this book, reprinted in Delaware in 1764, the editors consulted Native American healers and included this information in the recipes. For example, to treat a horse's wounds, they reported that Native Americans strongly recommended using the root of the "fringe-tree." If the root's bark was steeped in spring water and applied continuously to the wound, it would heal well even if ligaments and tendons were damaged. These texts were published for ordinary livestock owners as well as gentleman farmers. Text about herbal treatments, pamphlets, and almanacs were also popular in colonial North America and would have been widely used by both men and women to manage animal health and reproduction.

East and South Asia, the Middle East, and Europe

In considering circulations of animals and knowledge about healing, we cannot overemphasize the importance of the Muslim world in the late medieval and early modern periods (circa 1100–1500) and beyond. The great Ottoman empire encompassed many cultures, facilitating knowledge exchange. Many Muslim men (and some women) traveled to the Middle East on the *hajj* (pilgrimage to the holy city, Mecca). Others, such as the pilgrim Ibn Battuta, continued traveling for years, relying on the Muslim networks that spanned Africa, the Middle East, and Asia. Ibn Battuta's accounts of his travels (circa 1325–1350) survive today and give us a glimpse into the uses of horses and other animals during this time. For example, he described a thriving trade in horses between the ports of Yemen across the Indian Ocean to India (in return, Yemeni gardens received Indian betel-trees and coconuts). Although Ibn Battuta does not mention the standard Islamic texts, the *Bayṭara* or the *Hippiatrica*, the courts of his Islamic hosts during his travels would have included horse-masters because horses were the main mode of overland travel and an important military tool. Ibn Battuta's notes about animal feeding are particularly interesting: in a Yemeni port city, he found that the "beasts" were fed in part with fish; in the deserts of present-day Uzbekistan, the cattle ate the native "herbs" (which must have been sparse). From him we learn that princes and sultans across Asia and northern Africa were often the only people allowed to own and ride horses. They maintained large stables (where they would have employed professional animal healers familiar with classic veterinary texts) (Fig. 2.2). The common people cared for their own donkeys, goats, and (when they had them) cattle.

During the sixteenth through the eighteenth centuries, dramatic changes took place in the Old World's empires: the Manchus invaded northern China, ending the Ming Dynasty around 1644; the Ottomans under Suleiman the Magnificent made a final (unsuccessful) attempt to conquer Europe in the late 1600s; and under Akbar the Great's rule, the multicultural Mughal empire (Indian subcontinent) greatly expanded in wealth and size by 1600. The Mughals were well connected and constantly moving overland and across the Indian Ocean (where they met with the Ottomans and with Portuguese and other Europeans). As Muslims, Mughal rulers went on *hajj* to Mecca; and their diplomatic and trading networks were probably the greatest in the world. Overall, the Mughal Emperor Akbar encouraged tolerance and the incorporation of foreign knowledge and materials. But his armies' conquests and trading networks were built in part by wealth generated close to home: the elephants of Gondwana and conquering this mountainous region containing wild elephant herds was one of Akbar's first priorities. Along with the adoption of cannons and matchlock guns, Akbar's "Gunpowder Empire" could also be called the "Elephant Empire." Akbar's war elephants, once collected from the wild in Gondwana, were tamed and trained to charge and break enemy lines (Fig. 2.3). Their size and ferocity terrorized their opponents and enabled riders to fight from advantageous positions.

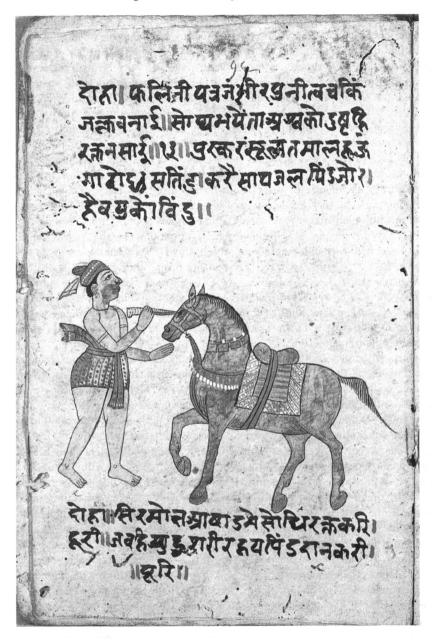

Figure 2.2 Eye operation on a horse.
Source: Shalihotra Samhita [treatise on horses] India eighteenth century. Courtesy:
Wellcome Library, London, Illustration and Text 18th Century Collection: Asian
Collection.

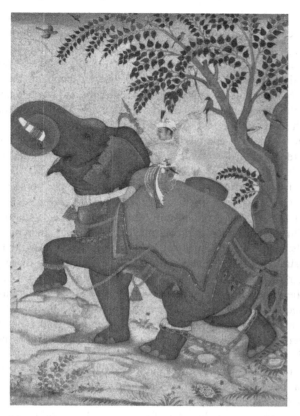

Figure 2.3 Emperor Akbar training an elephant. Miniatur der Moghulschule, Indien, dated circa 1609–1610.
Courtesy: Staatliche Museen zu Berlin – Museum für islamische Kunst.

Mughal victories and stability in the conquered areas depended greatly on healthy animals. Important animals are featured in artistic representations of this empire. Besides the war elephants, every unit of the Mughal army maintained a cavalry of Arabian horses and used bullocks to transport artillery. Especially with the war animals, animal keepers and healers needed to be able to perform minor surgeries quickly and cleanly. In elephants, wounds often developed into abscesses that required draining and cleaning. Southeast Asian elephant keepers packed fresh wounds with sugar and applied maggots to clean out gangrene. Herbal treatments were also commonly used in elephants (in large doses, we surmise). Lameness in horses was treated with poultices or hot irons (cautery), while drenching was used in both horses and cattle to administer medications and to treat colic. But the most important medicine was prevention, especially maintaining proper feeding for optimal digestion. For all animals traveling far away from home territories, or working in difficult conditions, making sure that they had enough high-quality food was probably the most critical aspect of keeping them well. For an elephant, that meant locating about 600 pounds of digestible fodder daily; in some places and circumstances, this would have been a monumental task. Horses, on the other hand, were both more mobile and easier to maintain.

Mughal rulers traded animals (and knowledge about them) and fought over borderland territory with the Persians, who were based in what is now Iran. In the time of the Shah Abbas (the Great, 1571–1629), the Persian empire included vast territories north into the traditional horse-breeding regions of the Caucasus, east to the territories of the Uzbeks, and south to Kandahar in present-day Afghanistan. Abbas' court was a multicultural center, with Chinese ceramics and silk-makers, Armenian merchants, and English generals. Circassians, Armenians, and Georgians served in the military and as administrative officials, and scholars have found that these people contributed their own knowledge about animal healing. Circa 1600, Abbas probably had the largest cavalry in the world. Persian success was based not only on the conquests of Shah Abbas' armies, but also on his court's diplomatic connections with the English East India Company and other trading factions, bolstered by several diplomatic missions to Europe between 1599 and 1615.

Moving east, knowledge about horses circulated between the steppe peoples of Central Asia and Chinese horse breeders and veterinarians. Some of this knowledge was described in texts such as the *Qimin yaoshu* (Essential Arts of the Common People), an encyclopedia of Chinese culture and society attributed to Jia Sixie (circa 540 CE). Art historian Robert E. Harrist has argued that this text and others strongly influenced the early science of equine physiognomy, the study of bone structure, and its influence on the horse's temperament, performance, and value. Physiognomy was an important foundation for anatomy, in both veterinary medicine and in Chinese art. The great Chinese veterinarians of the sixteenth century, Yu Ren, Yu Jie, Yu Ben-Yuan, and Yu Ben-Heng, described clinical judgments and treatment as deriving in part from a horse's physiognomy. This is especially evident in versions of the authoritative treatise *Yuan Heng liao ma ji zhushi* (Ming Dynasty, ca. 1550). As Chinese historians have shown, the horse physiognomy texts demonstrated the underlying theory of perfection in the cosmos, through perfect measurements of the horse's body and perfect balance of the *yin* and *yang*. Knowledge about evaluating horses and addressing their illnesses and injuries was both practical and philosophical; and it owed its origins to the blending of East and Central Asian expertise.

We can also trace the interactions between Asians and Europeans in the eighteenth and early nineteenth centuries by focusing on the role of horses during the late Qing Dynasty in China. The Qing Dynasty (1636–1912) succeeded the Ming when the Jurchen (Manchu) people swept down from the north, allied with Mongol cavalry archers, and conquered northern China (although it took 40 more years to subdue southern China). During the Qing Dynasty, the tributary system brought not only money and goods but also people and animals into northern China from the hinterlands. In this way, the Qing were interconnected with the Russian empire and the kingdoms of Central and Southeast Asia while officially remaining an isolated culture by choice. However, with the increasing contacts made by Europeans during the 1700s, the Qing created cantons, or trading places, to keep the foreign influence under their control. From the surviving accounts of Europeans who lived there (and traveled into China), we get a good picture of their admiration for Chinese sciences and technologies (not only gunpowder and printing, but also metal shoes for horses and bullocks had been first developed in Asia). From Marco Polo to travelers in the 1800s, Europeans noted the similarities between Western and Eastern animal husbandry and healing practices. The British veterinarian George Fleming, visiting China in 1862, noted that Chinese and British farriers similarly used the twitch and stocks to restrain horses. Fleming did not lack the unfortunate European sense of superiority common to this time period; but he also recorded many details about Chinese animal healing practices that revealed his genuine interest and even sometimes his admiration.

Fleming described the *Yi-ma*, a type of northern Chinese horse-doctor, as "intelligent" and as having "the dignity and self-possession of a skillful practitioner, and a useful member of society" (Fig. 2.4). To Fleming, the *Yi-ma* was a curious blend of the learned veterinary surgeon and the "empirical farrier." While the *Yi-ma*, "like our own empirical farriers . . . has a lot of idle notions, vague traditions and mouldy recipes," he also often could quote "Choo-tsze" and "other learned authors of works on Chinese Veterinary Medicine published more than five generations ago." (Most British farriers of this time period could not have done this, nor would they have thought "book-learning" to be useful.) The *Yi-ma* was trusted by his clients, was familiar with many diseases, and "was very confident of being competent to contend successfully with them." He was a mainstay of the medical marketplace for animals in nineteenth-century China.[1]

---

[1] Fleming, G. (2010, 1863). *Travels on Horseback in Mantchu Tartary: Being a Summer's Ride Beyond the Great Wall of China* (Cambridge Library Collection – Travel and Exploration in Asia). Cambridge: Cambridge University Press. doi:10.1017/CBO9780511709531, pp. 402–403; "very confident," p. 406.

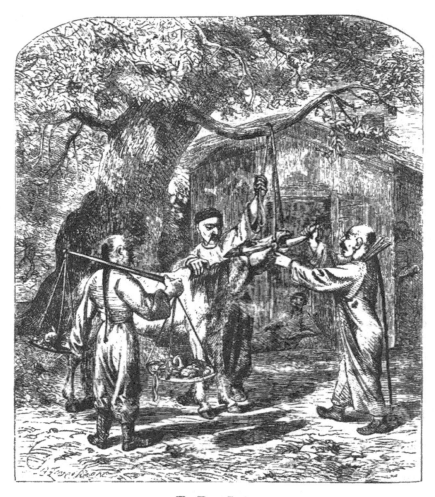

The Horse Doctor.

Figure 2.4 The *Yi-ma* or northern Chinese horse-doctor, Mantchu Tartary.
Note the use of drenching, using a horn to administer oral medication, while
the *Yi-ma*'s assistant carries the necessary instruments and ingredients.
Source: George Fleming, Travels *on Horseback in Mantchu Tartary* (London: Hurst
and Blackett, 1863) 406.

Today, we consider medical knowledge as something that should be freely
disseminated; but until the 1900s, political and mercantile considerations often
determined how knowledge traveled. A good example is Japan, which carefully controlled its contacts with China and the rest of the world in the

eighteenth and nineteenth centuries. The Japanese government restricted contact with Europeans to the Dutch, who had invaded parts of today's Indonesia and established income-generating colonies there. The Dutch East India Company was allowed to trade with the Japanese on the man-made peninsula Dejima during most of the Edo period. In the eighteenth century, this trading post became a center of knowledge exchange between Europeans and the Japanese, including medical and veterinary theories and practices. For example, Willem ten Rhijne (1647–1700), a Dutch medical doctor and botanist, visited Dejima in 1674–1676, where he introduced Western medical ideas and in turn learned about Japanese and Chinese medicine, including acupuncture and moxibustion. In 1683, he wrote the first account of acupuncture published in Europe and in turn imported Dutch anatomical atlases into Japan. The most popular Dutch booklet on horse medicine, written by the master farrier Pieter Almanus van Cour in 1688, was translated into Japanese in 1730. It is the oldest source on Western equine medicine in Japan. Each year the Dutch had to pay tribute to the shogun in Nagasaki, and the most important wish of the shogun was that the Dutch present him with horses imported from the Dutch East Indies. The shogun's court horse-keepers crossbred the Dutch horses with Japanese animals, breeding larger horses that could thrive on Japanese territory and also provide cavalry mounts for the military. Cavalry-building was an important part of the nation-building taking place in Japan during this early modern period of samurai rule.

In these examples and many others, the importance of animals to political and commercial power drove development and circulations of knowledge about animal healing in many parts of the world between the seventeenth and nineteenth centuries. Whether these knowledge circulations affected local practices throughout largely rural animal economies is still an open question. Nonetheless, during this time period the winds of change disturbed stasis in many quarters, including long-standing cultural beliefs and philosophies about the relationships/connections between animals and humans.

Competing Cosmologies and Beliefs about Human–Animal Relationships

An important theme of this book is that people treat animals according to how they value them: basically, for food and work, but beyond that, philosophically and ethically. In Chapter 1, we glimpsed some of these values and concerns within the sacred traditions associated with animal healing. In North America, for example, many of the Algonquian peoples understood animals and humans to possess equally the *manitou*, or spiritual life force. This moral framework linked humans directly to other animals and encouraged practices such as respecting the independence, autonomy, and power of animals. Many ancient belief systems incorporating shamanism (such as Tengrism in central Asia) attribute souls to animals as well as humans. The soul-connection structured human–animal interactions because human actions were *based on the animal's interests* – not just the interests of humans. This distinction shapes cultures of animal healing.

For centuries in the West, most scholars deemed human interests to be more important than those of animals. In ancient Greece, Aristotle believed that animals possessed a vegetative and a sensitive (animal) soul, but not a rational one or morals like humans. Therefore, animals were inferior to, and should serve, humans. Even observing and teaching about animals contributed to a logical system that subsumed them. Later, sacred Christian texts and beliefs maintained the Aristotelian hierarchy. In his theological works, Christian scholar Augustine of Hippo (354–430 CE) argued that humans could use animals at will but should treat them kindly because cruelty to animals led to cruelty to other humans. Likewise, the Christian scholar Thomas of Aquinas (1225–1274) wrote that animals needed no respect because they were not rational creatures as humans were. Only when human suffering could be avoided by treating animals kindly should the animals' interest be taken into account. This vision was challenged by Michel de Montaigne (1533–1592), French politician and philosopher, who advocated for the feelings and rationality of animals, including their unspoiled moral virtue. In 1580, he wrote: "When I play with my cat, how can I know whether she is amusing herself with me, rather than I am with her?"[2] De Montaigne and his successors believed that animals were wise and virtuous, possessed reason, and knew passions, love, hate, affection, jealousy, joy, sorrow, and pain. They asserted that animals lived consistent with nature, were morally superior, and, hence, served as an example for humans.

In the pre-modern Islamic treatises of the Ottoman empire, the moral imperative to learn about and care for horses was based on their exalted status as preferred weapons of Allah. Nourishing the horse as well as the devout rider was important to ensure success in *jihad*, the holy struggle on behalf of Allah; even angels were said to ride horses. Horses' temperaments and value (as well as their health) were evaluated according to the doctrine of the humors. Like humans, individual animals had a dominant humor, dictating the animal's behaviors and attributes. Even its color and conformation (external anatomy) indicated the mixture of the humors within its body. A horse with a generally hot and dry humoral disposition was well suited to training as a warhorse. Its particular personality and humoral disposition were paired with those of its owner or rider for the purpose of creating the most effective force for *jihad*. The Muslim holy book, the *Qur'an*, clearly stated that the beasts and birds

---

[2] Montaigne, Michel de; tr. Charles Cotton (1686). Apology for Raymond Sebond, *Essays*, Book 2, Chapter 12, paragraph 63.

were members of "communities, just like you" (humans); all were essential participants in the created world.

These are only very brief sketches of complex philosophical systems that changed dramatically over time. We have space to discuss in detail only one example, early modern European philosophy, to illustrate how changing moral dictates affected animal use and animal healing. During the seventeenth century, the writings of René Descartes (1596–1650) brought a new under-standing about the relationship between humans and animals. Descartes separ-ated humans from all other living things because only humans possessed the *res cogitans,* a special non-physical substance that today we might call aware-ness or consciousness. Based on his mechanistic model, Descartes explained that animals were irrational because they lacked language and a rational soul like humans, and, hence, could not be consciously aware of their sensations (including hunger, thirst, or pain). Animals were nothing more than soulless complex living machines, like a clock. Nevertheless, Descartes himself was not fully convinced of his doctrine on animals; it could not be proven if animals are able to think, because nobody could look inside the heart of animals.

French priest and rational philosopher Nicolas Malebranche (1638–1715) agreed with Descartes: ". . . in animals there is neither intelligence nor soul, as one ordinarily hears of it. They eat without pleasure, cry without grief, grow without knowing it; they desire nothing, fear nothing, know nothing. . . ."[3] However, this interpretation only represented a small minority of thinkers. Philosophers such as Henri More, Pierre Bayle, and John Locke protested that observation, reason, and common sense all argued that animals had thoughts and feelings. French medical doctor Julien Offray de la Mettrie (1709–1751) even argued that if animals were complicated machines, so were humans because the bodies of both followed mechanical laws and principles of the natural sciences. Still, these philosophical uncertainties meant that many people felt free to treat animals without any concern for their comfort or well-being during this time period.

The subsequent European Enlightenment period during the eighteenth cen-tury brought a change in philosophies, partly due to attention paid to earlier Islamicate and Hindu texts. For example, Jeremy Bentham (1748–1832), an English philosopher, economist, and theoretical jurist, advocated kindness to animals for their own sake because they could feel pain. In a footnote of his treatise *An Introduction to the Principles of Morals and Legislation* he referred to the "Gentoo and Mahometan religions'. . . interests of the rest of the animal creation," continuing with the oft-quoted rhetorical question: "The question is

---

[3] Malebranche, N. (1842; 1674). *De la recherche de la verité* in *Œvres de Malebranche,* vol. 2 (Paris: Charpentier), pp. 561–562.

not, can they [animals] reason? nor, can they talk? but, can they suffer?"[4] For both animals and humans, the greatest happiness for the largest number should be the basis for morality and laws of behavior, he wrote. This utilitarian approach meant that decreasing pain resulted in more pleasure and, thus, in more happiness for each individual. In terms of how animals should be treated, Bentham saw them as part of a larger moral system that should be encoded in the laws that affected women and slaves as well. For instance, he advocated slaughtering animals for meat quickly and without pain. Then these animals would be better off than if they had died a slow and painful death in nature.

Bentham's radical break with Cartesian ideas on differences between humans and animals, and his utilitarian plea for kindness to animals, didn't change the treatment of animals overnight. Nevertheless, it did fit in a general societal movement of increasing opposition against cruelty toward animals. Historians have demonstrated how English elites developed close emotional relationships with animals, particularly with their horses and dogs, during the sixteenth through the nineteenth centuries. Although we have less evidence about poorer people's attitudes, empathy toward animals and condemning animal abuse were not uncommon. The German philosopher Immanuel Kant (1724–1804) also condemned animal abuse but for a different reason: those who were cruel to animals would also be cruel to humans. For Kant, treating animals in a humane way was in the self-interest of humanity because animals existed to serve humans (a widespread belief in popular cultures).

These philosophical debates influenced the developing sciences and education in European societies. For example, Immanuel Kant's philosophical position justified experimentation on living animals. He argued that vivisectionists' goals benefited humankind and thus their cruelty to animals could be justified (although cruelty for sport was not justifiable). On the other side of the Atlantic Ocean in 1799, the American physician Benjamin Rush told his medical students that they should also learn how to treat the diseases and injuries of domesticated animals. Not only were these animals valuable, but humaneness toward them would encourage the same feelings toward human patients – thus making the students better physicians. Finally, he argued, philosophers and theologians disagreed about whether animals had souls, as humans did. In case animals *did* have souls, physicians must treat them as their own patients or risk God's wrath.

These developments promoted the rise of animal protection movements in the late eighteenth century and legislation to protect the interests of animals during the nineteenth century. For example, the British Parliament approved the Cruel Treatment of Cattle Act in 1822, which mandated humane treatment

---

[4] Bentham, J. (1789), Introduction to Ch. XVII, *An Introduction to the Principles of Morals and Legislation* (London: Payne), p. cccviii.

of animals being driven to market. Two years later, the British Society for the Prevention of Cruelty to Animals was established, receiving its royal charter from Queen Victoria in 1840. In Germany, it was a priest, Albert Knapp, who founded the first animal welfare society and established an animal shelter in Stuttgart in 1837. In the next 20 years, animal protectionists formed societies and worked to establish new legislation against animal cruelty in several other European countries. By the 1800s, these changes in philosophical and ethical attitudes toward animals, however, often came into conflict with the practices of natural philosophers determined to understand how human and animal bodies functioned.

How Bodies Functioned in Health and Disease: European Physiology

From antiquity, people have sought to understand the fundamental life processes of animals and humans. How did the body work? Did human and animal bodies work in similar ways? What made a creature alive? Ayurvedic and Chinese philosophies had a long tradition of understanding vital processes, especially how energy moved through the body and functions of the internal organs. In the West, Aristotle and other ancient philosophers – and their successors during the next 2,000 years – speculated about how the body processed food and maintained the spark of life. Galen (c. 129–207 CE) dissected animals, both dead and alive, and he offered anatomical and physiological explanations of what happened in the healthy and diseased human body. For example, he noticed that urine was produced in the kidney and not in the urinary bladder. He discovered the recurrent laryngeal nerve and introduced physiological theories on health and disease and wound healing. According to him, the normal bodily function depended on spirits (*pneuma*) instead of humors. He developed a model of human physiology in which he explained the elaboration and distribution of the natural, the vital, and the animal spirit in the liver, heart, and brain, respectively. Although he vivisected and dissected pigs, apes, and other animals and extrapolated what he discovered to humans, his model of human physiology remained the standard for more than a thousand years.

In the thirteenth century, Islamic scholars reexamined the ideas of Galen and revised them dramatically based on their own observations. Ibn al-Nafis (1213–1288), an Arab physician educated in Damascus but working in Cairo, wrote a *Commentary* on Avicenna's anatomical treatise. This treatise discussed Galen's belief about the circulation of blood: that it formed and acquired a vital spirit in the liver, flowed to the right ventricle, and then moved into the left ventricle through invisible *pores* (openings) in the interventricular septum. However, no one had ever seen these pores; and based on his own observations, Ibn al-Nafis corrected Galen by stating that pores did not exist in the interventricular septum. Instead, he argued, the blood could only travel from the right ventricle to the left by circulating through the lungs. Blood was heated in the right ventricle, mixed with *pneuma* (air) in the lungs, and then entered the left ventricle where it was infused with the vital spirit and sent out to the body. Ibn al-Nafis speculated that there must be some kind of passage between the pulmonary artery and pulmonary vein. Unfortunately, his treatise was not translated into other languages until 1547, but after that it influenced Europeans. The Swiss natural philosopher Michael Servetus (1511–1553) quoted Ibn al-Nafis' explanation and agreed with it, saying that the blood was refined by passing through the pulmonary circulation. Because his radical ideas offended religious leaders, Servetus and his writings were burned at the stake in Geneva. He was followed by the much more well-known Andreas Vesalius (1514–1564) and William Harvey (1578–1657), both of whom followed Ibn al-Nafis by arguing that blood was exchanged in the pulmonary circulation.

In Europe between about 1500 and 1850, natural philosophers applied chemical and mechanical principles to the functions of living human and animal bodies, and these approaches were foundational to the nineteenth-century development of the modern science of physiology. In trying to analyze life, various physiological processes such as digestion, growth, movement, and reproduction were systematically studied using early chemical and physical principles. The Swiss Paracelsus (c. 1493–1541), for example, considered chemistry a way to explain how the human body works and also as a source of drugs to cure disease. He and his followers, the iatrochemists, began using mercury and arsenic as medications. They saw digestion as a chemical process, while the advocates of mechanistics, the iatrophysicists, believed the body digested food by mechanically crushing it. Iatrophysicists compared the organ systems of the body to levers, pulleys, and gears. Later, the theories of British natural philosopher Isaac Newton (1642–1727) influenced physiologists who tried to measure muscular contraction and other bodily functions using Newtonian ideas about matter and force. This stimulated physiological research on living animals in the seventeenth and eighteenth centuries. Experiments, increasingly performed in special locations such as laboratories, revealed measurable and repeatable anatomical, chemical, and physiological data to support medical knowledge. For example, the Swiss polymath Albrecht von Haller (1708–1777) performed many experiments on living animals to observe the external stimuli on muscles and sensitivity of nerves.

Recalling the mechanical philosophy of René Descartes, the French medical doctor Julien Offray de la Mettrie (1709–1751) wrote in his treatise *L'Homme machine* that humans and animals were both complicated machines. For Offray de la Mettrie, both the human mind and body followed mechanical laws and principles of the natural sciences. His treatise was part of an ongoing philosophical debate about the differences and similarities between humans and animals. He was inspired by his teacher Herman Boerhaave (1668–1738), a professor in medicine at Leiden University who taught the principles of organ function and the sensitivities in the tissues of the human body. (Boerhaave's other famous pupil was Albrecht von Haller.) Along with philosophical debates, it was research on integrated physiology, then generally called animal economy. This research brought the bodies of humans and other animals closer together in natural philosophy and institutionalized the practice of using animal bodies for experiments and demonstrations.

This had some unintended consequences. European Enlightenment principles of the eighteenth and nineteenth centuries encouraged the recognition of suffering, both animal and human, and social principles that would maximize happiness and humanitarianism. By establishing similarities between humans and animal bodies, natural philosophers contributed to concerns about animal suffering and its effects on humans. Conducting public or semi-public demonstrations about animal physiology, such as suffocating birds and small animals in Robert Boyle's air-pump apparatus, inadvertently brought their own observational and experimental methods under broader scrutiny. Was vivisection justifiable? Even Albrecht von Haller found his animal experiments to be gruesome, and he questioned whether they were justified on moral grounds. It is important to remember, also, that these new ideas were seldom accepted right away – especially if they contradicted long-standing medical practices, since most experimenters were philosophers or physicians.

The eighteenth and nineteenth centuries also witnessed a debate between those scholars who felt that the known mechanics of chemistry and physics would eventually explain the difference between life and non-life and "vitalists" who argued that the processes of life could not be reduced to such mechanistic processes. Vitalism was based on the conviction that living organisms have a non-physical element, a vital principle, called life force, energy, spark, elan, or soul, that distinguishes them from non-living organisms. (This concept, however, should not be confused with divine spirits. Although some proponents of vitalism were religious thinkers, this was a different concept that did not necessarily depend on a supernatural creator.) Neither vitalistic nor mechanistic ways of thinking could answer all questions, and both continued to be important throughout the nineteenth century. For example, in 1828 Friedrich Wöhler challenged the vitalist hypothesis when he synthesized urea from inorganic compounds, but this didn't mean the end of vitalism. Even Louis Pasteur, in his famous rebuttal of spontaneous generation, stated that fermentation was a "vital action." Only with the development of biochemistry in the twentieth century did vitalist explanations slowly decrease. Nevertheless, living organisms were more than simply machines; and they did more than mechanically react to external stimuli.

Explanations of bodily functions as vital physics and vital chemistry changed theories about understandings about health and disease in humans and animals alike. However, just as with the new human and animal anatomy of Vesalius and Ruini, the development of new thinking about physiology in the seventeenth–nineteenth centuries did not essentially change medical and veterinary healing practices. For example, Alexander Numan (1780–1852), a Dutch physician and professor at the Veterinary School of Utrecht (1822–1850), operated according to theories of vitalism and humoralism, combined with an early form of comparative physiology. Sickness was an individual manifestation that Numan characterized according to his own nosology, organized by organ systems and informed by vitalism as well as chemistry. Practitioners had many theories from which to choose. Most of them probably worked like Numan did, by combining parts of different theories with their own training, observations, and experiences.

By the mid-1800s, veterinarians were important contributors to physiological research, especially in France. For example, the career of Jean-Baptiste August Chauveau (1827–1917) demonstrated a remarkable range of investigation. Chauveau was an accomplished comparative anatomist and authored an important veterinary anatomy textbook. At the École Nationale Vétérinaire de Lyon, he taught comparative anatomy and physiology to veterinary students for decades. Along with his more well-known contemporary, experimental physiologist Claude Bernard (1813–1878), Chauveau was a pioneer in physiological research. He studied the spinal cord and electrical potentials of spinal nerves, and he joined Bernard in demonstrating glycogenic functions of the liver. He invented instruments used to measure the pressure and blood velocity in the arterial circulation and was the first to achieve successful cardiac catheterization (on a horse). In the mid-1800s, especially in France, anatomy, physiology, and pathology were not completely separate disciplines. Although Chauveau's accomplishments were extraordinary, it was not unusual for a scientist to investigate questions that crossed species and disciplines. This is important to remember as we turn now to discussing pathology, the science that explained how exactly disease disrupted the body's normal physiology and anatomy.

The Science of Suffering: European Pathology

Historian of medicine Jacalyn Duffin noted the Greek origins of the word "pathology": *pathos* (suffering) and *-ology* (science of). Pathology is the study of mechanisms of disease and disability in humans and animals. Duffin listed four purposes for pathology: to explain suffering; to diagnose or name the abnormal condition; to predict an outcome for the patient (prognosis); and to guide therapy. Pathology in animal healing has a long history of asking questions to fulfill these purposes. Pathology has also been comparative: animal bodies served as the most common sites of understanding pathological mechanisms for both human and animal diseases. Probably the most venerable type of pathological belief is that suffering results from supernatural intervention. Because the disease or suffering is caused by the displeasure or whims of gods, the appropriate therapies lay in the realm of priests and oracles. The best treatment was the one that would bring the sufferer back into a good spiritual relationship with the supernatural power. Animals could be sufferers but also often served as sacrifices to placate the spirits or gods. In many parts of the world today, spiritual understandings of disease and suffering continue to play an important role in healing both humans and animals.

In Ayurvedic and traditional Chinese medicine, as we have seen, the basis for pathological explanations lay with the body's life force. Suffering and disease resulted from imbalances within the body; diagnosis followed from understanding how signs of disease corresponded to these imbalances; and the healer decided upon therapies (such as herbal medications, acupuncture, or moxibustion) to rebalance the body both internally and within its environment. This individualized understanding of bodily processes has guided healing even as thinking about pathology has become increasingly generalized during the past 400 years. By generalized, we mean a *nosology*: a set of principles and disease classification that applied to *every* patient. A patient's disease was not only theirs, but part of a category such as "cold illness" or "purulent fever." The disease could be expected to progress in predictable ways once it was identified, and its identification also narrowed the appropriate therapies from which the healer could choose. Ayurvedic and traditional Chinese systems of classifying and understanding diseases continue to be used successfully in human and animal medicine today.

The third way of understanding suffering and disease is that of *materialism*: understanding how signs and symptoms relate to changes in material components of the body (blood, urine, tissues). This, too, has a long history. In Chinese traditional medicine, for example, a very finely detailed examination of the patient's pulse was (and is) conducted because the pulse often reflects changes in the pattern of the life force, the *qi*. In Egypt, priests conducting ritual sacrifices carefully examined bodies before and after death to ensure that the healthiest and most handsome animals were offered to the gods. In many healing systems, the body's excretions – urine, feces, blood – also provided material clues to the causes and progression of suffering. Recalling the development of anatomy, dissections of diseased animal bodies revealed organs and fluids that appeared to look (and smell) different from those of healthy animals. Some anatomists began to gather their observations and even to relate them to the symptoms of disease during life. The Italian physician Antonio Benivieni (1443–1502) has been called a father of pathology for conducting autopsies on humans and relating changes in the internal organs to the symptoms during life. Benivieni's remarkable treatise *De abdibis morborum causis* (1507) summarized over 100 cases of human disease that he was able later to autopsy, including *canis rabiosi*, or canine rabies. Benivieni and his contemporaries dissected animals, of course; but we do not know whether he associated animal diseases with material changes in the animal's body after death.

In Europe, materialism slowly became the major basis for the development of early modern pathology in animal as well as human medicine in the early 1800s. The ideas of vitalism did not disappear, of course, but took on more materialistic forms as they affected thinking about disease. For example, William Harvey wrote in 1653 that contagions (such as plague and leprosy) came from outside the body; but they caused disease dynamically, by reacting with the body's internal vital processes. Early physiologists sought to understand these processes, and comparative physiology (comparing how the same bodily functions worked in different animal species) was a foundation of pathology.

Comparative anatomy also contributed to the development of pathology, although, as Duffin points out, knowledge of anatomy did not strengthen physicians' ability to treat diseases in most cases. But by the late 1700s, *comparative* anatomy (the study of different species of animals as well as humans) had become a powerful way to explore underlying general principles of how living creatures were constructed. As historian Abigail Woods has argued, important sites of investigation for comparative anatomy were specimens in museums (often associated with medical education) and menageries and zoological gardens, which were home to many different species of animals. Animals in zoos and menageries, exotic and valuable, received medical care from their keepers, physicians, and occasionally veterinarians; and they were often dissected after death. In this way, the many species of animals present made the zoo an excellent location to test ideas about the biological unity of animal bodies' structure and function.

Dysfunctional and suffering bodies generated material signs of distress, and this was particularly evident in animals. Sick animals may not have complained of their suffering in the same ways that sick humans did, although animals' behaviors often indicated that they were not feeling well. Without an overt psychological component in animal patients, healers probably placed more emphasis on material signs such as weakness or lack of appetite and exterior signs, lesions, or exudations to help them diagnose disease. Moreover, an animal's anatomy was often more easily observed after death and correlated to specific signs of disease. Veterinarians, with easy access to large numbers of (living and dead) animals, were uniquely positioned to link anatomy, physiology, and pathology and to correlate form, function, and dysfunction.

Veterinary medicine, particularly in France, provided an important milieu for the establishment of modern comparative physiology and pathology in the late 1700s and early 1800s. Historian Lise Wilkinson has even argued that "medical research adopted the veterinary approach, including animal experiments, to study ... diseases."[5] Veterinary schools and active scientific societies nourished observation, experimentation, and discussion on a wide variety of topics (Chapter 3 details the establishment of French veterinary schools). Jean-Baptiste August Chauveau (mentioned above) graduated from veterinary school, investigated questions in comparative anatomy and physiology, and became interested in the developing cross-species approach for pathology. At fifty years of age, Chauveau completed his second degree, in human medicine, with a thesis on *vaccinia* and the relationships between horsepox, cowpox, and smallpox in humans. In 1865, he plunged into research on such questions as what made vaccine matter virulent and the prevention of rinderpest (then raging in England). After hearing Chauveau's paper on vaccinia at a meeting of the French Academy of Medicine, Louis Pasteur encouraged Chauveau to expand his investigations in comparative pathology. Chauveau then developed his famous diffusion technique to separate out components of the blood (white blood cells, red blood cells, and unidentified particles). He showed that glanders and sheep pox could be transmitted only by these particles and not by a type of toxin dissolved in the serum of sick animals (see Chapter 4).

Although most histories of pathology point to the laboratory and dissection theater as the sites of pathological discovery, the best place to observe large numbers of bodies before and after death was the abattoir, or slaughterhouse. Animals such as cattle, pigs, and sheep arrived alive and could be observed for signs of illness, then killed and their internal organs examined. Curious professional slaughterers and butchers, who observed hundreds of animals every year, thus joined natural philosophers as collectors of anatomical knowledge and how it might relate to signs of disease. Recognizing this, the German physician Rudolf Virchow (1821–1902) frequented abattoirs to make observations and collect samples of diseased tissues and organs. Virchow, who was also a champion of meat hygiene, came from a family of butchers (which was at that time, in Germany, a humble but respectable trade); for him, the abattoir was a familiar place. Virchow supported the development of veterinary pathology as well as the profession of veterinary medicine in Germany (see Chapters 3 and 4). Virchow is also famous as a proponent and elaborator of cell theory.

For Virchow, elucidating the general principles of pathology and medicine was a comparative project. Virchow's comparative pathology explicitly linked theories and methods of understanding human and animal diseases in the service of establishing normal and abnormal for tissues and organs. This natural philosophical agenda fit hand in glove with Virchow's social agenda of science in the service of public health. A member of the German Parliament, Virchow tirelessly advocated for the "scientific" linkages between animal

---

[5] Wilkinson, L. (1992) *Animals and Disease: An Introduction to the History of Comparative Medicine* (Cambridge: Cambridge University Press), p. 148.

health and human health, especially in food hygiene. In the late 1850s, his research on the life cycle of the parasite *Trichina spiralis* connected this nematode with the cysts formed in porcine muscles and the parasitism of humans eating undercooked pork. Virchow advocated inspection of meat by professionals trained to find the parasite, a process greatly aided by low-power microscopy. Although microscopes had been used by natural historians before the mid-nineteenth century, technological advances and falling prices made these tools much more widely available by 1850 and increased the resolution with which people could observe insects, parasites, and even microorganisms. Microscopic pathology contributed to changing notions about what caused diseases (as we discuss in Chapter 4), thus helping to reorient the science of suffering from individual bodies to groups and populations of animals. Indeed, the suffering of whole populations – epidemics – became a major feature of the globalizing early modern period and continued during the nineteenth century.

Trade and Conquest: Responding to Animal Disease Outbreaks

Today we believe that many zoonotic diseases emerged because animals, humans, and microorganisms co-evolved over thousands of years as part of the process of domesticating animals. Increasingly dense populations of animals created fertile conditions for the development of *epizootics* (epidemics of animal diseases), and these local epizootics spread to new areas with pastoralists, traders, and armies. This brings us back to the ecological exchanges of the 1500s–1800s, with which we began this chapter. Most historical research has focused on human diseases. In Europe, diseases such as smallpox, measles, and tuberculosis had already been introduced centuries before through trade with Asia and Africa. Over centuries, the theory goes, people evolved some resistance to these and other diseases, thus rendering them far less lethal. When Europeans traveled to new lands, they carried these diseases with them. (Scholars believe, however, that tuberculosis was already endemic in the Americas.) When such diseases were introduced for the first time to Native Americans with no resistance, the effects on these populations were catastrophic. Depending on the location, 30 to 90 percent of Indigenous peoples died, and the resulting sociocultural disruptions destroyed their civilizations. This invasion of diseases was a crucial factor in the success of European invasions of the continents and isolated islands of the Western Hemisphere.

By 1800, marauding Europeans had relocated peoples and animals over long distances, especially from the west coast of Africa to East Africa, India, the East Indies, and South America. Animals and their products became important parts of an expanding international trade, especially with the increasing use of steamships in the mid-1800s. When animals moved from one place to another, their microenvironment moved with them: new microorganisms and parasites, and often new plants, accompanied the insects, rats, cats, dogs, sheep, horses, and cattle that invaded new places (usually accompanying humans). Today we understand these biological invasions, along with diseases, as weapons for conquest. Animals served as shock troops, with feral domesticated animals often preceding human invaders. We know that European domestic animals transmitted diseases among indigenous American animals: bovine tuberculosis from European American cattle spread to bison and other wild ungulates, for example.

Zulu Disease Causation Theories

These global exchanges were the broadest manifestation of well-established local and regional patterns of disease: diseases had homelands, from which they spread throughout regions. For example, animals traveling between different disease environments presented a threat that was well understood by pastoralists in Africa. The region inhabited by the Zulu, in southern Africa, is a good case study. The Zulu people had been raising cattle for centuries before their homelands began to be encroached upon by European colonists. Between 1836 and 1838, the Cape Colony farmer Louis Tregardt kept a diary during the time he and other *Boers* (farmers) emigrated to Zululand in the interior of South Africa. There, he recorded several types of cattle diseases, including a highly lethal disease called *nagana*, which the Zulu believed was spread by the tsetse fly. (Tregardt did not describe some of the other diseases he mentioned, such as the "stop disease" of oxen and the "thick disease" of calves, which are unknown to us today.) The local names for cattle diseases hint at a well-defined indigenous nosology already in place when Europeans arrived.

If the Zulu homelands are any guide, groups of African pastoralists in the early 1800s already recognized that the activities of trading, raiding, and invasion facilitated the travel of animal diseases and the tsetse fly. Moving cattle from other places to (or through) tsetse fly regions was understood to be dangerous and to be avoided if at all possible. Besides harboring tsetse flies, KwaZulu-Natal (today's name for Zulu homelands) also harbored ticks that could kill cattle, especially young animals. Knowledge about animal disease environments and the transmission of parasites and microorganisms probably guided treatments and preventive measures (such as restricting contact between animals), and much more historical and anthropological research is needed on this topic for the many cultures and nations of Africa. But it is clear that Indigenous Africans understood these animal diseases as related to moving animals between environments – and that they characterized some environments as unhealthy and dangerous to animals.

Zulu beliefs about healthy and unhealthy places also appeared in the writings of the British scientist David Bruce, who worked in Zululand in the 1890s. He wrote that the Zulu believed nagana was indigenous to places that harbored the tsetse fly; places without the fly were healthy districts. Dogs, horses, and cattle that were moved from healthy districts to unhealthy places soon became ill. Dogs and horses suffered acute nagana, with signs of emaciation, extreme weakness, and swelling under the belly and in the lower legs. Cattle experienced a more chronic disease course, but most still died within a month of the signs first appearing. Bruce respected the Zulu belief that *where there is no game [wild animals], there is no nagana.* The Zulu therefore attempted to kill or drive away all the large wild animals as a preventive measure against nagana in their domesticated animals. This reduced fly populations and restricted transmission from wild to domesticated animals, which the Zulu clearly understood as the source of nagana.

The Cordon Sanitaire

Nagana is only one example of diseases understood to be enzootic (always existing) in certain places and environments, and whose spread was linked to moving animals from place to place. Within Europe, the early modern period witnessed the rise of the northern and eastern cattle trade. The overland or overseas transport of huge numbers of cattle connected remote agricultural production areas with new markets for beef cattle in urban populations in Western European societies where consumers wanted more meat in their diet. Drovers (herders) conducted long-distance cattle drives from the fourteenth century onward from production regions in Denmark, Romania, and Hungary to Central and Western Europe along fixed routes, over distances sometimes exceeding 1,000 kilometers. To avoid spreading disease, contact with the local human and animal populations was avoided as much as possible at the inns and during the purchase of fodder from local farmers, and drovers stayed away from the main state roads.

In the second half of the eighteenth century, a special veterinary police service was established in Austria to regulate the flow of drovers and animals across the border and prevent the importation of diseases. As part of a *cordon sanitaire* (literally in French: a thick cord fence, a sanitary fence, or protecting closure ring), these mounted civil servants patrolled the long eastern border to prevent illegal livestock imports. Unfortunately, we do not know how (or if) herders and drovers provided veterinary treatment or therapies to these traveling livestock. Drovers were paid for each animal that arrived at the destination, and while this suggests some attention to health care it also sometimes meant cruelty. Drovers whipped, stabbed, and prodded animals to keep them going, even if sick. These long-distance livestock drives in Europe and elsewhere continued until railroad transport replaced them in the second half of the nineteenth century.

By raising large numbers of cattle in Denmark, northern Germany, and on the Hungarian and Romanian plains, Italians, French, and other Western Europeans were able to access unprecedented supplies of animal protein without sacrificing their own arable land. In addition, imported oxen were crucial for traction and plowing as agricultural output increased. Hence, important economic interests were threatened when epizootics decimated livestock. Farmers, traders, and authorities were well aware of the potential disease threats to local livestock populations and cattle markets posed by military action, colonization, cattle drives, and international livestock trade. Perhaps the most devastating – and feared – livestock disease of the seventeenth–nineteenth centuries was what we know today as rinderpest.

Epizootic Diseases: Rinderpest, Foot and Mouth Disease, and Sheep Pox

Rinderpest, a highly contagious viral disease lethal to cloven-hoofed animals with no exposure to it, had many names: *Pestis bovina* (Latin), *taoun* (Arabic), *cattle plague* (English), *peste bovine* (French), *sadoka* (Swahili), *miljan/myalzan* (Mongolian), and *tachi* (Japanese) are only a few examples. In this book, we will use the term *rinderpest* for convenience. It is important to remember that the causes and symptoms of diseases in the past, and how people understood them, may differ from those of today. Therefore, it is often difficult, if not impossible, to diagnose rinderpest or any other epizootic that occurred in the distant past. Instead, historians work to study epizootics from the point of view of the people who lived through, and reported about, those often-disastrous events. We know much about the history of rinderpest because the measures taken by authorities to prevent spreading of this disease and to deal with the socioeconomic implications have been fairly well documented in many places. Rinderpest led to major state interventions in rural society and played an important role in the development of veterinary medicine (including as a stimulus to establish veterinary schools in some countries; see Chapter 3). In addition, because it was so highly contagious and lethal (killing 60 to 90 percent of infected animals), rinderpest played an important role in ecological imperialism during the seventeenth–nineteenth centuries. Its history as a disease in motion, entangled with both trade and conquest, is well worth focusing on here (the rinderpest story continues in Chapter 4).

Rinderpest, the Cattle Killer

The first account of rinderpest is described in first-century Roman sources. More is known about mass outbreaks that occurred at the beginning of the ninth century during the reign of Charlemagne and around 1300 as a result of raids from Asia into Europe by the forces of Chinggis (Genghis) Khan. Europeans believed that this disease was imported to Europe, a notion reflected in the name "steppe murrain." Steppe murrain supposedly originated from the steppes between Asia and Europe, from where it regularly spread eastward to the Pacific and westward toward the Atlantic along with cattle trading, ox carts, and Central Asian invaders (such as Chinggis Khan's soldiers). Apparently, cattle from the steppe had an innate resistance and could infect cattle and buffalo

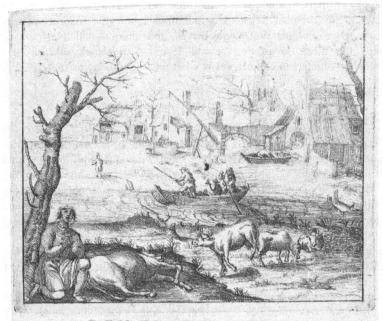

DEN KLAGENDEN

HUYSMAN,

SChrik Neerland, fchrik, op deeze droeve maar,
Die ons in d'ooren klinkt dit eerfte van het Jaar;
Is dit 't begin, wat zal het eynd' dan wezen,
Wie zal, ô Chriften menfch, aan Gode nooyt volprezen,
Afbidden deze Straf, die zynen Toorn ons zend,
Op dat hy die, helaas! ten goede van ons wend.
Hoe woed het Oorlogs-vuur, in onzer Buuren Landen,
Een ander Oorlogs-vuur komt in ons Land ontbranden
De fterfte onder 't Vee, een voorbood dat de dood,
Ons op de hielen volgt in dezen droeven nood,
Hef dan, ô menfch! met my uw hert en hand tot God,
Op dat hy ons niet zend een nog veel erger lot;
Maar dat wy mogen zien, dat alles weer herleven,
En dat wy Gode dank, en eere daar voor geven.

Gedrukt by ETIENNE ISAAC CAILLAU, Boekver-
koper in de Stilfteeg, het derde huys van de Blommarkt,
en zyn ook te bekomen by den Autheur.

Figure 2.5 New Year's print about rinderpest. Amsterdam 1745.
Courtesy: Rijksmuseum Amsterdam, RP-P-OB-83.843, public domain.

herds in the invaded countries without showing clinical signs. Once local herds became infected, international cattle trade routes caused further spreading, for example, from Ukraine and Hungary into Italy, Austria, and southern Germany, or from Denmark, Northern Germany, and the Netherlands into England. In East Asia, the Japanese compendium on cattle, *Gyuka Satsuyo* (1720), mentions mass outbreaks of a highly contagious disease which killed 80 percent of cattle in Korea (in 1541, 1577, 1636, 1668) and Japan (1638, 1672). Because of the reported signs and symptoms, historians believe this disease was probably *tachi* (Japanese for rinderpest). Rinderpest spreads by invasion, conquest, and war, as well as trade; and this fact often shaped responses to epizootics. For example, an outbreak of rinderpest in the 1740s was the sequel of the Austrian War of Succession when infection moved from Hungary into other European countries.

In the eighteenth century, Europe was struck three times by waves of mass outbreaks of rinderpest: around 1713, 1744, and 1768. The disease became endemic and reappeared regularly, killing millions of cattle. These outbreaks affected large areas, but smaller local outbreaks also occurred over this time period. The consequences – loss of food, animal power, transport, and wealth – were deeply felt in European societies, and rinderpest was greatly feared. There were many theories about what caused these outbreaks, and how to respond to them, but these were religious societies. Confronted with these disasters, religious authorities organized meetings of public prayer and public processions asking God for help. Livestock owners requested spiritual remedies, exorcism, and blessings of herds and stables. In Figure 2.5, a translation of

---

Figure 2.5 (*cont.*)
The complaining houseman

> Fear, Netherlands, fear, this sad story,
> Which sounds in our ears, this first of the year;
> If this is the beginning, then what will be the end,
> Who shall, oh Christian, to God unsurpassed,
> Pray away this punishment, sent to us by his wrath,
> So that he will turn it to our favor.
> How rages the fire of war in our neighboring countries,
> Another fire of war comes to ignite in our country
> Death among cattle, the foreboding that death,
> Is following us on our heels in this sad need,
> Raise then, oh man! with me your heart and hand to God,
> So that he will not send to us a much worse lot;
> But that we may see, that all will revive,
> And for that we give God gratitude and honor.

a Dutch religious appeal compares rinderpest to war and urges people to pray for the disease to end. Until well into the eighteenth century, outbreaks of rinderpest were considered a divine punishment for a sinful population. The end of the outbreak was celebrated with a day of thanksgiving in all churches. Superstition also played a role: in Denmark, a calf from each herd was buried alive, or livestock were driven through a fire to prevent infection. Next to prayer, songs about disasters such as floods, earthquakes, insect plagues, and rinderpest were common in the early modern time period. This genre is an important source to understand how people in the past coped with such catastrophes. Such songs were used to spread the news, to interpret them as signs of God's vengeance and warning to repent in order to prevent new disasters. They could shape a shared sense of solidarity and religious or geographical identity.

Lancisi's Principles

Believing this disease to be contagious, local, regional, and national author-ities took measures to prevent the spreading of the disease. These included embargoing cattle imports, closing livestock markets, banning transhu-mance and animal transport, quarantining infected areas, disinfecting stables, and burying or burning dead livestock. Such measures hindered the spreading of cattle plague to some extent. More effective was the systematic and rigorous culling of all infected livestock, a method applied for the first time in Italy in 1711 on the authority of Giovanni Maria Lancisi (1654–1720), personal physician of the pope. He had studied the outbreak among the papal herds and concluded that rinderpest was due to a fer-mented substance released by the bodies of sick cattle. The contagious agent, he wrote, consisted of very small deadly particles that could pass from one animal to the other via mucous membranes and direct skin contact. Consequently, Lancisi drew up eleven recommendations to prevent infection, including killing all infected animals, which became law by papal edict (see Box 2.1 for one of Lancisi's recommendations). These measures seemed to help rid the Papal States of rinderpest; but they were put into effect only under threat of severe penalties. Livestock owners who would lose their valuable animals protested and often attempted to hide sick animals from officials trying to control the disease.

The same approach was advocated by Thomas Bates, surgeon to King George I of England, when the first pandemic struck England in 1714. Bates was ordered to study and control rinderpest. He knew Lancisi's work from a period spent as a naval surgeon in Sicily, and

---

Box 2.1 **Recommendation 4**

Before treating sick animals, the veterinarian (*marescalchi*) should put on a waxed overall. After the treatment, the overall should be left *in situ* and the veterinarian should wash his hands and face with vinegar before going to look after the animals in other cowsheds, or later returning to the same place. It would, however, be better to kill the infected cattle rather than to treat them, since veterinary intervention may increase the risk of contagion.

Recommendation 4 (out of 11) made by Giovanni Maria Lancisi to Pope Clement XI in 1715 to prevent the spread of rinderpest to the Papal States.

Bates applied the same control measures as those used in the Papal States. However, instead of severe penalties, he followed a policy of indemnifying (paying or compensating with money) the unfortunate farmers. After a campaign of three months, rinderpest had disappeared in Britain. Continental countries without a strong central government did not implement such cull-and-slaughter campaigns, and nor did Britain when it was struck by the second wave of rinderpest mass outbreaks in 1744 – and many more animals died.

The pattern of each epizootic was the same. The disease spread rapidly after introduction and killed most animals in the first two years. Mortality then quickly decreased because fewer animals remained, most of which had developed immunity (which we now know to be lifelong). The disease prevailed in the high-density livestock areas. Reintroduction of rinderpest remained low as long as trade barriers were maintained by official measures. In various countries, committees were established in which agriculturists, medical doctors, clergymen, and civil servants were appointed to advise local and national governments on how to control cattle plague. Numerous recipes for medicines to prevent and to cure the disease were published in edicts, decrees, and pamphlets. The veterinary police, established in some European countries, also supervised quarantine measures at the borders (although some drovers found ways to evade them). In the beginning of the nineteenth century, a German veterinarian described how seemingly healthy livestock imported from Russia and Ukraine still infected cattle populations in East Prussia and Poland. In many European countries, rinderpest appeared again as soon as the ban on cattle imports was lifted, infecting young and susceptible animals. This pattern proved very hard to break for social as well as epidemiological reasons.

Controlling Rinderpest

Epizootics were social crises, causing tensions between farmers and local authorities and between local and central governments. The outbreaks called for severe state interference; however, local farmers often considered the imposed measures to be too draconian. Their opposition is understandable. Forced to slaughter their cattle, sometimes even healthy-looking animals, some farmers became so poor they could not feed their families or lost their farms. State interference, including military *cordons sanitaire* and mandatory slaughter, also challenged the customary rural self-sufficiency in animal husbandry. On the other side, consumers faced skyrocketing meat prices. After the epidemic slowed down, recovery in animal populations took a long time. In some areas, for instance, in southern France, it took years for livestock husbandry to be reestablished. Arable farming became difficult in places that had relied on oxen for farm labor. Outbreaks also led to temporary or permanent land abandonment, and the victimization of farmers by unscrupulous money lenders and cattle "insurance" salespeople. Other regions were more fortunate. Farmers who were able to keep a few animals profited from higher meat and dairy prices and temporarily shifted to cheese production, sheep breeding, fattening of calves, or arable farming.

Outbreaks of rinderpest also influenced the development of veterinary treatments for individual animals. Recommendations focused on isolation of sick animals and general hygiene of stables, disinfection of cow sheds, and providing nutritional food and fresh water. In Denmark, farmers burned tobacco leaves in stables to keep out infection. All kinds of (folk) remedies were applied, particularly the administration of various kinds of potions and herbs. In Bavaria it was recommended to administer theriaca (special mixtures of various herbs and medicinal substances) dissolved in wine. In Hungary, healers used a mixture of sulfur, antimony, gentian, and juniper. An alternative was adding two spoonsful of salt and sulfur to bread soaked in human urine and feeding it to sick animals. These are but a few examples of remedies applied to sick animals by animal owners and professional healers alike.

Although these folk remedies and sacred remedies (such as prayer) continued to be important, the control of rinderpest in the course of the eighteenth century increasingly focused on animal *populations*. Population-level treatments varied from quarantine measures and hygiene to polypharmacy to mass slaughtering. Around the middle of the eighteenth century, researchers of rinderpest agreed on one empirical finding: animals that had survived rinderpest were able to resist further infection. It was known that in China and Turkey people tried to protect themselves from smallpox infection by previously infecting themselves artificially with pustular material from a patient with a mild infection: so-called variolation. Inspired by this practice, European researchers tried to protect healthy animals against rinderpest by preventively infecting them with an attenuated form of the disease (inoculation). Many experiments with inoculation were conducted in various countries. These were based on the observation that the mortality rate of naturally contaminated cattle was about 85 percent, while many fewer died when they were inoculated on purpose with blood, saliva, or secretions taken from the mouth or nose from animals that had survived initial infection. The inoculation experiments contributed to the knowledge of active immunization against infectious diseases. The technique of variolation famously inspired the English physician Edward Jenner (1749–1823) to develop and apply vaccination against smallpox in humans. (He derived the term "vaccine" from the Latin word *vacca* = cow.)

Despite these early attempts to vaccinate individual animals to create effective disease control, regions hit by rinderpest emphasized population-level treatments in this period. This was due to several influences. First, municipalities and regions needed to stop the epidemic as quickly as possible to prevent the social crisis that usually resulted. If animals could not be moved or exported, huge amounts of money would be lost. Draconian stamping-out (slaughtering all animals in the affected region, even if not sick) was the quickest method. Second, stamping-out was also probably the most reliable method. In spite of some isolated successes, inoculation against rinderpest did not stop the outbreaks. Despite the protests of farmers, damage to agriculture, and the risk of social crisis, governing officials quickly learned to attempt to stop the disease as soon as possible. As we discuss in the next chapters, rinderpest would not be under control around the world until the late twentieth century.

The domain of veterinary empiricism was a mixture of popular and learned cultures; eighteenth-century almanacs and other published sources played a role in knowledge transfer between these two cultures. To us today, the recommendations and treatments of that time appear very primitive. However, one should not judge the degree of efficacy of the interventions from a present-day (veterinary) point of view, but rather measure their scope within the functioning of a society confronted with a major crisis. Nevertheless, is it striking that long before the development of germ theories in the late nineteenth century and the discovery of vaccines against some of these epizootic and zoonotic diseases, people found ways to control the disease such as stamping out and strict quarantine. Still, it is estimated that more than 200 million cattle perished from the rinderpest in eighteenth-century Europe. This disease would continue to challenge European authorities until the 1860s and also to devastate the parts of Africa and Asia to which European animals traveled (see Chapter 4).

Foot and Mouth Disease and Sheep Pox

If rinderpest was the rapid killer of cattle, vesicular diseases were often more chronic and insidious. Vesicular diseases (causing vesicles or blisters) usually did not kill the animal immediately. Instead, the animals refused to eat, lost weight, and gave little milk, thus decreasing their market value. These contagious diseases spread rapidly; today, we know that viruses cause foot and mouth disease (FMD, or *aphthae epizooticae*) and most other vesicular diseases. The symptoms of FMD familiar to us today appear in ancient texts: blisters and ulcers on the feet, around the lips and inside the mouth; hypersalivation, difficult swallowing, loss of appetite; and low mortality in adult animals (2 to 5 percent). Along with bovines, camels, goats, and swine, the disease was sometimes reported to affect horses (which are resistant to FMD). Moreover, since our categorizations of diseases today are different from those of history, we avoid diagnosing disease outbreaks of the past and simply consider them "FMD-like" based on their historical descriptions. A detailed description of an FMD-like disease (according to present knowledge) was given by Italian physician Girolamo Fracastoro (1478–1553) in 1546: It was also in the northern Italian states of Piedmont, Venice, and Lombardy that an outbreak of *febre aftosa* (vesicular fever) occurred in 1799–1800. The highly contagious nature was then recognized, and officials implemented isolation measures for animals from infected areas to prevent the spread of the disease.

Nevertheless, the debate about whether these FMD-like diseases were strictly contagious or could be caused by other factors such as miasmas lasted until well into the nineteenth century. As with rinderpest and smallpox, early scientists tried inoculation experiments with matter from infected animals at least since 1810. However, most of these "aphtization" or inoculation attempts failed. Next to inoculation, veterinary healers treated the pustules by cauterizing them, followed by dressing them with salt and butter. Another common therapy involved extracting blood from the gingiva by leeches or by cupping glasses, followed by a mouthwash based on mallow roots, linseed, milk, or honey. Although animals usually recovered, they often did not gain weight, gave less milk, and remained weakened for the rest of their lives. The cost of feeding and transporting such animals was greater than the profit realized by selling them or their products (such as milk or wool). The highly contagious FMD-like vesicular diseases were greatly feared because they dramatically decreased the economic value of cattle and sheep and spread so rapidly from place to place.

Another disease that disrupted the international trade in sheep and wool was sheep pox (known today as a viral disease caused by *variola ovina*). Next to anthrax and foot-rot, it represents one of the main scourges of sheep production. Some historians claim that this disease killed almost the entire sheep population in England in the period 1275–1300. Sheep pox appeared repeatedly: France suffered in 1515 and again in 1819 (when one million sheep died), as did England (with a huge outbreak in 1862). Both nations had large textile industries that depended on the wool supply. Sheep pox–like diseases were also known to herders in northern Africa and were reported by observers in the Arabic and Turkic worlds. The disease was characterized by the formation of whitish and stinking cutaneous pustules, respiratory problems, and foul breath. Young sheep and lambs often died of sheep pox–like diseases.

In his *Traité de la Clavelée* (1822), veterinarian Louis Hurtrel d'Arboval (1777–1839) presented a detailed description of the various stages and clinical symptoms of sheep pox. German anatomist Friedrich G.J. (Jacob) Henle (1809–1885) classified sheep pox, anthrax, and rinderpest under the disease category of miasmatic origin, which could later develop to be contagious in its course. In cases of an outbreak, diseased sheep were isolated from the healthy ones. Healers tried to get the miasmatic "poison" out of diseased sheep by letting the animals sweat in an enclosed space, followed by bloodletting. Finally, this therapeutic regimen was finished by fumigating these sheep by burning horsehair, ground horn, or woolen rags.

An interesting fact about sheep pox is that it was one of the earliest animal diseases for which owners and herders attempted a form of inoculation. This may have been due to the disease's signs and symptoms, which were clearly a pox similar to smallpox in humans. The ancient Asian practice of inoculation, known to Arabic, Turkic, and northern African herders, was used against both smallpox in humans and sheep pox in ovines. In West Africa, a form of inoculation called "clavelization" was applied by Indigenous pastoralists long before the French invasion and colonization. They scratched open the skin of the animal's ear with a thorn, and inserted material from a sick animal's pustules under the skin. Similar to inoculation with rinderpest, Europeans tried to protect their sheep by subcutaneous clavelization or "ovination" with matter collected from the pustules. From the eighteenth century on, some of these inoculation practices seemed to prevent the disease to some extent. However, it seems that sheep pox clavelization was less successful than the prophylactic against smallpox in humans. To answer the question of whether sheep pox was a zoonosis, European physicians apparently carried out inoculation experiments on humans. They found that the infection could not be transmitted to humans either by direct inoculation or by eating meat from infected animals. The danger of sheep pox was its epizootic potential, with the deaths of almost all young animals in an exposed herd. This disease and others were feared for their potential to spread like wildfire through herds and between different geographical regions along with the international trade in live animals.

Disease of Trade: Anthrax

Anthrax (Latin), *charbon* (French), *Milzbrand* (German), *ántrax* (Spanish), *dalak ateşi* (Turkish for "spleen fever"), and сибирская язва (Russian for "Siberian ulcer") represents another feared disease that was already known in antiquity. The name of this zoonotic disease literally means "coal" due to the characteristic dark discoloration of the spleen and blood, and the blue-black eschars it causes on the human skin (*carbunculus* = little coals). Authors like Hippocrates, Galen, and Apsyrtos described an anthrax-like disease and confirmed its contagious nature. Within the humoral theory, anthrax was linked to heat (the carbuncles gave a burning feeling underneath the skin of infected humans) and to a surplus of black bile, which caused the evil ulcerations occurring with carbuncles. In southern India, *pinnadapan* (splenic apoplexy), with symptoms similar to anthrax, was described as one of the four fatal diseases.

In medieval Europe, many accounts were written of outbreaks of *ignis sacer* (sacred fire) anthrax in various countries, causing high mortality among people and cattle. The disease often occurred during and after particular climatic conditions and was believed to have arisen from infected pastures (*telluric*, arising from the soil). Herdsmen were familiar with this risk and designated certain fields as cursed. Traditionally, herders prevented animals from grazing on cursed fields for seven years. Sheep could obtain anthrax due to an abundance of thick blood. Medieval Arabic writers recognized two fatal forms of anthrax: *Dā el-Bakar* (cow sickness), with typical dark diarrhea, and *Zībah* (tumorous anthrax).

Many accounts of anthrax in cattle and horses were written in the seventeenth–nineteenth centuries in various European countries, but also in Siberia and the French West Indies. The disease was common in Siberian horses; western Russians believed that it originated there (thus the name "Siberian ulcer" in Russian). Frequencies of anthrax outbreaks were higher in certain years, for instance in 1682, 1732, and in the 1770s and 1780s in Western Europe. The written accounts often mention mass outbreaks and describe a highly contagious nature for anthrax. The disease appeared in certain places, disappeared, then returned in later years. Observers noticed that particular climate conditions favored development of the disease. Anthrax tended to appear after periods of heavy storms and rain that followed long dry periods in summertime. Today we recognize that this pattern was created by the storms stirring up existing spores of the causative bacillus in the soil; but until the late 1870s, no one knew why certain weather patterns could trigger anthrax outbreaks.

Anthrax was widely known to be transmissible to humans. It was recognized as a professional disease posing a higher risk of infection for herdsmen, butchers, knackers, tanners, and veterinary healers. Contamination and infection could occur via direct contact between animals or animal products and a person's skin. In Turkey, a specialized branch of human medicine dealt exclusively with anthrax infections, spread by handling wool, hair, and hides from infected animals. The *dalak*-doctors could prevent severe effects and death from the disease if an exposed person received treatment early in the disease course. In Europe, a well-known case of anthrax transmission was that of a German knacker (slaughterer) who consulted the physician F.A.A. Pollender (1800–1879) in 1841. The knacker had carried the bloody hide of a cow on his shoulder; unfortunately, the cow had died of anthrax. The knacker developed a carbuncle in his neck and died two days later. Pollender reasoned that the deadly infection had somehow been transferred from the cowhide, and his suspicion brought up the question of whether the meat from sick animals was safe to eat.

As with rinderpest, scholars and scientists disagreed about whether meat from animals that had died of anthrax was fit for human consumption. Many decrees ordered those carcasses and meat from animals with rinderpest and anthrax should be buried or burnt. Swiss physiologist Albrecht von Haller (1708–1777) believed that meat from anthrax-infected animals was deadly to humans. However, according to Dutch physician Petrus Camper (1722–1789), people who had eaten meat from anthrax-infected animals during food shortages suffered no ill effects to their health, particularly when the meat was well cooked. This was confirmed by members of the Paris *Conseil de Salubrité*, who declared that soldiers from Napoleon's *Grande Armée* had consumed meat from cattle presumed ill with anthrax and rabies without becoming ill. The safety of meat from anthrax-infected animals remained an open question.

It is often difficult to distinguish between animal diseases in the past or to associate diseases that occurred in the past to seemingly similar diseases of today. This is also the case with anthrax. Many descriptions of symptoms of anthrax given in the past remain controversial, because these were often confused symptoms of other diseases and clinical complications linked with anthrax. A typical example illustrating this is the buccopharyngeal form of anthrax, the so-called *glossanthrax*, which seems to have been far more widespread in the past than it is today. Glossanthrax, also called tongue-cancer or tongue-blister, was a type of disease that struck cattle and caused white blisters on the tongue that turned red, then black. The blisters enlarged and deepened into pustules, and at the back of the tongue the pustules ate away at the tongue until it literally fell out. Some gruesome accounts of this disease claimed that the fields were covered with tongues. Because of the blisters, glossanthrax was and is often confused with FMD or rinderpest. This is very doubtful in light of the facts that horses were also affected, and that various sources indicated that animals could die very quickly, within 24 hours. Therefore, from today's point of view, this disease was probably part of the anthrax complex. (Moreover, in the second half of the nineteenth century, biomedical scientists clearly delineated FMD with a different name and pointed out that FMD was far less lethal.) Why glossanthrax seemingly disappeared is still a mystery.

For centuries the opinion prevailed that anthrax was incurable. Animals died so quickly from this disease that it was confused with poisoning or lightning strike. Nevertheless, healers tried various treatments: bloodletting, the application of setons based on the root of hellebore, deep incision of the carbuncles followed by cauterization, and the administration of various herbs and potions. During the 1682 and 1732 epizootics of glossanthrax in Western Europe, healers, cow-doctors, and farmers treated affected animals with tongue-scrapers, which were supposed to prevent the disease from killing the animal. This instrument consisted of a handle with a sharp point on one side to open the blisters and a blade comb with silver teeth to scrape off the pustules until bleeding. Then the tongue should be rubbed with salt and wine vinegar and smeared with honey. This treatment probably did not save the animal's life, but it was a way for livestock owners and veterinary healers to take some action against this dreadful disease.

As historians, we cannot impose today's definition of diseases onto historical outbreaks, but we can try to understand how people of the past thought about them. Anthrax is one of the oldest known diseases, and it is an excellent example of how curious natural historians (and microbiologists, later) classified the same disease differently in different times and places. Our twenty-first-century classification of anthrax as the disease caused by *Bacillus anthracis* is remarkably different from that of the 1700s. In France circa 1700, for example, there were two distinct diseases that we might call *anthrax* today: "malignant pustule" (skin or cutaneous anthrax); and "splenic fever" (a fever disease of the whole body). Beginning in the 1770s, these two different diseases were connected to each other, based on the patient's history of exposure to anthrax-infected animals. Figuring out ways to use government powers to prevent anthrax outbreaks took even longer. This was due to the soil-borne nature of infection, which caused confusion about the direct transmissibility of anthrax between animals and from animals to humans. In addition, the two forms of clinical expression and the similarities of symptoms with other diseases such as rinderpest, blackleg, and glanders made it hard to diagnose.

Disease of War: Glanders

Finally, we will discuss a disease that caused serious problems for solipeds (horses, mules, donkeys) in transportation, agriculture, and especially the military, namely, *Malleus* (Latin) *glanders, farcy* (English), *Rotz* (German), *morve* (French), *ruan* (Turkish), and *can* (Russian). It is one of the oldest known horse diseases. The symptoms of this disease – ulcerating lesions of the skin and mucous membranes, coughing, fever, and the release of nasal discharge – were first described in antiquity. Although the highly infectious nature was well known, disputes about exactly *how* the disease was transmitted continued into the nineteenth century. In hindsight, this can be explained by the various expressions and symptoms of the acute or chronic course of glanders, which were confusing and not always clearly related to each other. In 1797, the Danish veterinarian Erik Viborg (1759–1822) proved that glanders could be transmitted by inoculation or by putting infected and healthy horses together.

Glanders is zoonotic, although the incidence of animal to human transmission is low. But when humans do get infected, mortality is high. Therefore, this disease was long feared among blacksmiths, farriers, flayers, hostlers, soldiers, and veterinarians. Among animals, infection usually occurs by intake of contaminated water or feed or direct transmission. Transmission to humans takes place through direct contact with infected animals (including handling dead animals), or by inhalation. Only a relatively small exposure to contaminated material is necessary to cause infection. This fact was known for centuries, and infection with glanders is considered one of the first biological weapons during warfare. Of course, horses were crucial to warfare and an outbreak of glanders would incapacitate an army. Therefore, armies tried to infect horses of the enemy with glanders by sending infected animals to the enemy camp or leaving them during retreat. It is quite certain that during various wars, great numbers of horses died due to this disease. Along with disease, another major killer of horses during military campaigns was injuries, wounds, and infections. At this point, we briefly review the crucial role of horses and their healers in the history of warfare – a major factor in the development of veterinary medicine and surgery in the early modern and modern periods.

Warfare and the History of Veterinary Surgery

War Animals: Horses

Horses, mules, and donkeys have been used for cavalry, artillery, communication, reconnaissance, and supply; at times, they have even provided food for armies. Central and mounted warfare was revolutionized by the introduction of saddles and stirrups; horse saddles with trees were first used in Asia around 200 BCE. After their invention in China in the first centuries CE, stirrups spread west and south through the nomadic peoples of central Eurasia and east to Japan. The Avars introduced the stirrup to cavalry in Europe in the eighth century, enabling horsemen to mount more easily, sit more tightly in the saddle, handle the lance, and stand up to use the bow and arrow. Due to these advantages, cavalry replaced infantry in Carolingian France and contributed to the rise of Samurai rule in Japan. By the early 1300s, these technologies had spread throughout the Muslim world. For example, the Malian ruler Sunjata demonstrated the power of cavalry in overcoming enemy armies and establishing a vast empire in Western Africa.

Since domestication, people have tried to protect horses' and mules' hooves from wear, and this was particularly crucial during long military campaigns. In ancient Asia, hooves were wrapped in rawhide, leather, or other materials for both therapeutic purposes and protection from wear. The first widely used iron horseshoes probably originated with metalworkers in central Asia, where the art of blacksmithing and farriery traveled east into China. The Romans used a type of horseshoe and mule-shoes. These so-called hipposandals consisted of leather boots, reinforced by an iron plate. Evidence for the use of nailed horseshoes in Europe is relatively late, first known to have appeared around 900, indicating a transfer of blacksmithing knowledge from Asia to Europe around that time. Protection for animals' hooves was crucial to successful long-range military actions, during which the distances traveled would wear down the hooves and cause lameness. In the sixteenth-century Ottoman treatise *Tuhfet'ül-mülûk ve's-selâtîn*, the author summarized a great deal of existing knowledge about hippiatry because horses were essential to Islamic Holy War and were God's own weapons. Sections of the treatise instructed readers on defects of the forefeet, how to nail horseshoes, common horseshoeing mistakes, and the symptoms and treatment of lame horses. These practical instructions, interspersed with religious commentary and sections on training horses for battles and competitions, were intended for the *nalbantlar* or farriers doing the daily work of horse care.

While specializing in the care of horses' hooves, farriers provided other health-care services as well. While traveling with an army or working in encampments, farriers worked with horses who went lame. They treated animals with diseases (such as glanders, which was probably the most common disease problem) as well as parasitic infections. Without healthy horses, armies were incapacitated: supplies and artillery could not be moved, and military leaders lost the significant advantages of cavalry units. Military operations depended on horses, elephants, mules, camels, and other war animals until the early twentieth century. In the fifty years leading up to the end of World War I, the farrier's role in keeping the army moving transitioned into an official attachment of a veterinarian or veterinary surgeon to cavalry and infantry units (see Chapter 5). Finally, the use of horses in warfare helped to stimulate the development of veterinary surgical techniques and practices

Quick, Clean, and Kind: Surgery in Animal Healing

Healers have practiced surgery since ancient times. Every culture throughout history has used its own methods and, of course, those methods have changed over time; but the need to treat traumatic injuries and external conditions has been constant throughout the history of human–animal interactions. Treating wounds, injuries, and external infections was hands-on work that involved manipulations of the body, cutting or lancing, cautery (burning or searing wounds), and applying salves, oils, and bandages. In ancient India, the 2,500-year-old text *Sushruta Samhita* details *shalya-chikitsa*, the Ayurvedic surgical practices (see Fig. 2.2). The text describes learning surgical skills and anatomy from dead animals. Since Ayurvedic principles were applied to both animals and humans it is likely that surgeons worked on living animals as well as humans. Procedures included tooth extractions, eye operations, draining abscesses, and cauterization (searing the wound, usually with a hot iron rod). Early Chinese surgery was likely based on a combination of practical skills (such as bone-setting) and the theory about the flow of the *qi* (essential energy). The essential redirection of the *qi* in cases of illness and injury required treatments such as acupuncture, placing slender needles in the skin to direct the *qi*, and moxibustion, burning herbs on the skin at critical locations to stimulate the flow of *qi*. These treatments would be used for diseases, pain, and injuries. Over time, Korean and Japanese medical cultures also developed their own medico-surgical systems based in part on that of China.

In the Middle East and Europe, surgery developed according to simple experience and principles articulated by Hippocrates, Galen, and the other ancient thinkers. Surgical practices were, generally, slow to change over time; but it's essential to remember that surgeons were very practical and probably individually creative and innovative. In this section, we will describe the surgical marketplace, with many different types of animal surgeons available from which to choose. We also discuss how surgical care helps us to see how closely human and animal bodies were thought to be related. If the body reacted by generating inflammation or pus, for example, this was interpreted in similar ways for animals and humans over time. In general, we see surgical ideas and practices on humans deriving in part from experiments on animals. Knowledge about *human* surgical treatments, and the related topics of pain relief and anesthesia, then informed developments in veterinary medicine. Many types of treatments were used, and we trace some of the developments in animal surgery, 1500s–1700s, here. Surgical practices were slowly adapted to three goals over time: to be quick, clean, and kind. "Quick": lacking effective anesthetic methods, surgeons needed to work quickly. "Clean": Increasingly during this time, surgeons developed ways to avoid deadly wound infections using cleanliness and antisepsis. Finally, "kind" surgeons over the past two centuries have shifted from a belief in dramatic and destructive treatments to being taught to treat tissues gently and kindly for better healing.

Although veterinarians practice both surgery and medicine today, many groups of specialized surgeons, each performing a narrow range of procedures, existed in the past. There were castrators, dentists, firers (used hot irons), cow leeches, and farriers, each of whom competed for clients. Over time, the social and professional positions of these specialists changed based on the society's needs and how people valued different types of animals. Surgeons held higher social positions during certain time periods, for example, in ancient Egypt and for a time in the European Middle Ages. However, these were exceptions, and historically the social status of human and veterinary surgeons reflected surgery's emergence from the lowly barbers and knackers. In contrast with educated and learned physicians, surgeons trained by apprenticeship and dirtied their hands setting bones, cauterizing wounds, extracting teeth, removing skin warts and tumors, applying leeches to remove blood, and amputating limbs. During military action, their duties also included euthanizing soldiers and animals wounded too badly to survive

Surgical practices reflected how people of the past understood the similarities and differences between human and animal bodies. Inflammation looked similar in human and animal bodies, with swelling, heat, pain, and redness. An ancient concept dating at least to Hippocrates (fifth century BCE), a certain amount of inflammation was considered a necessary component of healing after injury. Surgically, inflammation was a localized condition often accompanied by bodily secretions. In both humans and animals, if inflammation was not properly managed, it could advance to wound putrefaction, gangrene, and loss of function or death. Both Ayurvedic and traditional Chinese medicine used (and still use) herbal decoctions to reduce the heat of inflammation; these decoctions were made from plants such as *huáng lián* (*Coptis chinensis*) and *huáng qín* (*Scutellaria baicalensis*), which also effectively stopped bleeding. In the European tradition, healers since at least the twelfth century had carefully watched the formation of pus in a wound. "Laudable" pus, the thick, yellowish discharge from a wound, was viewed as helpful to healing, and some practitioners encouraged its formation by applying irritating substances to the wound. A wound discharging thin, reddish-tinged pus, on the other hand, was not healing well and might progress to gangrene. To prevent gangrene, animal and human healers both used poultices containing honey, butter, clay, herbs, and plant extracts. Additionally, the Arabic practice of cauterizing wounds was used to stop bleeding and to combat suppuration of wounds, both in humans and animals.

As always, violence and war stimulated the development of new surgical knowledge and techniques. From the 1500s onward, the most important change in warfare around the world was the adoption of gunpowder-based weapons. The injuries resulting from these weapons were complex: they often involved both soft tissue (muscles) and bone and caused burns from the powder or shrapnel wounds and concussive head injuries that required trephination (drilling a hole in the skull to relieve intracranial pressure). Once the Chinese techniques of gunpowder-based weaponry spread to

Europe, surgeons began to consider how to treat these new types of wounds in both humans and animals (usually horses, although elephants, mules, oxen, and other animals were also used in warfare). They first tried traditional cautery, using boiling oil; then during the 1536 siege of Turin, surgeon Ambroise Paré realized that soldiers treated with healing ointments instead of the boiling oil actually recovered more quickly and fully. Surgical knowledge about humans influenced veterinary practices, in part because animal bodies were thought to function like those of humans in surgical terms. An excellent example pointing to this mode of thought is the use of standard diagrams in surgical treatises from the seventeenth–eighteenth centuries: the "Wounds Man" and his veterinary counterpart, the "Wounds Horse" (see Fig. 2.6). These diagrams showed the most commonly injured parts of the body during battles and warfare, and the representation of the "Wounds Horse" was clearly borrowed from that of the "Wounds Man."

Until the development of antisepsis in the early 1800s, a wound to the interior of the body (thorax or abdomen) was usually fatal in both humans and animals. The ideas of cleanliness and dressing wounds to keep out dirt and insects made practical sense to many surgical practitioners. But cleanliness did not address the basic problem of healing: the imbalance of the *qi* or the *doshas* or the humors that created out-of-control inflammation. By the 1700s, some physicians and surgeons used bandages dipped in wine to cover wounds. In a rare example of women healers appearing in the historical sources, Frenchwoman Geneviève d'Arconville (1720–1805) has been credited with using mercury chloride in the 1760s to keep wounds clean. However, to most human and animal surgeons, a "clean" wound was one free of foreign bodies, cauterized, and perhaps with its edges debrided and brought together and bandaged. Surgical instruments played an important role: there were dozens of different types of cauterization irons, forceps, bone saws, trocars, trepans, scalpels, and lancets and fleams for bleeding. Interestingly, some surgical instruments looked like or were named according to animal species, for example, "alligator forceps." (This originated with traditional medicine in India; the texts of *Samhita* and later *vedas* discussed the merits of animal-shaped tools that invoked spiritual forces to assist the surgeon.) While the shapes of basic surgical tools used in veterinary medicine have not changed dramatically over the past several hundred years, the late 1700s and early 1800s witnessed a growing interest in wound cleanliness and antisepsis, which we discuss in the next chapter.

Lacking sufficient anesthesia for surgical patients, surgeons had to be "quick" as well as "clean" and "kind." Although anesthesia and analgesia were not discussed much in historical veterinary texts, the lack of effective pain relief is clear from frequent descriptions of the best ways to restrain animals. Ropes for casting livestock (throwing the animal to the ground), the

XVII

¶ Wiewol ich bin vol straich vñ stich/   Doch hoff ich Gott/künstlich ärtzney
Zermo=est/verwundet jämerlich/   Schylhans der werd mir helffen frei.

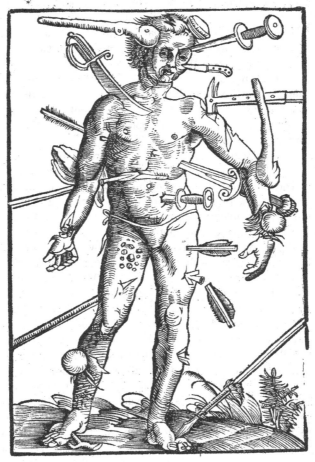

Eyn

Figure 2.6 Representations of battle wounds in veterinary texts were modeled after those in books about human medicine and anatomy. Above is the "Wundenmann [Wounds Man]," Strasbourg, Germany, 1530.

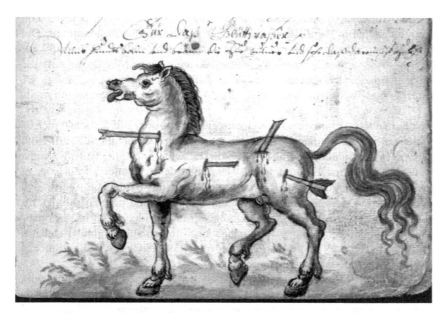

Figure 2.6 (*cont.*) "Wundenpferd [Wounds Horse]," Germany, 1683.
Source: "Wundenmann [Wounds Man]," Hans von Gersdorff, *Feldtbuch der
Wundartzney* (Augsburg, H. Stayner, 1542) 17; public domain. Source: "Wundenpferd
[Wounds Horse]," Johannes Carlyburger, *Rossarzneihandschrift* 1683. Courtesy:
Dr. Veronika Goebel, Bibliothek des Instituts für Paläoanatomie,
Domestikationsforschung und Geschichte der Tiermedizin der LMU München,
IPGTM Hs germ. 1, p. 63.

twitch (twister for the horse's nose), and many other mechanical techniques
speak to surgeons' difficulties with animal restraint during operations.
Nonetheless, *materia medica* for pain relief existed (although we have little
evidence that these compounds were routinely used on animals). A famous
historical physician-surgeon, Hua T'uo (died c. 200 CE), developed an anesthetic from opioids and wine; performed abortions, castration, and other
operations; and used moxibustion on human patients. (We do not know if he
treated animal patients.) Opium and alcohol have long histories in many
cultures, but these were mainly used for humans. They were expensive, and
in larger animals the dosage needed to have an effect was cost prohibitive. The
plant henbane, which contains active anticholinergic properties, was used in
China and the West for pain relief.

Finally, the use of analgesia and general anesthesia for animals depended on how the people of that historical time and place viewed pain in animals. Did animals feel it as humans did, and, if so, was pain helpful or harmful for healing? Was it morally necessary to alleviate animal pain? We do not have the space to adequately address the topic of pain relief in animals, although we return to this discussion in later chapters. Much more historical research needs to be done on the topic of how different cultures viewed animal pain. Clearly, both humans and animals endured treatment we consider brutal today (such as cauterization). In humans, setting fractures, limb amputations, and tooth pulling were conducted without anesthesia even after the British dentist William Morton made his famous 1846 public demonstration of ether as an anesthetic. Although anesthetic agents such as nitrous oxide, chloroform, and carbon dioxide were tested on experimental animals and pets (as proxies for humans) in the early 1800s, these agents were not widely used in veterinary practice for another century – and then only for smaller animals. Debates within the veterinary profession about the uses of analgesics and anesthetics continued into the late twentieth century.

By the 1800s, surgical care for animals began to be incorporated more with medicine, although this was an extremely slow process that varied from place to place. In some cultures, in the modern period veterinarians have been called "veterinary surgeons." Bringing together veterinary medicine and veterinary surgery and reducing the importance of the surgical specialties (castrators, dentists, and the like) were components of the professionalization strategy for veterinary medicine. For veterinary medicine to be a valued, recognized profession in the modern era, veterinary leaders sought to control the veterinary marketplace through education, regulation, and licensing. How they accomplished these goals and the unintended consequences of their strategies are our topics for the next chapter.

Conclusions

From this very brief survey of several centuries, we can conclude that:

1. The domestication of elephants, horses, poultry, bovines, and other animals supplied animals for food, transport, power, and cultural status.
2. Ecological exchange, international trade, and wars resulted in global spreading of animal diseases.
3. Beliefs about human–animal relationships determined the position and use of animals in various cultures, as well as methods of treating diseased animals.
4. In Europe, humoralism continued as the dominant theory to explain disease causation in humans and animals. In Asia, similar theories

centered on balance and/or energy in the body were used to explain diseases. Treatment corresponded to disease causation theories.

5. The 1700s and early 1800s witnessed the rise of knowledge about how bodies functioned in health (physiology) and disease (pathology).

6. Mass outbreaks of rinderpest continued into the 1700s, increasing in scope due to increasing globalization. In many places, observers considered this and other livestock diseases (such as foot and mouth disease and sheep pox) to be a divine punishment.

7. The most effective responses to reduce the spread of infectious diseases included isolation; quarantine; a ban on trade, markets, and transport; and a cull-and-slaughter policy for infected herds. Using these measures, livestock diseases could be contained without knowledge of pathogens.

8. In the course of the eighteenth century, inoculation and vaccination were introduced to contain rinderpest, foot and mouth disease, and sheep pox. These new ideas in healing and medicine were quickly incorporated by some societies and more slowly by others.

9. Anthrax is a zoonotic disease associated with trade; glanders is a zoonotic disease that has long been associated with horses used in wars.

10. Because they inflicted an endless variety of wounds on people and animals, violence and war have stimulated the development of new surgical knowledge and techniques. Surgical practices reflected how people of the past understood the similarities and differences between human and animal bodies.

11. Surgical ideas and practices on humans derived in part from experiments on animals.

12. By the 1800s, surgical care for animals began to be incorporated more with medicine, although this was an extremely slow process that varied from place to place.

Question/Activity: Find examples of how your region or nation contributed to knowledge about animal disease, medicine, and surgery, circa 1700–1850. How did the people of your region or nation keep animals alive and well, especially during times of stress or war?

3   Formal Education for Animal Healing

From Riding Schools to Veterinary Schools, 1700–1850

Introduction

Historians often date the official beginning of the veterinary profession or the start of veterinary science to the first permanent veterinary school founded in Lyon, France (École Vétérinaire de Lyon, 1762). They argue that Lyon and other European schools made veterinary medicine "modern" and "scientific," implying that veterinarians could heal animals much more effectively. But there are problems with this founding myth. Although the rise of veterinary schools in Europe represented an important step in the history of veterinary medicine, the education was not quite scientific (from today's point of view), and it didn't change veterinary practices much either. Professional veterinary healers had already existed for centuries, and these healers cannot all be disqualified as ignorant empiricists or dangerous quacks; after all, their practices were very similar to those of more "educated" animal healers. Nor were veterinary educational institutions new in the late 1700s. As we have seen, veterinary schools teaching the most up-to-date information had existed in ancient China, India, and many other advanced ancient medical cultures for centuries. The Islamic madrassas trained veterinarians who practiced, wrote texts, and trained apprentices. These practitioners were esteemed in their own times for their education, knowledge, and experience, just as the graduates of eighteenth- and nineteenth-century European schools expected to be.

In this chapter, we reconsider the significance of these European veterinary schools, which were the most recent in a long history of educational innovations in animal healing. We argue that, like the Chinese, Ayurvedic, and Islamic systems of education that preceded and coexisted with them, European veterinary schools grew from particular contexts: the intellectual developments of the European Enlightenment; the competition within the veterinary marketplace; and the expectations that professional animal healers would support the military, colonial, and agricultural goals of national governments and empires. The development of veterinary educational and professional institutions was greatly affected by major events in Europe and around the world: the aftermath of the Black Death, political and religious turmoil, the increasing continental circulation of animal diseases, and European and Ottoman imperialism. New theological and secular philosophies shaped European veterinary education just as they had during the height of the Islamic schools. The needs of the state dictated the types of animals treated by veterinarians, and those treatments in 1762 looked a lot like the ones available in 1500.

Still, the question remains how a professionalization process took place in Europe, from animal healing practiced by all sorts of empiricists, to the increasing importance of veterinarians trained according to particular principles developing in a rapidly growing number of similar schools. Much of today's infrastructure of professional veterinary medicine is descended from the institutions and regulatory framework of the eighteenth–nineteenth centuries. Veterinary education in the modern period developed against the background of competing traditions and turfs, and we follow this story as it developed in Europe and spread with imperialism to many parts of the world. Why did these schools start in France, why in the 1760s, and why did similar institutions multiply and spread to other nations and continents? We begin with the specific circumstances in eighteenth-century France: veterinary education's philosophical roots in the intellectual developments of the European "enlightenment." We present an overview of the market for veterinary services with demand and supply from various animal healers around 1750, and how the graduates of the new veterinary schools tried to obtain their share of the veterinary marketplace from then on. We show how, increasingly, the enlightenment ideals built into the early years of French veterinary education bent to more pragmatic concerns: physiocrat economics with its emphasis on the value of agriculture (including animals); the challenges of disease outbreaks; and the need for healthy army horses. Subsequently, we outline the institutionalization of graduate veterinarians alongside shoeing-smiths and farriers in armies against the background of wars, the process of industrialization, and the growth of empires.

Building on the recent work of a new generation of veterinary historians, we consider why the French model of veterinary education and professionalization spread widely, and how other nations and territories adapted it. We treat the development of the eighteenth-century European veterinary regime as a product of its times, arguing that it succeeded in spreading because it fulfilled crucial social, political, and cultural needs during subsequent decades of increasing industrialization and imperialism affecting the globe.

How Veterinary Education Emerged from the "Enlightenment" in France

The Natural History Tradition

To answer the question, "why were European veterinary schools first established in late eighteenth-century France?" we begin with the Enlightenment period in Europe (c. 1700s–1800s). The way in which people treat animals depends on how they value them and think about them, and this period witnessed a change in how animals were considered: from objects of intellectual curiosity, animals also became subjects of the state. First, we define what we mean by the Enlightenment and its ideals: overall, it was a set of major changes in ideas and social institutions that moved away from older sacred traditions, with a greater emphasis on the agency of humans to alter their environment. Historians have characterized this enlightenment period as a transition from strictly theologically based societies to more tolerant and secular ones, increasingly focused on rationality and pragmatic ways to solve specific problems. European intellectuals gathered observations and knowledge, applied strict rationales (modes of reasoning), and expected that increasing knowledge would lead to improved conditions for human life.

Enlightened principles proved useful to developing nation-states – for example, helping to consolidate power and wealth. Of course, this was a potential problem if the peasants also expected to reap the benefits of social progress; this problem contributed to the outbreak of the French Revolution in 1789, for example. Nation-states depended at this time on high-level agricultural production, and one of the greatest threats to agriculture in the eighteenth century was the *peste bovine*, or rinderpest, which killed large numbers of European cattle for at least 70 years. Consolidating agricultural wealth meant harnessing knowledge about animal health. A vibrant print culture, the growth of medical knowledge, and royal (later republican) governmental sponsorship enabled formal veterinary education to grow quickly in France. The appreciation of reason, the study of nature, and the development of cosmopolitan knowledge were closely linked to their practical uses. (Cosmopolitan knowledge is knowledge that successfully traveled and took hold in many places, albeit adapted for local use.) Historians have characterized France as an important center of the European enlightenment, and this context explains why veterinary education first developed there. (Of course, the presence of strong individual leaders and some luck also contributed.) We have begun this chapter by reviewing "the enlightenment" because these developments shaped the first permanent modern-era veterinary schools: the French École Vétérinaire de Lyon and École Vétérinaire d'Alfort. Both were products of the enlightenment period, and specifically of the French Enlightenment.

Consider the work of Claude Bourgelat (1712–1779), who instigated the establishment of both Écoles and served as the first director of the Lyon school. With extensive experience in horsemanship, access to high-ranking royal officials, and as a member of Paris' Academy of Sciences, Bourgelat had already contributed to French enlightenment knowledge about animals with his text, *Élémens d'hippiatrique* (Lyon, 1750–1753). For Bourgelat, an animal (such as the horse) should be studied using newly articulated principles of natural history, mathematics, and statistics. For example, Bourgelat developed

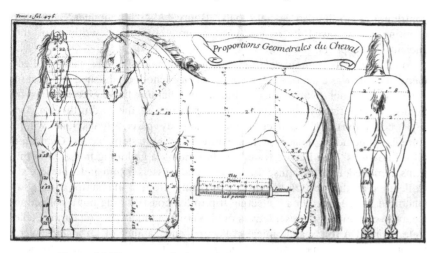

Figure 3.1 The geometrical proportions of the horse.
Source: Claude Bourgelat, *Élémens d'hippiatrique* (Lyon: H. Declaustre and les frères Duplain, 1750–1753), Vol. 1, 476.

the "hippometer," an idealized set of measured proportions of the horse's body based on the length of its head. The ideal horse should comply with these geometrical proportions (Fig. 3.1). This type of mechanistic explanation of the animal body was new, and it fit well within the methods and ideals of the French enlightenment. Bourgelat was influential: he had the ear of the king and he corresponded with the celebrated thinkers of his time, including Voltaire and Frederick the Great, King of Prussia. Moreover, Bourgelat contributed 235 chapters on horses, horsemanship, and animal diseases to the most influential contemporary collection of natural history knowledge: Denis Diderot and Jean d'Alembert's *Encyclopédie ou Dictionnaire raisonné des sciences, des arts et des métiers* [Encyclopedia, or Classified Dictionary of Sciences, Arts, and Trades, 1751–1772]. This 28-volume compendium of knowledge covered the whole world in a systematic way, and historians characterize it as the classic enlightenment text. Bourgelat was asked to write the veterinary chapters because he was a friend of d'Alembert and considered France's greatest enlightenment thinker on the subject of domesticated animals. The content and style of Bourgelat's contributions were in line with the free spirit of the enlightened philosophers: he based his work on the study of nature while ignoring most of the older literature. His focus was on preserving the health of animals and improving them. His "hippometer" was meant to be used, to accumulate the evidence of observations on animals and analyze its contributions to human social goals. Bourgelat's "hippometer," and his resulting ideas, owed its authority to nature, not to the writings of the ancient philosophers.

Another way to accumulate observations about animal bodies was to collect them, and this was a major goal of the veterinary school established at Alfort in 1765. The school owned one of the largest natural history collections in France, considered by some to be superior to that of the Jardin du Roi (the royal collection). This collection included body parts, organs, and whole animals – including anatomist Henri Fragonard's masterpiece *Le Chevalier* (also known as "The Flayed Rider"), a boy riding a galloping horse, with the skins removed and the muscles, nerves, and vessels exquisitely preserved. Collectors at the school acquired everything from a llama to a dolphin (acquired by students on a collecting trip to the coast), filling out a collection meant to encompass representatives of all known animal types on earth. École Vétérinaire d'Alfort's anatomical collection and cabinet of curiosities were famous in its own time (and still today). Collecting specimens was a foundation of natural history and natural philosophy, the central enlightenment-era studies of life on earth. At Alfort, the collection was the basis for veterinary students' study of comparative anatomy, not just for horses but also cattle, sheep, pigs, goats, and others. Reflecting Bourgelat's military expertise and interests, horses dominated the students' education at Lyon and Alfort; but the king's treasurer also expected that students be trained in controlling economically devastating livestock diseases (especially a concern in the agricultural areas around Lyon). Both schools combined natural history with the more practical training in horse husbandry and livestock diseases. The example of Alfort, especially, demonstrates that early French veterinary education grew in part out of Enlightenment philosophy and shared its goal of generating cosmopolitan knowledge about animals from around the world – not just the local domesticated animals

The mission of veterinary schools changed, however, becoming more attentive to the practical problems of epizootics and keeping military animals healthy. Lyon and Alfort had begun as institutions generating knowledge about all life on earth (natural history) as well as providing medical care for domesticated animals; indeed, these two intellectual goals were seen as interlinked. However, after 1789, government officials separated natural history (and human medical) education from that of veterinary students. Gone were the days of learning natural history broadly and traveling to the French coast to collect aquatic animals for the collection. After the French Revolution, officials of the new government split up Alfort's collection, leaving only the specimens from cows, horses, and other domestic animals. Now, the veterinary schools' mission would focus on domestic animal health to increase the nation's wealth. By 1800, this shift to a narrower, economic focus allied veterinary education more firmly with agriculture and another philosophical trend during the enlightenment: the pragmatism of the physiocrats.

Enlightenment Pragmatism: The Economic Value of Animals

Physiocrats believed that a strong nation depended primarily on its agricultural wealth. Physiocracy developed within the setting of the mainly rural societies of eighteenth-century Europe and was influenced by the world's largest economic system, namely, that of China. Most physiocrats believed that government policy should not interfere with natural economic laws, and that land and agrarian labor were the sources of all wealth. Similar to Chinese agrarian politics, the nation's wealth derived from the land development and (high) prices for agricultural products. The most important early representative of this group was François Quesnay (1694–1774). He advocated productive work as the only true source of value and wealth for the state, in contrast to mercantilism in which merchants traded goods produced by others and the value was determined at the market. In order to achieve national wealth and planning of long-term economic growth, rulers and their administrators needed statistical data on trade, population, and agricultural output (especially for livestock and horses). These quantitative data on a national level facilitated the growing power of centralized state control from the 1760s onward.

The rise of rational planning principles and the physiocrat economy with its emphasis on the value of agriculture drew more attention to livestock production, farmers, and veterinary medicine. Veterinary education should be oriented toward the needs of the nation's farmers and livestock raisers, a belief only underscored by repeated, long-lasting outbreaks of rinderpest in cattle (Chapter 2), which severely decreased agricultural growth. Next to healthy livestock, the nation demanded equine medicine as the number of horses – the motors of society and the army – increased during the eighteenth and nineteenth centuries. The final reason for veterinary schools to shift toward a more practical education for their students was the cut-throat competition they faced upon graduation. What was the status quo of professionals active as animal healers at the time of the foundation of the first French veterinary school?

Competing for a Position in the Veterinary Marketplace

Every Man His Own Veterinarian

Around the world at this time, animal owners were the foundation of the veterinary marketplace: they often treated their own animals, and they decided when to call in a healer. Europe was no exception. Literate animal owners got significant help from the popular literature published cheaply in the eighteenth century. Numerous booklets of recipes for ointments, drenches, and other treatments circulated, particularly in the countryside. Anyone could write (or reproduce) booklets, such as the long-lived collection of horse remedies written by the "uneducated" Meister Albrant. The most well-known examples are booklets called *Every Man His Own Farrier*, published in French, Italian, German, English, Dutch, and other languages. On the frontispiece typically, a drawing of a horse is presented in the center, surrounded by lines, figures, or letters illustrating and describing the locations of all known diseases, and – often – with recommended locations to apply bloodletting. Another common image is a drawing that includes the names of multiple defects and diseases illustrated on the body of one horse (*Défauts du cheval*, French; *Fehlerpferd*, German; *"Defective" horse*, English) (Fig. 3.2). Such images were mostly copied from earlier comprehensive books on hippology (knowledge about horses). The figures or letters correspond with short descriptions of the disease in the booklet with recommended remedies and recipes. Similar booklets were published on diseases in cattle as well.

Travel journals, guild regulations, annals, feudal accounts, almanacs, and recipe books derived from popular books also provide information on who practiced animal health care and healing and how. These sources also give an impression of known infectious diseases such as cattle plague, sheep pox,

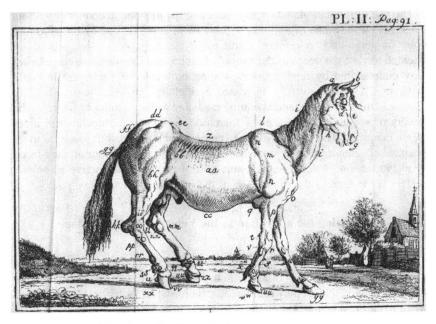

Figure 3.2 Image of the "defective" horse.
Source: L.W.F. van Oebschelwitz, De Nederlandsche stalmeester ('s Gravenhage: Van Kleef, 1763) 91, plate II.

anthrax, vermin, rabies, and glanders, and mention disorders like laminitis (inflammation inside the hoof), numbness, blood clotting, tumors, sprains, and lameness. Smiths were occupied with horseshoeing, but later broadened their surgical skills with bloodletting, firing, castrating, and tail docking. Next to administering purgatives they treated illnesses such as the glanders, the botts (a parasite), or lameness. Next to bloodletting, standard treatments were attaching a seton, *Sèton* (French), *Haarseil* (German), that is, making two incisions in the skin using a long needle and putting a cord of hair under the skin to stimulate bad humors to discharge from the body together with pus; root-sticking, that is, sticking a part of hellebores root under the skin of the ear or tail; scarification or cauterization of the skin around chronically diseased joints and subsequent anointing with irritating turpentine, mustard, and the like to provoke healing. Trepanation was a specialized skill consisting of drilling a hole into the bones of the skull to relieve pressure (Fig. 3.3). A very crude

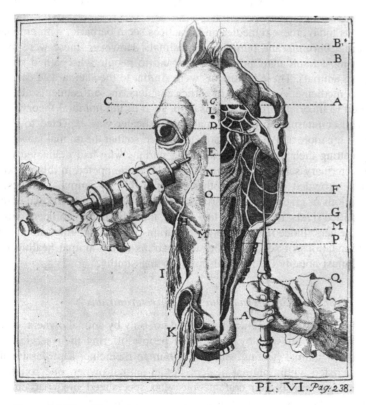

Figure 3.3 Plate illustrating trepanation of the *sinus maxillaris*, which became a regular surgery in the eighteenth century.
Source: L.W.F. van Oebschelwitz, *De Nederlandsche stalmeester* ('s Gravenhage: Van Kleef, 1763) 238, plate VI.

surgery known since antiquity until well into the nineteenth century was the removal or cauterization of the membrane under the tongue, the lyssa, to prevent or treat rabies in dogs.

Next to the application of opium, mandrake, and other *materia medica*, and the Islamic influence from the thirteenth century, cauterization became common in surgery. Hot burning irons with their dry and hot fire were used to burn and dry out cold and wet diseases such as abscesses, ulcers, and spavin exostoses. To keep horses calm during simple operations, an assistant or groom used a twister or twitch on the upper lip. The Hippocratic idea that prevention was better than treatment remained very important in the early modern period, for humans but also for animals. General advice to maintain animal health included not overworking them and providing a warm and dry place to sleep, clean water, and appropriate feed for each season. However, magic and superstition with centuries-old incantations, prayers, and blessings survived antiquity and was adjusted after Christianization to remain during the early modern era.

To us today, these remedies and practices seem barbaric, with emphasis on bleeding, burning, and purging sick animals. However, these were the treatments most familiar to animal owners and to people who earned money for treating animals. These treatments were similar to the standard of care used in human medicine. As we saw in earlier chapters, these treatments also corresponded to theories of disease causation, such as the humoral theory. Like his medical counterpart, a professional animal healer was expected to *do something* – the more active or dramatic, the better, so that the animal's owner knew they getting their money's worth. Veterinarians who had graduated from the new veterinary schools at the end of the 1700s competed in this marketplace already crowded with many other manipulators of animals' bodies. Later generations of graduate veterinarians condescendingly looked down upon their unqualified rivals; but until the late 1800s, they still had to compete with those other healers. Indeed, European veterinarians built their professional roles on the foundations of several earlier occupations in the animal healing marketplace, most notably the marshals and shoeing-smiths.

Shoeing-Smiths and Other Proto-veterinarians

Folk veterinary medicine was performed not only by animal owners, herdsmen and shepherds but also by an array of people offering their services on the market for animal healing. Similar to human medicine, a professional hierarchy existed within animal healers. As an animal owner, one could choose between generalists and craftspeople who specialized in a particular area. These included shoeing-smiths, castrators, tail-dockers, obstetricians, horse- and cow-leeches, medicine-mixers, flayers, executioners, and others. Wealthy owners with valuable animals often employed a full-time caregiver for their animals (especially horses). In Europe, this caregiver was called a *marshal*, *maréchal/maréchaux*, or *Marschalk* (the word originates from the Gallic *marahskalks*, meaning horse and servant). The horse marshal was the first-line healer, although he could call in a specialist if necessary. The status of marshal had increased during the late Middle Ages: if an animal was ill, the marshal made the diagnosis, while the practical work was left to the specialist, groom, or shoeing-smith. Some marshals obtained a military rank; a few even rose to the select (often royally appointed) post of equerry (*équier*), at the very top of the hierarchy. Historians have pointed to the role of horse marshal as a direct precedent for the role of veterinarian in Europe, along with the farrier or shoeing-smith, an occupation with a long history (see Chapter 2). Shoeing-smiths were important members of each local community in many parts of the world (Fig. 3.4).

After horseshoeing's introduction to Europe, the two roles of horse marshal and shoeing-smith slowly merged into one occupation: the *farrier* (English), *maréchaux-ferrant* (French), or *Hufschmiede* (German). Farriers were usually tradespeople who learned their craft through an apprenticeship and practiced on a gentleman's estate, in a village or town, or in the military cavalry (as the marshal had). Their practical knowledge was supplemented by popular vernacular literature such as printed booklets, manuals, and almanacs (also available to animal owners). The term "farrier" originated from the Latin *ferrarius*, meaning "of iron," and farriers were an organized profession. As early as 1356, the mayor of London requested that farriers within a seven-mile radius of London should establish a guild to regulate their trade and improve their practices. Guild control of the animal healing marketplace emerged slowly in England, however. The most powerful guild, the Worshipful Company of Farriers, was not granted a charter until 1674. In Germany, the guild system was common for many occupations, including the *Hufschmiede*. Guild rules protected the farriers and their customers from poor workmanship, overcharging, and loss of employment.

Another very important precursor to the role of professional veterinarian in Europe was the *albéytare* in Spain. As we have seen, this word derives from Arabic and reflects the key importance of the Islamic tradition of animal healing in Spain. Indeed, Islamic knowledge's influence remained considerable long after 1492, and this knowledge formed the basis for professional equine medical guilds in Spain. Like physicians, surgeons, and apothecaries, albéytares had to pass an official state examination. This examination, overseen by the *Tribunal del Protoalbeyterato*, was established in 1500 and remained active well into the nineteenth century. In preparation for this examination, students used the *Libro de Albeyteria* from Francisco de la Reyna (c. 1520–1583) as the textbook. Once a student passed the examination

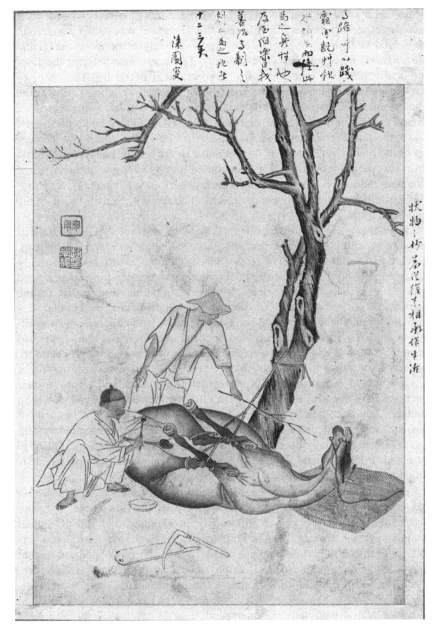

Figure 3.4 Shoeing-smith, Korea, eighteenth century. Painting by Cho Yong-Seok (1686–1761).
Courtesy: Prof. Myung-Sun Chun, College of Veterinary Medicine, Seoul National University, Korea. National Museum of Korea, Seoul, reg. no.: Dogwon-2307.

(after a period of study and apprenticeship), they had the right to the title of *albéytare* or horse-doctor and could practice their profession. The *albéytares* were known and admired throughout Europe. For example, in 1563 the German politician and businessman Markus Fugger traveled to Spain with his marshal, a man named Seuter, to buy horses for his stud. Fugger was very impressed by the Spanish horse farms and the fact that in Spain, horse-doctors (*albéytares*) were practicing animal healing instead of shoeing-smiths. He consulted *albéytares* to conduct examinations of his horses before he purchased them, as these horse-doctors were also specialists in buying and selling horses.

Justifying Veterinary Education: Military Horses and Warfare

The development of surgical knowledge and practices was greatly stimulated by warfare, with its horrific wounds to the bodies of soldiers and their animals. In Europe, medieval surgeons occupied their own social niche: the "barber-surgeons," whose hands-on work was disdained by the higher social orders occupied by learned physicians. These surgeons did various operations: setting bones, cauterizing wounds, extracting teeth, removing skin warts and tumors, applying leeches to remove blood, and amputating limbs. For instance, a remarkable archeological finding (the Netherlands, thirteenth century) shows a broken and later-healed sheep bone fixed with a nail. During military actions, their duties also included euthanizing soldiers and animals wounded too badly to survive. Both animals and humans endured treatments we consider brutal today. This included not only cauterization but also setting fractures and conducting amputations without anesthesia. This led to the need for surgeons to do their work quickly while their animal patients were restrained with ropes and hobbles. As with the earlier surgical traditions discussed in Chapter 2, surgical knowledge about humans influenced veterinary practices.

Aristocratic and Military Use of the Horse

Since domestication, horses have had great socioeconomic, military, cultural, and recreational meaning for human society. This is reflected by the (estimated) tens of thousands of books and treatises that have been published about horses. Topics include breeding, feed, care, healing, and specialized training (such as dressage and equitation). A chronological analysis of these writings clearly mirrors the different phases of professionalization of horse medicine. Many old books about horses in veterinary library collections deal with hippology. Within this theme, the art of horse riding represents a separate subcategory. This is not surprising, given the fact that horse riding belonged to aristocratic court culture and the appearance of power (hunting, tournaments, splendor parades, marches, etc.). Until mechanization, horses were indispensable in agriculture and transport. Of course, horses were essential in warfare as cavalry mounts, beasts of burden, and sources of traction.

During the Roman and Byzantine eras, horses were increasingly specially bred and trained to fulfill different tasks. This process continued in the ensuing centuries, when horses represented an essential part of court culture and military campaigns. The high social position of knights at estates and courts required horses to carry them during hunting, hawking, jousts, parades, and tournaments. On the battlefield, horses proved to be a most effective and significant weapon of the cavalry. With their speed, swords, and lances, mounted knights increased the military capabilities of an army significantly. Knights needed more than one horse and, appropriate to their warrior status, they rode stallions, not mares or geldings. A specific and expensive type of horse (not a breed) a knight used in warfare or tournaments was the destrier. These strong horses supported fully armored knights and were trained to withstand the noise of combat and the shock of charges by other horses in frontal collisions. However, for all other types of transportation, knights used palfreys as ordinary riding horses. Palfreys were lighter than destriers and trained for smooth gaits and endurance. Finally, knights owned sumpter horses, mules, or donkeys. These beasts of burden were cheap but essential for transporting equipment and armor. Obviously, these different types of warhorses needed veterinary knowledge for successful breeding, feeding, shoeing, and health care.

Between 1522 and 1648, Europe was the scene of religious wars with battlefields everywhere as a result of conflicts between Protestants and Catholics. The need for warhorses increased, as did the demand for professionals to maintain their health, particularly since a well-trained military horse cannot be quickly replaced. (The production and training of a horse requires at least five or six years.) During the Middle Ages and early modern times, European nations did not have standing armies. The commander was the owner or assembler of the regiment, and the horses were privately owned. Some regiments employed shoeing-smiths, saddle-makers, *maréchaux*, and sometimes knackers to care for horses. For soldiers in the mercenary armies, war was a way to make money, but only if their horses remained healthy. European armies were a melting pot of nationalities, and this was one way that veterinary knowledge circulated. Horse owners and animal health practitioners exchanged knowledge about horse diseases, injuries, and treatments, which is reflected in the veterinary writings of those days.

Riding Schools

Within the tradition of Xenophon, many books were written on the art of horsemanship. In his instruction for the horseman, Xenophon described the training of riding horses for military use. Translated into various languages, this treatise was applied as standard for many centuries. In the sixteenth century the number of books on horse riding increased, because the use of new weapons (gunpowder, guns) required new riding styles and combat tactics. Quick and dynamic maneuvers became very important in fights between riders. Training was thus focused on various intricate turns and half-turns of horse and rider, which required advanced training. These new insights were taught to the aristocracy at riding schools that were established in Europe, especially in Italy. The Naples riding school attained international fame. The main representative of this school, Federico Grisone, described the new training methods in his handbook *Ordini di cavalcare* (Venice, 1550). Via various translations, this new hippological knowledge spread to other countries where stable masters, *marechals*, and riding masters gratefully exploited it.

Foreign pupils who had stayed at the Naples riding school for a longer period spread their knowledge on horsemanship further into Europe. A well-known example is Antoine de Pluvinel. After his stay in Italy, he established an *Academie d'Équitation* in Paris in 1594. Ingratiating himself with the French court, Pluvinel won the position of equestrian tutor to the dauphin, later King Louis XIII. From these lessons, Pluvinel wrote a beautifully illustrated book: *l'Instruction du roy, en l'exercice de monter à cheval* (Paris, 1625). As French ambassador to the Netherlands, Pluvinel spread his methods to the Dutch court and beyond with the military. In his *Instruction*, he called for the establishment of royal academies where horsemanship and the art of war were taught. With their combination of theory and practice, such royal academies, which were effectively founded in France in the seventeenth century, became excellent breeding grounds for the further development of horsemanship (hippology) and equine medicine (hippiatry). They produced several influential *écuyer* (stable masters).

The first books on horsemanship published in England were Thomas Blundeville's *The fower chiefest offices belonging to horsemanshippe* (1565) and John Astley's *The Art of Riding* (1584). Examples of other famous equerries who directed riding schools are Jacques de Solleysel, William Cavendish, François de la Guérinière, and Gaspar de Saunier. De Solleysel (1617–1680) was director of the Royal Academy in Paris. In 1664 he wrote *Le parfait mareschal* (The perfect marshal), which became an international best-seller with 33 editions. Cavendish (1592–1676), duke of Newcastle, was the husband of the philosopher and poet Margaret Cavendish. This monarchist couple was exiled from England and lived in Paris and Antwerp (Belgium). Inspired by de Solleysel, Cavendish began research in horsemanship and started his own riding school in Antwerp. His book, *New method for horse dressage*, was published in 1658. The book is famous because of its wonderful 42 illustrations. These copper engravings in Baroque style were made by

Abraham van Diepenbeke, the horse painter in the atelier of famous artist Peter Paul Rubens.

De la Guérinière (1688–1751) was royal stable master in France and is considered the founder of modern horse riding. His dressage methods, of which the tradition is continued in the Spanish Riding School for Lipizzaner horses in Vienna today, were outlined in his *École de cavalerie* (Paris, 1733). After a career in France, Gaspar de Saunier (1663–1748) became riding master at the universities of Utrecht and Leiden (the Netherlands). In Leiden he worked on his book *La parfait connaissance des chevaux*, which was published in The Hague in 1734. The first part covers diseases and therapy, and the second part deals with horse anatomy. In 1756 he published *l'Art de la cavalerie*, in which different chapters were dedicated to warfare training. For a long time, the riding schools remained centers for the sophisticated equitation required by the military and prized by the aristocracy. Next to the nobility, the well-to-do-class started recreational horse riding in the eighteenth century. Horse riding no longer remained reserved only for gentlemen; ladies riding sidesaddle became a common phenomenon in riding centers. The same period witnessed the rise of horse and trotting races, which formed a further stimulus for the development of equine medicine.

Justifying Veterinary Education: The Great Animal Plagues, Revisited

Along with the needs of the military for healthy horses, governments' other urgent concerns about the health of cattle and other food-producing animals only increased during the 1700s and early 1800s. This reflected a surge in the spread of animal diseases, due to accelerating transnational trade of animals and animal products. The most destructive diseases were rinderpest, foot and mouth disease, and contagious pleuropneumonia in cattle; vesicular diseases and sheep pox; and anthrax. Of course, glanders in horse populations (especially in armies) continued to be a major problem; but the economic impact of food–animal diseases increasingly stimulated regional national governments to seek solutions. These solutions, however, did not obviously point to the establishment of formal veterinary training. The most effective means of disease control were bureaucratic, involving the police powers of the governments. Quarantines, the control of animal movements and trade in animal products, and slaughter of sick and exposed animals remained the most important methods of disease prevention and control.

Rinderpest, which spread from its reputed homelands in the Russian empire to Europe and beyond, is an excellent example. Major outbreaks of rinderpest hit Europe in the 1710s, 1740s, and 1760s–1780s. City-state and national government officials had sophisticated knowledge about these waves of the disease, which they accurately traced along the trade routes. Differing from country to country, the need to control rinderpest in order to secure the supply of food of animal origin represented potentially important reasons to establish institutes for formal veterinary education. Although livestock diseases with their disastrous effects on the animal economy were explicitly mentioned in the founding charters, this target often faded into the background once the early schools were established.

There was rhetorical value inherent in mentioning the specter of the great epizootics, such as rinderpest, as a reason for monarchs and private benefactors to fund formal veterinary schools. School officials certainly sounded like they were concerned about this important problem. However, a close look at the activities of the early European veterinary schools shows that they were focused on the treatment of valuable horses. Little attention was paid to studying diseases of food-producing animals (such as rinderpest). Likewise, in the veterinary historiography, later historians who casually cited the great livestock epizootics as the only (or major) reason for establishing veterinary educational institutions often overestimated its actual importance. The promise of trained veterinarians' ability to control the eighteenth-century outbreaks of rinderpest was a hopeful idea at best because they had no tools (vaccines, etc.) besides quarantines. As a final point, we note that most schools were established after the third wave of European rinderpest outbreaks (1768–1786) had ended.

As we will see, even the earliest French schools (established during the third wave of rinderpest) were mainly concerned with injuries and diseases of horses. This fact disappointed many students, particularly those who had been sent by other nations to study veterinary medicine in the service of disease control. As in the French schools, students complained about the lack of attention to nonequine epizootics at the early German schools. Equine medicine for horse breeding for economic and military purposes was the main focus of curricula for the early schools. This probably reflected the fact that the schools' founders themselves were most interested in horses (especially for the military) and that horses were the most valuable of all the domesticated animals. For example, in 1821 when the Utrecht veterinary school opened its doors, compare the average value for a horse (115 guilders) to that of a milk cow (37 guilders), a pig (25), and a sheep (5). To protect their valuable investment, horse owners would be more likely to pay for veterinary care. Cattle, although less valuable individually than horses, were subjects of what we today would call a type of "herd health" or "veterinary preventive medicine." In large numbers, cattle obviously represented a notable percentage of the national wealth. But bureaucratic functionaries – not country veterinarians – usually controlled the few tools available against cattle epizootics. As we will see, these practical considerations eventually slanted the training available at formal veterinary schools toward equine medicine, surgery, and farriery.

The high value of horses was only one of the factors that shaped the development of formal veterinary educational institutions. These schools developed within particular contexts, especially the learned and philosophical developments of the "enlightenment" period. The earliest schools reflected their founders' interests in, and the patronage of, the military, which was focused on cavalry horses. The veterinary marketplace, which included a variety of healers, shoeing-smiths, and horse marshals, also influenced formal veterinary training. To demonstrate how this system of contemporary veterinary education developed, we next make a detailed examination of the founding of the first two schools, at Lyon and Alfort in France.

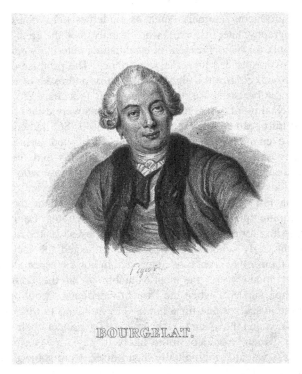

Figure 3.5 The competitors: above, Claude Bourgelat (1712–1779); below, Philippe Étienne Lafosse (1738–1820).
Source: stipple engraving by François Pigeot, Courtesy: Wellcome Library London Digital Image no. 1298i. Philippe Étienne Lafosse (1738–1820). Source: Line engraving by Michel after Harguinier, Courtesy: Wellcome Library London Digital Image no. 5197i.

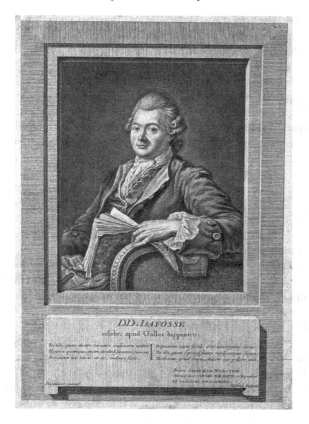

DD. LAFOSSE
celebr: apud Gallos hippiatro:

Figure 3.5 (*cont.*)

Establishment and Spread of Veterinary Schools

1762: Lyon, France

The story begins in the city of Lyon, 470 kilometers south of Paris, which was a center for economics (banking) and silk production. Lyon was not an obvious choice for locating a veterinary school, but it was the home of the Royal Academy of Equitation and its director, Claude Bourgelat (whom we met earlier in this chapter) (Fig. 3.5). Bourgelat envisioned a new kind of institution, a college for veterinary education based on the model of the Academy of Equitation, but he could not make his vision a reality without Henri-Léonard Bertin. Bertin was King Louis XV's Controller General of Finances and Secretary of State for Agriculture – he controlled the money necessary for the new school. How Bourgelat and Bertin shaped this veterinary school and defended it against its competitors is an interesting story.

Although trained as a lawyer, Bourgelat was far more interested in equitation and the proper care of horses. Besides directing the riding school, Bourgelat began studying equine anatomy and hippiatry. Between 1750 and 1753, Bourgelat published the three volumes of his *Élémens d'hippiatrique*, which he wrote in the form of questions from a young apprentice and answers given by an experienced master. With this innovative style, Bourgelat tested some of his own educational ideas and made these books particularly useful as texts for students. The content was innovative. Bourgelat was an educated rationalist, and he stressed observation and experiment while expressing doubt about traditional therapies such as bloodletting (still very popular at the time). His publications and his social connections helped Bourgelat to become a corresponding member of the French Academy of Sciences and a contributor to Diderot and Alembert's *Encyclopedie*, which made him a member of the highest ranks of the French intelligentsia.

Bourgelat used his reputation, broad social network, and communication skills to sell the idea of an *école vétérinaire* in Lyon to Henri-Léonard Bertin. Along with being head of the French treasury, Bertin oversaw an agricultural reform program established in 1761 that was primarily aimed at controlling rinderpest, and he envisioned the new school as a center for education and research about agricultural diseases. In contrast, Bourgelat's vision focused entirely on horses: he planned a school based on horse husbandry and farriery, with theoretical lectures on medical subjects given by professors from the medical school. Bertin told Bourgelat that the French government would pay to establish a school if it included investigations into the diseases of cattle and other livestock. Seizing his opportunity to gain royal patronage for the school, Bourgelat agreed (in principle). In this way, the rhetorical reasons for establishing the Lyon school fit within the scope of the physiocratic movement to improve livestock production, as well as within the enlightenment approach to solving larger societal problems (protecting the food supply and the animal economy). Bourgelat's *école vétérinaire* opened its doors on January 1, 1762, in a former tavern building. (Perhaps this explains veterinary students' longstanding enthusiasm for social activities.)

The Lyon veterinary educational model had a few similarities and some important differences with that of contemporary medical education (for physicians and surgeons). As with physicians' formal medical education, the students were expected to memorize and be able to recite the lectures. Bourgelat instructed students to write down every word, exactly as he had dictated. For this purpose, Bourgelat later wrote *Élémens de l'art vétérinaire, zootomie ou anatomie comparée, a l'usage des élèves des écoles vétérinaires*, a textbook that was published in Paris (1766–1769). Like their medical counterparts, Bourgelat's veterinary students began with anatomy. Here the differences become apparent: veterinary students were destined to combine the traditional roles of physician and surgeon, by both understanding the theory and carrying out the practices. Like traditional country physicians, veterinarians could expect to see a wide variety of medical and surgical problems, but in multiple species and working with their boots in the mud of the barnyard. Veterinary students had much more access to bodies for dissection and clinical material than their medical counterparts. In Bourgelat's school, veterinary students received an admirably hands-on education. Following their professors' theoretical lectures, students moved on to demonstrations and practical training on dissections, botany, horseshoeing, and preparing medicines. Under supervision of their teachers, students carried out consultations and cared for hospitalized animals. They were housed internally in the school, had to wear uniforms, and had regular clean-up duties – which were part of Bourgelat's intent to teach them "proper" professional behavior. In 1777, Bourgelat published a detailed set of instructions for how to run a veterinary school, *Règlemens pour les Écoles Royales Vétérinaires de France* (*Rules for the French Royal Veterinary Schools*). The procedures and curriculum of the Lyon veterinary school became a model for similar schools that were established around Europe and in other nations during the following decades.

Bourgelat had initially considered a background in human medicine as ideal for potential veterinary students. However, he soon downgraded this demand, in large part because it greatly limited the pool of students. In most areas, physicians earned more money than veterinarians did; why would a physician or surgeon spend time and money to become a lower-paid veterinarian? Most young men interested in becoming veterinarians were primarily interested in animals, and many had grown up in families of farriers, horsemen, or livestock owners. Bourgelat considered the traditional practices of farriers and shoeing-smiths that were educated by experience and long family traditions to be backward and inefficient. But he quickly realized his school would fail if he could not attract the children of the common folk, the sons of honest farmers or farriers of the "better" type (in other words, able to read and write). Bertin, the French agricultural minister, agreed with Bourgelat on this point, since his major interests lay with educating veterinarians who would work with France's large agricultural populations of livestock (mainly cattle and sheep). Bourgelat compromised by admitting farriers' and farmers' sons, and then educating them as rigorously as possible in theory and philosophy as well as hands-on practice. In 1765, Bourgelat established a second veterinary school, based on the Lyon model, just outside Paris: the *école vétérinaire d'Alfort*. Bourgelat then asked for, and obtained, the title "Inspector-general" of all veterinary education in France. This title empowered Bourgelat to make his veterinary school model the only one approved by the French government. However, Bourgelat immediately encountered opposition to his plans.

There were other successful models of veterinary education in France and other European countries. Compared to Bourgelat's school, most of them were based less on theory and more on practical skills. Bourgelat's model broke with traditional farriery and with shoeing-smiths' guilds to create a new kind of practitioner of a specialized profession. This resulted in a clash between social classes and also between the long hippiatric traditions and the newer ways of developing veterinary knowledge. Bourgelat was confronted with fierce criticism, particularly from his most important opponent, farrier Philippe Étienne Lafosse (1738–1820), heir of an old and well-respected family of Parisian *maréchaux* (horse marshals) (Fig. 3.5). This meant the onset of a long-lasting debate about the monopoly of equine medicine between farriers and equerries, in which Bourgelat represented the small upper-class group of equerries and Lafosse the much larger (and lower in the class structure) guilds of shoeing-smiths.

Philippe Étienne Lafosse learned horseshoeing in the blacksmith shop of his father, Étienne Guillaume, who was also a well-known horse anatomist. Philipp Étienne was not merely a crude apprenticed horseshoer, however; he was also a learned man. He studied human and animal anatomy by visiting slaughterhouses and observing dissections in hospitals. Furthermore, he followed advanced studies at the Academy of Sciences, investigated anthrax, and was educated in the art of horse riding. He joined the army as a horse-doctor in 1758. There he wrote a treatise on glanders (1761) and recommended measures to control this highly contagious scourge of military horses. After the French defeat in the Seven Years' War, Philipp Étienne Lafosse joined the medical faculty of the Paris university. In 1764 the Minister of Foreign Affairs and War asked his father, Étienne Guillaume Lafosse, to draw up an instruction manual for an "École militaire d'hippiatrie pour les maréchaux des regiments de cavalerie." This school for shoeing-smiths would support the military and focus on cavalry horses. One year later, the senior Lafosse died. Philipp Étienne Lafosse then attempted, but failed, to get an appointment as an instructor at the Lyon and Alfort veterinary schools. This made him an enemy of Bourgelat.

Instead, Philipp Étienne Lafosse started his own public courses in hippiatry for interested individuals in 1767, and this sparked a debate about the social attributes and purposes of veterinary education. Lafosse believed veterinary education should grow out of the farrier tradition, focus on horses, and primarily support the military. Bertin disagreed and opposed Lafosse's type of veterinary school. Bourgelat, eager to stifle a rival, protested that Lafosse's school was merely a type of lower-class trade school entirely lacking in the newer philosophical approaches. By taking Bourgelat's side, Bertin ensured that the French style of veterinary education did not grow primarily out of farriers' guilds, with their lower-class origins and narrow focus on horses.

Under political pressure, Lafosse had to close his public school in 1770. After that, he was only able to provide private lectures.

Nevertheless, the courses of Lafosse attracted many students, from Alfort as well as from abroad; and his competition with Bourgelat eventually led to formal national regulations about who could legally call himself a "veterinarian." Lafosse may have bested his rival Bourgelat in attracting students, but he was not able to obtain political support for veterinary training aimed at the horse alone. The competition between Lafosse and Bourgelat was finally settled by the king, who issued an official veterinary certificate ("Privilégiés du Roy en l'art vétérinaire") in December 1766 that could be attained only by graduates of Bourgelat's veterinary schools in Lyon and Alfort. This was the first modern national regulation about who could be a professional veterinarian. This decision was crucial for the initiative to obtain a higher level of education for professional animal healers beyond that of shoeing-smith or farrier. It provided advantages for graduates of the approved veterinary schools, thus encouraging students to attend them. It was an early example of later regulations, in multiple countries, to elevate the graduates of certain veterinary schools into a higher position in the veterinary marketplace. By restricting the title of "graduate veterinarian" to the few graduates of approved schools, governments essentially endorsed a particular model of veterinary education and stimulated students to choose it above the older apprenticeship and guild models.

However, the older models did not immediately decline; and Philippe Étienne Lafosse's continuing career is a good example. As a reaction to Bourgelat's trilogy *Élémens d'Hippiatrique*, Lafosse chose to spend his own private fortune to compete in the same arena: he published *Cours d'hippiatrique, ou traité complet de la médecine des chaveaux* in 1772. This unique edition of 70,000 copies (bound in a very expensive folio) – in which Lafosse tried to show his superiority over Bourgelat – is generally considered the most prestigious, accurate, and complete study of equine anatomy; locomotion; nervous, digestive, and reproductive systems; diseases; and advanced stable management in the eighteenth century. Lafosse also did not hesitate to openly criticize Bourgelat's work in numerous footnotes. Reflecting his own higher learning, Lafosse chose to structure his folio according to the anatomy and physiology of organ systems, a format that is still used in veterinary textbooks today. Bourgelat's vision for veterinary education won the competition mainly because Bourgelat was able to get royal patronage in return for a promise to economize for the French government by saving the lives of its valuable animals. But Lafosse's influence, with its focus on practical equine medicine and surgery, also continued to be important for two centuries or more.

Due to their rivalry, both Bourgelat and Lafosse have influenced and stimulated the development of veterinary medicine on a national and international level for the past 250 years. Some historians claim that veterinary medicine would have developed faster (and could be more socially authoritative) if Bourgelat and Lafosse and their followers had cooperated with each other. However, observed from a model of conflict – not uncommon within science – one could also argue that the rivalry between these two giants in veterinary history reflected social/cultural attitudes toward animals and generated a broader scope for veterinary activities. It certainly stimulated several influential early veterinary publications and trained the profession's early leaders to recognize different roles for veterinarians.

Bourgelat died in 1779, having won his battle with Lafosse; but at this time, the political situation began to deteriorate for the French monarchy. Philibert Chabert (1737–1814), a skilled farrier who became the horseshoeing instructor at Alfort in 1766, succeeded Bourgelat as director of the Alfort school in 1779. Like his predecessor, Chabert was committed to the broader philosophical educational ideal; but he also recognized the increasing importance of supplying graduates who could truly solve practical problems. France sacrificed vast numbers of horses to the Seven Years' War; the royal stables alone lost 5,000 animals. Military veterinary medicine, mainly for horses, was an important concern of the king, who regularly brought visiting heads of state to the Alfort school, boasting that the school would advance French military power. Farriers, and the art of horseshoeing, remained crucial to the cavalry, as did equine health. Therefore, these remained core subjects for the curriculum at the veterinary schools.

Of course, animal disease outbreaks (especially rinderpest in cattle) provided the other justification for establishing veterinary schools. Bourgelat's school at Lyon had only been open for six months when it faced its first major test: controlling an epizootic among horses and cattle in the Dauphiné region in July 1762. Accompanied by seven of his new students, Bourgelat was sent by the government to investigate and control this epizootic with orders to save as many animals as possible. Bourgelat was well aware of the fact that the government expected the school to deliver practitioners who could control epizootics, and fortunately, the mission was successful (in large part because the disease was already declining when Bourgelat arrived). Bourgelat wrote a positive report, including statistics, which was a useful boost for the young veterinary school. This helped Bourgelat's school succeed in gaining a royal charter in 1764. Ten years later, the third wave of rinderpest hit France and continued for two years. This time, however, Bourgelat and his successors in Lyon and Alfort failed to control the disease. The timing was unfortunate for French agriculture, which suffered during the late 1770s–1780s from heavy taxation and several years of bad harvests. Food shortages, also due to a very harsh winter, contributed to political unrest, which culminated in the French Revolution in 1789. During a decade of violence and chaos, the veterinary educational model established in the 1760s barely survived. Lafosse, Bourgelat's old enemy, took part in the Revolution, and other veterinarians' fortunes rose or fell depending on their social connections and religious and political beliefs. (For example, Johann Gottlieb Wollstein, who established the school at Vienna, was imprisoned for his sympathy to French Protestant revolutionaries in 1792.) Nonetheless, veterinary education on the model of the Lyon and Alfort schools survived in France. The Lyon school, under France's next major leader, Napoleon Bonaparte, became first an "Imperial School" and finally a "National School," and this model of training professional animal healers spread throughout Europe and beyond.

The Veterinary "Meme": How French-Style Veterinary Education Propagated around the World

We have detailed the development of the early French veterinary schools because, as veterinary historian Robert Dunlop has argued, French-style institutions became the dominant model of contemporary veterinary medicine that spread around the world during the past two centuries. Dunlop proposed the concept of the *veterinary meme* to explain the emulation of the Alfort and Lyon educational model throughout Europe, Asia, the Americas, Australia, and Africa. (See Appendix A for a list of selected schools.) The "meme" concept, as described by geneticist Richard Dawkins, was defined and used by Dunlop as a "cultural element" transmitted from one culture/place to another by imitation or emulation, as if this cultural element was "infectious."[1] Of course, this very general concept is not sufficient to explain the complexities of each school's foundation. In every region and nation, the types of animals needing care, the local economy and culture, and the political complexities all determined the shape of veterinary education. Some regions, especially those in South and East Asia, already possessed vibrant animal healing professions and educational traditions, so they did not need the European model. We also do not believe that this model worked well in every place it was transplanted. But as we will see, the French schools provided a basic plan for formal, state-sanctioned veterinary education that spread to many other regions and nations for over a century.

Our purpose is not to detail the founding and history of every veterinary school; indeed, that would be impossible in a concise book. Moreover, we do not have space to mention most of the schools established, after the "first" one (even identifying the "first" school is difficult, since more than one school may claim this honor in each nation). We list the first veterinary educational

---

[1] Dunlop, R.H. (2004). 'Bourgelat's Vision for Veterinary Education and the Remarkable Spread of the Veterinary Meme'. *Journal of Veterinary Medical Education* vol. 31, no. 4, pp. 310–322.

institution established in various selected nations during two centuries, 1762–1962, in Appendix A. Each nation has a proud history of veterinary education that should be taught to young veterinarians, and this book is only a general introduction to the linkages between these national, regional, and local histories. We will use the "veterinary meme" idea here in the broadest sense: to link the development of veterinary education institutions since the late 1700s with the broader movements of animals, ideas, and practices around the world. However, it is important to remember that the world's veterinary schools were *not* merely copies, or replications, of the French Enlightenment model. Each school was established *sui generis*, in its own time and place, with its own interpretation of the model or "meme" that included some aspects and rejected others. Some common elements that linked these early schools included an ambitious leader (well connected, energetic, and often with a cult of personality); an emphasis on teaching anatomy, *materia medica*, and botany, along with the practical arts of farriery, medicine, and surgery; royal, governmental, or agricultural association sponsorship; and a mandate to address disease outbreaks, military needs, and other concerns of the sponsors.

As the French style of veterinary education spread around the world, its sphere lay in pastures and stalls, not so much in the broader study of the natural world. Over time, the philosophical tradition of the European enlightenment largely yielded to the demands of the local marketplace and other more practical circumstances. The new schools were added to existing cultures of animal healing. Therefore, veterinary schools and their graduates had to compete in the existing marketplace for animal healing in their area. Without regional or national funding, formal veterinary schools could not succeed for very long. Students paid to attend veterinary school; but this was a problem if the school could not guarantee that its graduates would get their money back by earning a better living than their unschooled competitors. To solve this problem, most European veterinary schools established in the late 1700s and early 1800s (at least, those that survived more than a few years) relied on a combination of government (and military) support, wealthy patrons, or businesspeople who kept student fees low. Then they petitioned the government to award special status to graduates of their schools. The form of the French school that spread was not primarily the early form embedded in natural history and the philosophical ideals of the physiocrats; rather, the later, more practical "veterinary meme" disseminated beyond the borders of France.

French-style veterinary schools began to spread throughout neighboring countries in Europe almost immediately, at first due to a small number of individuals and eventually through a combination of power and imperialism, economics and global trade, and the need to respond to pandemics of animal diseases. Often, government or military leaders selected an outstanding individual and sent him to France to study, with the expectation that he would return home and establish a veterinary school in the French style. An early example was the Milanese Ludovico Scotti (1728–1806), a disciple of Bourgelat in Lyon, who moved to Vienna to open a horse hospital named *k. k. Pferde-Curen- und Operationsschule* ("Imperial-Royal School for the Cure and Surgery of Horses," 1767). In 1769, Turin was the first Italian city to open a French-style veterinary school. Its first director was surgeon Carlo Giovanni Brugnoni (1741–1818), who studied in Lyon and Alfort between 1764 and 1768. Peter Hernquist (1726–1808), a student of Carl von Linné (Linnaeus), professor in medicine and botany in Uppsala (Sweden), studied both in Lyon (under Bourgelat) and in Paris (under Lafosse). After his return home, he established a veterinary school in Skara in 1775, basing it on the French model but also training its students to address the problems of livestock in rural Sweden.

Danish medical student Peter Christian Abildgaard (1740–1801) was sent to Lyon by the Danish king with two other students to study veterinary medicine, particularly to obtain knowledge to control rinderpest. He started there in September 1763 but was very disappointed with the horse-focused three-year curriculum. Abildgaard supplemented his Lyon studies with visits to locations suffering outbreaks of rinderpest to see for himself which measures worked to control the disease. Abildgaard returned from France and founded a private veterinary school in Copenhagen (1773) that survived by becoming a state-funded and royally chartered school in 1776. A final example is Johann Gottlieb Wolstein (1738–1820), a German military surgeon selected by officials of the Austro-Hungarian empire, who attended both Bourgelat's and Lafosse's competing veterinary schools and then traveled around Europe to learn breeding techniques and medical treatments, and to observe how other nations responded to epizootics – all at the government's expense. Wolstein returned to Vienna to establish a new veterinary school, *k. k. Thierspital* ("Imperial-Royal Animal Hospital," 1777) and also assisted in planning the Hungarian school established at Budapest in 1787.

As historian Martin Brumme has shown, the main motives for founding the early veterinary schools in the Germanic nation-states resulted from the concerns of the schools' regional sponsors: the prestige, ambition, and social status linked to maintaining a stylish court or a powerful standing army. Landgraves and princes competed on a local or regional level. The first German node of veterinary education, however, arose in a university. The curator of Göttingen university sent one of his ambitious young lecturers, Johann Christian Polycarp Erxleben (1744–1777), to study at the Lyon school and travel in search of veterinary knowledge. Erxleben had medical training, and he had also already authored a treatise on veterinary medicine and education (*Betrachtung über das Studium der Vieharzneykunde* veterinary, Göttingen, 1769). Besides his French studies, Erxleben traveled to the

Netherlands to observe a rinderpest outbreak. He returned to Göttingen, where he was successful in obtaining a professorship in veterinary medicine in 1771 with ambitious plans to create a veterinary school. Unfortunately, he died young in 1776, and his *Tierarzt institute* was closed. In 1778 his school moved to Hannover. Erxleben is considered the founder of the scientific education of veterinarians in Germany. Other German towns where veterinary education was established included: Dresden (1774), Giessen (1777), Hannover (1778), Freiburg (1783), Karlsruhe (1784), Marburg (1789), Berlin (1790), Munich (1790), Würzburg (1791), Schwerin (1812), Jena (1816), and Stuttgart (1821). However, only five of these schools survived, reflecting the difficult start of many veterinary schools during these initial decades. Several authors published literature about the goals, contents, and types of veterinary education. Wilhelm von Humboldt (1767–1835), brother of the explorer and natural philosopher Alexander von Humboldt, was perhaps the most well known. This German language scholar, philosopher, diplomat, and educational reformer strongly advocated veterinary education and the incorporation of veterinary schools within university faculties. However, other writers found this too ambitious for such a modest field, instead recommending smaller private schools.

Other European nations, such as Spain, Portugal, Finland, and England, sent young men to France to study at the French schools, return home, and establish new institutions. Examples are Bernardo Rodríguez (1749–1819), who studied in Alfort and founded the veterinary school (under military control) in Madrid in 1793. Carvalho Villa and António Filipe Soares studied in Alfort in the 1820s at the expense of the Portuguese government. They became professors of the *Escola Militar Veterinária* established in Lisbon in 1830. Gabriel Bonsdorff (1762–1831), a Finnish physician and biologist, was sent to Hernquist and Abildgaard, both graduates from the French schools, to learn veterinary medicine. Upon his return in 1786 he was appointed professor in this field at the University of Turku. In these direct and indirect ways, the schools in Lyon and Alfort became a model for about 30 veterinary schools founded in Europe during the period from 1765 to the 1820s.

Imagine that *you* were one of these students, selected to travel, learn, and establish this new "veterinary meme" in your own country. You perhaps already had some medical education, which usually meant a few months (up to two years) of formal schooling. You probably were already interested in natural history and animals and had experience with livestock or military cavalry training. Perhaps you had even published a treatise or book on animal care and healing or horsemanship. You needed a keen intellect, good connections at home, and sponsorship to pay for your travels. In addition, you needed to be young, healthy, and willing to live in foreign countries and bear the stresses of traveling. No matter your native language, you needed to be fluent in French, and – most important of all – energetic and full of ambition. Knowing that you were expected to return home and start your own veterinary school, not only did you work hard to learn the basic scientific information, but you also paid attention to how the school was organized, its buildings, its faculty, and its financing. All this knowledge was essential to success in establishing a new school. Consider the example of the Danish student, Peter Christian Abildgaard: he read 7 languages, owned more than 2,000 books, revolutionized the art of horseshoeing in Denmark, and successfully controlled rinderpest outbreaks. After hearing about Edward Jenner's discovery that inoculation with cowpox protected people against smallpox, Abildgaard ordered the vaccine from England and conducted the first human vaccination trials in Denmark. Abildgaard was truly extraordinary, and not all students could boast of so many accomplishments. But each student went to France with a mission to absorb as much knowledge from the French style of veterinary education as possible, and to fulfill the confidence placed in him by his sponsors at home.

Governments were not the only sponsors for veterinary students; in many countries, local or regional agricultural societies were established between 1750 and 1800. These societies' membership consisted of wealthy gentlemen and farmers who were very interested in veterinary medicine and scientific agriculture. Some of these societies sponsored promising students who were sent to veterinary schools abroad, then expected to return home and teach or practice for some years in a certain district. Some recruited veterinarians from France. In Britain, for instance, the Odiham Agricultural Society held a meeting in 1785 at which it resolved to help elevate the education of farriers according to "rational" scientific ideas. Six years later this appeal, which was supported by the aristocratic horse racing fraternity and the leading physician John Hunter (1728–1793), resulted in the founding of the Veterinary College in London. Hunter favored comparative human and animal medicine, believing that veterinary and medical students should learn from both disciplines. (A few years earlier, Hunter had sent the young field surgeon William Moorcroft [1767–1825] to Lyon to study veterinary medicine. Moorcroft arrived in France in the revolutionary year of 1789 and became the first Englishman to qualify as a veterinary surgeon; we will discuss his subsequent career in British India later in this chapter.)

The history of the London Veterinary College illustrates some of the obstacles faced by early proponents of veterinary education, as well as the ongoing tension between the goals of controlling livestock epizootics and maintaining healthy military horses. This Veterinary College's first director was Frenchman Charles Benôit Vial de St. Bel (1753–1793), who had graduated from the Lyon veterinary school. After his graduation, he became associate professor at Alfort. However, soon he got into an argument with Bourgelat (who considered him incompetent and arrogant, although the feeling was probably mutual). St. Bel then worked as a professor at the university of Montpellier. After the French revolution began, he fled into exile in London. There he helped to plan and establish what became the Royal Veterinary College, which opened its doors in February 1791. As director, St. Bel instituted the French model: a three-year curriculum, beginning with anatomy and general sciences, and continuing with lectures, demonstrations, and practical courses for students in medicine, surgery, and farriery. St. Bel, a keen anatomist, dissected hundreds of animals. Unfortunately, from one of these dissections he caught glanders, suffered terribly, and died in August 1793 at a young age. The death-mask of his face showed the horrible disfigurement from this feared zoonotic disease.

St. Bel's tragic death was only the first in a succession of misfortunes for the young veterinary profession in England. St. Bel's school had been supported by the eminent physician and surgeon John Hunter (1728–1793), and after St. Bel's death Hunter made sure that the veterinary students could attend lectures at nearby medical schools free of charge. Unfortunately, Hunter died just two months after St. Bel. St. Bel was succeeded in 1794 by Edward Coleman (1766–1839), a physician without veterinary training who had little interest in the profession's progress in England. Coleman discarded St. Bel's rigorous curriculum in favor of a short course of three months' duration. Coleman dropped the admissions requirements, which meant some students could not read or write well. The level of students' social class dropped, aligning veterinary medicine less with medicine and more with the trades. In highly class-conscious Britain, this effectively demoted veterinary medicine socially as well as intellectually. Coleman believed that the ambitions of the London Veterinary College should be limited to training military farriers, focusing on the massive loss of horses in warfare. He was rewarded with the appointment as Principal Veterinary Surgeon of the British Cavalry in 1796.

Until his death in 1839, Coleman's school provided the bare minimum of training for military farriers; and historians have argued that Coleman seriously hindered the development of British veterinary medicine by abandoning the French veterinary model. They have plenty of evidence from contemporary observers. For example, Carl Heinrich Hertwig (1798–1881), professor at the Veterinary School in Berlin, visited the London veterinary school in 1828. Shocked by the lack of lecturers and discipline, Hertwig declared the educational level to be deplorable. Coleman was apparently not concerned by criticism; he viewed the school as a moneymaking proposition for himself (each student paid tuition of 20 guineas per term). Coleman believed that veterinarians needed little education and were best suited to be farriers. In fact, this history of the London Veterinary College could be seen as a return to the earlier battle between Claude Bourgelat and the Lafosse family in the

1760s. It reminds us that Bourgelat's model, although we see it today as the more progressive one, was not the inevitable winner of debates about veterinary education.

One interesting parallel between veterinary education and the history of (human) medicine is the importance of Scotland (the nation to the north of England). In the late 1700s, the cities of Edinburgh and Glasgow were home to important medical schools, such as the University of Edinburgh Medical School (established 1726). Established during the Scottish Enlightenment, this school was considered the best medical school in the English-speaking world. Edinburgh attracted top students from many nations, creating a rich cosmopolitan culture that would also benefit the development of veterinary medicine there. William Dick (1793–1866), ambitious son of an Edinburgh farrier, studied at Coleman's London Veterinary College and also with the anatomist John Barclay at the Royal College of Surgeons in Edinburgh. Dick, aided by the administrative talents of his sister, Mary Dick, won a grant from the Highland Society and founded a veterinary school with high standards in 1823. Dick's veterinary school collaborated closely with Edinburgh's medical establishment: students also attended lectures at the University of Edinburgh medical school and the Royal College of Surgeons; and graduates were examined by the city's strict medical examiners. In this way, the Edinburgh model remained independent from (and superior to) that of Coleman's school in London. Another veterinary school was founded in Glasgow in 1863 by James McCall (1834–1915), a graduate of Dick's college. These two schools trained many of the founders of veterinary education in other Anglophone countries, such as Australia, Canada, and the United States.

Veterinary Education Moving beyond Western Europe, 1800–1850

By the late 1700s, the French schools had provided a basic plan for formal, state-sanctioned veterinary education, which their graduates transmitted to other countries. As mentioned above, by the 1820s almost 30 new centers of veterinary education had developed in Western Europe, of which 20 proved to be sustainable. Another 20 schools were established in the first half of the nineteenth century, spreading farther across Europe. Veterinary education diversified as it spread, and each of these schools modified the original plan to suit its local social, political, military, and agricultural context. Consequently, in the absence of local qualified veterinarians, medical doctors trained in veterinary medicine also played crucial roles in establishing veterinary instruction, for instance, in Kraków (1804), Bern (1805), Vilnius (1806), Utrecht (1821), and Bucharest (1861). In Switzerland, it was the German physician Carl Friedrich Emmert (1780–1834) who extended the medical faculty of Bern Academia with a veterinary school. In the Netherlands, physician Alexander Numan (1780–1852) became the founder of veterinary medicine, as did Frenchman Carol Davila (1828–1884) in Romania in 1861. Just as Lyon and Alfort had served as training places for founders of veterinary education abroad, so did Vienna, Berlin, Madrid, Lisbon, London, Utrecht, and Edinburgh decades later. The first example is the Germanic veterinary school's transmission of veterinary education within the Habsburg empire and to the Russian empire.

Hungarian Paul Adámi (1739–1814) studied medicine in Vienna and was appointed full professor in medicine and epizootiology in Vienna in 1775. Between 1804 and 1809, he occupied the newly established chair in veterinary medicine in Kraków. Veterinary instruction in Budapest started in 1787 with the appointment of Sándor Tolnay (1748–1818), a former medical student and graduate of the Vienna veterinary school. He taught lectures in Latin, German, and Hungarian. Instruction in veterinary medicine at Lviv University (then belonging to the Habsburg empire, now Ukraine) was established in 1784 by three graduates from the *k. k. Tierspital* in Vienna (A. Krupinski, G. Chmel, and the Frenchman Balthazar Hacquet). From these histories, we can see how graduate veterinarians created transnational networks of veterinary education that expanded rapidly.

In Russia, a sophisticated folk-healing tradition based on careful empirical observations guided local healers who provided most veterinary care. Books and pamphlets on animal anatomy and physiology, the preparation and use of *materia medica*, and the prevention and treatment of diseases were widely available. Many were translations of texts from other European languages. Russians' early familiarity with texts in French and German probably helped the spread of the Western European veterinary educational model into Russia. In 1803, rinderpest (enzootic in parts of Russia) returned and began decimating cattle herds. In response, the minister of the interior sent six Russian veterinary specialists and students to the veterinary schools in Berlin and Vienna to study. After returning, some of them (including I.D. Knigin and A.I. Yanovsky) helped to establish the Veterinary Division of the Medico-Chirurgical Academy (MCA, which became the Military Medical Academy in 1881) in St. Petersburg in 1808. The Veterinary Division included departments of anatomy, surgery, and therapeutics, all headed by professors trained in the Germanic tradition. Under the orders of the imperial government, veterinary professors focused on the diseases of cattle, sheep, and other livestock, as well as horses. This is a good example of how different places adapted the original French plan for veterinary education, transferred through the Germanic schools, into a new national and imperial context.

It is also interesting to note that, in tsarist Russia, studying livestock knowledge within universities was well supported (different from the Western European tradition, which was often based on private schools). The first official veterinary educational program (including professors of livestock husbandry and medical treatment) in the empire, established at Kharkov University (Ukraine) in 1805, was set up by the German veterinarian Martin Pilger. In 1806, German physician and naturalist Ludwig Heinrich Bojanus (1776–1827) began lecturing at Vilnius University (Lithuania) after being appointed professor in veterinary medicine. Before beginning his professorship, he had followed courses in veterinary medicine at Alfort, London, Berlin, Hannover, and Vienna. In central Russia, the Moscow State University had a "Department of Cattle Treatment" in 1807, led by a physician. Therefore, in Russia, Ukraine, and the Baltic region, the foundation for specialized veterinary institutions lay within higher education and emphasized animals beyond only the horse, unlike the first French model based on equine medicine and farriery. By 1850, the St. Petersburg school taught anatomy, physiology, pathology, surgery, epizootology, hygiene, pharmacology, and therapeutics. The veterinary department at Vilnius moved to the University at Dorpat (now Tartu, Estonia) in 1843. This department was based on the Germanic schools, employed some German professors, and even taught in German as well as Russian.

The establishment of veterinary education in Turkey, at the center of the Ottoman empire, is an example of exporting knowledge from Berlin, London, and Alfort and adapting it to local needs. In 1841, the German veterinarian Godlewsky went to Turkey to introduce veterinary instruction at the Military School in Constantinople (now Istanbul). This mission was part of a request from Sultan Mahmud II to Prussia, with the goal of building up a new army. Godlewsky obtained the diploma "Veterinarian 1st class" in 1837 in Berlin and had been a brigade horse-doctor in the Prussian army. Next to education, his task was also to set up and lead a veterinary institute at the barracks in Constantinople. The first three-year course started in 1842 with 12 students. Next to language problems, a drawback was that the religious beliefs of the Islamic students opposed postmortems of animals, which made teaching anatomy and pathology difficult. From 1845 onward, Godlewsky taught his lectures in Turkish.

In 1847, the Military School moved to another location, and there it was also influenced by British and French graduates. Turkish student Ahmet Pasha was sent to London and graduated there as a veterinarian. Upon his return, he was involved in the extension of the curriculum to four years in 1849. In the same year, French military veterinarian Daniel Dubroca (c. 1810–1853), a graduate of Alfort, went to Constantinople to work on the reorganization of veterinary education at the military school, of which he became head. The French influence became stronger than the Prussian because France acted as an ally of the Ottoman empire during the Crimean War (1853–1856). Later, veterinary academic staff from France and Belgium were imported to establish a civilian veterinary school in Turkey in 1889. The French model of scientific veterinary education was strengthened when Turkish students returned from their training in Alfort in 1895. Military and civilian veterinary education merged in 1921, at the end of the Ottoman empire. Overall, this history demonstrates how Turkish officials created a new and unique structure for veterinary education during the mid-1800s by selecting and combining the most useful aspects of German, French and English veterinary knowledge.

The Imperial Veterinary Education Model in Northern Africa and the New World

Formal veterinary education also traveled with European colonialism, but usually very slowly. The veterinary schools still supplied very few of the actual practitioners available to heal animals in the late 1700s. This was true in many places around the world (including much of Europe). Graduate vets were rare even in the military stationed in the French colonies, despite the fact that a military commission was one of the best positions available to the growing number of veterinary school graduates. (This would be true, later, in the British colonies as well.) For example, most animal healing in St. Domingue (today's Haiti) was conducted by enslaved healers, the *gardiens de bêtes*. These veterinary specialists used traditional African knowledge, including herbs and other materials along with spiritual rituals, to heal injuries and treat diseases. The colonial government used quarantines and slaughter of infected horses, cattle, and dogs to control epizootics of glanders, anthrax, and rabies. The first graduate veterinarians arrived in St. Domingue in the 1780s, but they concentrated on military animals and enforcing colonial epizootic control. The enslaved *gardiens de bêtes* did most of the healing for individual animals during the colonial period and afterward.

In northern Africa, animal healers were joined by a few graduate veterinarians after the first European-model veterinary school was founded in Egypt in 1827 under the government of Mehmet 'Ali. Although an epizootic in bullocks was the urgent reason for its founding, this school was also directly connected to the French model after the Napoleonic expedition to Egypt (1798–1801) and the subsequent departure of Egyptians to study and observe French methods. Mehmet 'Ali also sent for two French veterinarians: Pierre Nicolas Hamont (1805–1848), who studied at Alfort and became an army veterinarian, and Auguste Prétot, also an Alfort graduate, who died within a few years of his arrival. Hamont began training students from the military academy, then successfully campaigned for a new veterinary school to be built near Cairo in 1831. Incorporating military veterinary medicine for cavalry horses increased the school's enrollment despite its rigorous curriculum: four years that included anatomy, surgery, pathology, physiology, internal medicine, diseases, and the French language. Following graduation, Mehmet 'Ali's officials sent veterinarians around the country to agricultural regions. Veterinarians were also needed by the military, which was expanded during the 1830s when Mehmet 'Ali invaded Syria and parts of Anatolia.

As historian Alan Mikhail has shown, Egyptian veterinarians worked within a remarkably centralized and active bureaucratic structure during the 1830s (much earlier than many other areas). Government officials deployed veterinarians to certain places; sent equipment, supplies, and reports from Cairo out to them; and expected them to report animal health problems arising in the provinces. This veterinary bureaucracy changed methods of animal breeding, how animals were fed and housed, and their work conditions. It also changed the relationships between individuals and their animals by instructing them how to care for animals as components of the national wealth. Although this first Egyptian veterinary school was closed in the 1840s by Mehmet 'Ali's grandson, Egyptians were still sent to France to absorb European knowledge about how to prevent epizootics and maintain cavalry horses. In turn, the Egyptian veterinarians took their knowledge and practices with them to remote provinces and other parts of the empire.

Across the Atlantic Ocean in the Americas, official and missionary reports of early Spanish and Portuguese settlements described diseases of humans and animals and their treatment. Spanish conquerors mention pre-Colombian professional healers taking care of wild mammals and birds in Moctezuma's menagerie at Tenochtitlan (Mexico). They were also impressed by the wide variety of medicinal plants the indigenous populations used to treat human and animal diseases. In the early colonial period, veterinary activities included shoeing, meat inspection, and the breeding of newly introduced species. On Columbus' second voyage and on all later expeditions, Spanish livestock (horses, donkeys, pigs, sheep, goats, rabbits, hens, etc.) were taken along to feed the colonists, but three-fourths of these animals died before arrival. Only a few Iberian *albéitares* and blacksmiths went to the Americas, mainly focusing on equine medicine, since horses were crucial instruments of war. The first *albéitar* who worked in the New World between 1495–1498 was Cristóbal Caro. Another, Fernán Gutiérrez, introduced cattle into Peru in 1537. The Spanish and Portuguese method of cattle ranching was exported to New Spain (the Americas). From there sprang the greatest cattle empire in world history, from the vast Argentine pampa north to the plains of Wyoming (United States). Horses had been long extinct in the Americas; the arrival of European invaders brought these entirely new species of equids. The descendants of those first European horses multiplied abundantly in the open grasslands, where Indigenous peoples such as the Comanche began using horses successfully for hunting and warfare.

One problem for the early conquistadores was the lack of horseshoes, causing many hoof injuries and lesions. Supposedly, due to the lack of iron, silver and even gold horseshoes were used during the conquest of Peru. Juan Suárez de Peralta (1541–1613) was the first *albéitar* born in the Americas (Mexico); he probably learned by apprenticeship. Another interesting figure is Félix de Azara (1746–1821), a Spanish soldier and probably also veterinarian, who studied natural history and animal husbandry in Paraguay. The Spanish veterinary schools at Madrid (1793), Cordoba and Saragossa (1847), León (1852), and Santiago de Compostela (1882) took the school at Alfort as their model (and in turn provided founders for new schools in the colonies). In 1821 the Spanish government made plans to erect schools overseas in Mexico, Lima, Santa Fe de Bogotá, Caracas, Buenos Aires, and Manila (although some of these schools were never established or were short lived).

The first veterinary school in North America was established in Mexico City in 1853. Frenchman Eugène Bergeyre (1829–1880), a graduate of the Veterinary School in Toulouse in 1850, emigrated to Mexico in 1853 and became head of the stables of President Santa Ana. Bergeyre also became the first professor of veterinary medicine (including meat inspection) at that school in 1856. Other European emigrants included farriers William Blake (since 1810) and Edinwaldo Adges, who were employed in the army of Simón Bolívar (Venezuela). A famous veterinarian in Bolívar's army was German Otto Philipp von Braun (1798–1869). Braun qualified in Hanover, emigrated, and was made commander of the Hussar Battalion of Bolívar's army in 1823. From 1830 until 1839 he also became one of the most successful generals in Bolivian history, repelling an Argentinean invasion in June 1838. After 1850, more veterinary schools were established in the Americas, and we return to them in Chapter 4. Not until the end of the 1800s did a substantial number of graduate veterinarians from Spain, Italy, France, Britain, and the young American schools accumulate in North, Central, and South America.

Professionalization of Veterinary Medicine in the Industrial Era

Although the establishment of formal veterinary training was important, it was only one of the necessary steps in the slow and gradual professionalization process, which characterized the rise of modern veterinary medicine. Education, training, and professionalizing are dynamic processes. The position of even established professions is not unassailable. Institutionalization and legitimation of a profession are continuing processes, while the domain of professional activities is continuously evolving. Consensus and cooperation play a role in these processes, as do discord, competition, and conflict. The successful continuance of a profession thus depends on different factors. Therefore, it is worthwhile to evaluate the different processes and factors involved in the genesis of a profession. Professionalization can be defined as the process by which members of a profession use their special knowledge and the value of their skills to attain a powerful social position. When the duties of a particular profession are largely described by the law, the position of that profession is mainly determined by negotiation with the government. Internal and mutual competition between the members of the group as well as external competition (mainly by empiricists) are unfavorable for the negotiation value of the group. Veterinarians' social power and ability to negotiate remained low until the era of microbiology, due to a lack of effective therapies. A successful professionalization process also depended on collective power: the solidarity and the influence of a group. A high degree of organization in associations, coalition with other groups, and public relations are effective ways of increasing this power as well as improving political influence. From the eighteenth century onward, members of the professional group also took external factors into account when using a particular strategy. Factors such as legal, socio-economic, and technological developments, as well as – in the case of veterinary medicine – epizootics and zoonoses all contributed to their choice of strategies.

Beginning in the middle of the nineteenth century, Western European society rapidly modernized. The need for people with specific professional expertise increased as a result of industrialization, division of labor, and democratization of society. The process of advancing differentiation in society was associated with a change in university education. New disciplines like economy, agriculture, technical sciences, and veterinary medicine were introduced. Education focused more on practical applications and the societal benefits derived from scientific knowledge. Clinics and laboratories become important in human and veterinary medicine as well as in the application of the natural sciences. The newly upwardly mobile occupations imitated the model of the older professions. Medicine was the first discipline in the nineteenth century to move toward academic professionalization and diversification. Urbanization, concern for the poor hygienic standards in the rapidly growing cities, and a rise in per capita income favored the growth of the medical profession. Influenced by the thinking of the Enlightenment, the physiocrats, and the French Revolution of 1789, profession building of both physicians and veterinarians had begun in Western Europe in the eighteenth century.

The crucial role of higher learning in the emergence of professional culture, as well as in the process of professionalization, is obvious. Within this process, three factors play an interactive role: the profession with its practitioners and organizations, the state as regulator and certifier, and institutionalized higher education as a training ground. Higher education affects professionalization primarily in terms of admission (selection), curriculum (knowledge), and examination (credentialing). The interaction between higher learning and professionalization also varied with political and social traditions. In Great Britain and the United States, the professionalization model was liberal and characterized by a strong professional organization and autonomy, even in professional training. The same goes for a country like the Netherlands, which lacked a powerful centralized bureaucracy and followed a liberal doctrine of free trade and restriction of state interference. The state established a formal educational system in 1821, but the State (*sic*) Veterinary School was financed by a cattle fund for almost 30 years. Furthermore, until 1874, veterinary healers without formal training were allowed to practice veterinary medicine. In Germany and Russia, the model followed the bureaucratic tradition, depending heavily on state regulation and licensing because professionals, officials, as well as professors revolved around government.

When we take a closer look at the emergence and the sociology of professions, different factors and processes can be distinguished. According to sociological theories, three processes – differentiation, legitimation, and institutionalization – have to be completed to validate the definition of a profession. Differentiation is completed when certain activities are concentrated and routinely conducted by skillful persons. Legitimation and institutionalization occur when these persons are faced with problems resulting from these activities and jointly try to find solutions. The process of legitimation is completed when other groups – the authorities, principals, and customers – accept and approve the specific professional activities. Institutionalization is divided into social institutionalization and institutionalization of the domain. The latter occurs when the field of activities claimed and defined by the practitioners themselves is recognized by the legal system. Social institutionalization represents the degree of acceptance of the professional group by the society. One big problem for the acceptance of the emerging veterinary profession was the significant competition by uneducated veterinary healers. One of the main objectives of the early veterinary associations founded in Denmark (1807), Switzerland (1813), the Netherlands (1862), the United States (1863), Spain (1865), Romania (1875), and Britain (1882) was to remove this competition. In addition, these associations for veterinary advocacy pursued legislation and published a professional journal. Conflicts arising between the different empiric craftsmen and the new professions that pursued academic acceptance were common in the medical professions. During the long professionalization process, such conflicts between barber-surgeons and medical doctors, apothecaries and pharmacists, tooth-pullers and dentists, and farriers and educated veterinarians were typical.

Regarding the professionalization process of educated veterinarians, important phases can be distinguished (Table 3.1). Such a scheme could also be drawn up for other medical and paramedical professions, thereby enabling a comparison between different phases in the origin and development of these professions in various countries to discover whether similar patterns occurred globally.

Table 3.1. *Phases of the professionalization process of educated veterinarians*

1	Formal education and (state) legislation regulating the veterinary curriculum
2	Professional journals established
3	Professional activities become full-time jobs
4	Professional associations established
5	Veterinary state supervision of livestock diseases (such as Cattle Acts) with veterinary civil servants responsible for design and implementation
6	Legal protection of the title "Veterinarian" (veterinary surgeons acts) only for graduates of accepted schools; this minimized competition from competing animal healers
7	Provision of effective therapies such as vaccines against epizootics, based on (laboratory) scientific research
8	Elevation of veterinary colleges to institutions of higher education, to the level of a department or faculty in a university
9	The right to write and defend academic veterinary dissertations (doctoral status)
10	National laws for quality control of food of animal origin under veterinary supervision
11	Professional code with its own disciplinary law, as well as professional conduct toward the outside world

Using this general scheme, we can compare the professional development of veterinary medicine in various countries. We can also understand the criticism toward the early schools and their graduates. One problem was the development of scientific veterinary medicine, which lagged behind the development of formal education, journals, associations, and state supervision. Often, governments instituted formal education, thereby legitimizing the status of "scientifically" trained veterinarians, long before these graduates and the schools could meet the desired expectations by clients. This also explains why uneducated healers continued to dominate veterinary practice for decades. In many countries, empiricism continued to flourish throughout the nineteenth century and into the twentieth. Animal owners preferred to have their animals treated by skillful and often cheaper animal healers rather than by qualified veterinarians who might be well educated, but therapeutically less experienced. After all, even graduate veterinarians felt powerless against the most dreaded diseases: rinderpest during the 1700s and 1800s and contagious bovine pleuropneumonia from the 1830s onward. For individual animals, economics were usually the only criteria used to determine who was called in to treat a sick animal.

This status quo is confirmed by a nationwide government survey on veterinary services in the Netherlands in 1846 (25 years after the establishment of the first veterinary school). By that time, there were about 121 educated veterinarians and 771 other animal healers active within the country. Almost all municipalities saw no added value in qualified state veterinarians, and they did not want to support them. They preferred to maintain the services of the majority of available healers – the private empiricists. This outcome led to a radical reorganization of the veterinary school at Utrecht in 1850.

The further development of veterinary sciences and the veterinary profession in the period 1850–1900 will be analyzed in Chapter 4. But another important theme, and one of the reasons to establish veterinary schools, was the need for horse veterinarians for the army. This justification continued to be an important one for formal veterinary education because the decades around 1800 witnessed many battles, conflicts, and wars in which horses were crucial. The armies needed shoeing-smiths, army farriers, and army veterinarians to keep their numerous horses healthy.

Animals in Warfare, Late 1700s–1850

Napoleonic Wars and Veterinary Education

The veterinary schools in France were reorganized during the French Revolution of 1789. Due to political reform, the organization of veterinary education became a matter of national concern and attempts were made to unite veterinary and human medicine. The French veterinary schools had a difficult time, but they survived independent of medical schools. The need for healthy horses in the expanding French army, particularly when Napoleon came into power, played a role in this respect. Napoleon Bonaparte (1769–1821) was a general and dictator during the last governments of the French Revolution. In 1799, following a coup, he ruled as First Consul until 1804 when he crowned himself as Napoleon I, emperor of France. He kept that position until 1814 and again briefly in 1815 until his final defeat at the battle of Waterloo (Belgium). Napoleon built a large empire dominating continental Europe for more than a decade. As one of the greatest commanders in history, with a brilliant strategic understanding, he won most of his battles and the so-called Napoleonic Wars in which he led France against a series of coalitions. Napoleon, like so many military rulers before and after him, was highly dependent on a huge army of healthy horses, mules, and donkeys. In the second half of the eighteenth century, significant changes occurred in the roles of horses within the cavalry, mounted infantry, and the new horse artillery units in European armies. In addition, Napoleon introduced the concept of a supply train, a horse-drawn logistical transport of artillery, engineer forces, and forage. Adequate provision of these materials was crucial for combat forces in the field, but bringing all these supplies to the armies required vast numbers of horses.

Under these political and military conditions, the emerging veterinary schools could profit from the increasing demand for shoeing-smiths, army farriers, and army veterinarians to keep army horses healthy. Previously, governments had contracted private shoeing-smiths and farriers who were responsible for shoeing army horses and providing general care. At the end of the eighteenth century, governments established military veterinary services to counter the continual heavy losses of horses during the military campaigns. These military veterinarians were recruited from the newly formed veterinary schools. Shoeing-smiths and farriers who were employed by the armies were sent to veterinary schools around Europe, thereby representing a significant influx of students and a steady source of revenue for the schools. Between 1804 and 1812, the number of veterinarians in the French army increased from about 100 to 250, for example.

Living in the twenty-first century, it is hard to imagine what life must have been like for army smiths and veterinarians, as well as for the animals they tried to keep healthy. Imagine the challenges and logistical problems of mobilizing, feeding, and watering more than 100,000 horses without modern technology. In peacetime, the European armies planned to have one horse per seven soldiers; but in wartime, the ratio increased to one horse per four soldiers. Veterinary physiologist Peter Bols has calculated that 5,000 horses at rest (during peacetime) consumed 175,000 liters of drinking water; 15,000 kilograms of hay; 15,000 kilograms of straw, and 15,000 kilograms of concentrated feed every day. (During battle and at higher temperatures, these figures would be much higher.) Five thousand horses would also leave 35,000 liters of urine and 200,000 kilograms of manure in the encampment. Planning for the needs of these animals while on military campaign must have been a huge challenge. History shows what happened when military leaders failed.

In the summer of 1812, Napoleon took about 175,000 horses with him on his campaign to Russia, while the French army counted 450,000 troops overall and the Russians 400,000. Napoleon's Russian campaign was disastrous for the French. They spent time and energy traveling to Russia and attacked during the harsh Russian winter, for which they were not prepared. Cunning Russian commanders took full advantage of the French army's logistical problems. The French army was poorly equipped and lacked adequate forage for the horses (insufficient and bad quality), leading to immense suffering for the animals. Huge numbers of horses died due to hardship (dust, heat, thirst, hunger, cold, deadly wounds) and diseases (colic, diarrhea, and contagious diseases). The scourge of horses, glanders, raced through the army's animals (and probably sickened soldiers, also, since it is a zoonotic disease). Unfortunately for the French, Philibert Chabert, director of the veterinary school at Alfort, taught his students that glanders was not contagious between horses (or between horses and men). This mistaken doctrine cost the French armies dearly during the Napoleonic Wars. Descriptions of the withdrawal of the French army from Moscow during the harsh winter are horrific. About 140,000 horses were lost.

The cold and hunger drove soldiers insane. They cut pieces of muscles from their dead but even still living horses, put it on their bayonets, roasted it above fires and spiced it with gunpowder. They even ate cats and dogs to survive. A soup of horse blood, melted snow, flour, and a little gunpowder for the taste was considered a feast.

After the failure of the Russian campaign, Napoleon blamed the *maréchaux-ferrants* (shoeing-smiths) and *artistes vétérinaires* (veterinarians) as one of the scapegoats for his defeat. He considered their shortcomings to keep the army horses healthy a proof of lacking education and, therefore, decided to reform veterinary education in the so-called decree of Moscow of January 15, 1813. In this imperial decree (*Décret impérial sur l'enseignement et l'exercice de l'art vétérinaire*) he determined that henceforward there would be five veterinary schools in his empire: one of the first category in Alfort and four of the second category in Lyon, Turin (occupied Italy), Aachen (occupied part of Germany), and Zutphen (occupied Netherlands) [the latter two were never established]. All schools would provide a three-year course leading to the diploma of *maréchaux vétérinaires* (veterinary marshals). Only at Alfort would a supplementary two-year, more in-depth course be given to deliver fully qualified *médecines vétérinaires*. The Alfort school should also account for the training of professors who would teach at the second-category schools. Veterinary inspectors were appointed who were responsible for veterinary care of large cavalry groups. In this way, Napoleon broadened the job opportunities for veterinarians. However, in practice it was only gradually that specially trained military veterinarians took over the veterinary tasks of the traditional army shoeing-smiths. Moreover, this reform could not prevent the final defeat of the Napoleonic regime at the battle of Waterloo in 1815 (again, thousands of horses died).

These military details may seem insignificant to us today; but this was not the case in the long nineteenth century because horses were essential to all military activities. This included the role of military forces in invading, conquering, and settling new territories. "Imperialism" is defined as a country exerting power and influence over other countries or regions through diplomatic and military activities. Within the time period covered by this book, European imperialism through military activities was a major force in world history. Often-violent takeovers of lands, peoples, and resources spread Europeans to Asia, Africa, the Americas, and islands throughout the world. Veterinarians and models of veterinary education and regulation spread with the armies and settler colonialist regimes of the late 1700s and 1800s.

Veterinary Medicine and Imperialism

Imperialism during the 1700s dramatically increased contacts between Asia and Europe, expanding on a centuries-long interchange of goods, people, and ideas. Global trading, diplomacy, religious pilgrimages and missions, and military incursions had all brought medical knowledge from one part of the world to another, especially from Asia to Europe, for centuries. How did these circulations of knowledge about animal healing affect local practices? Adoption of novel healing practices depended on social context, not only on how well the therapy worked. Animal owners in a society subjected to imperialism, for example, often viewed "foreign" healing practices with suspicion and hostility. However, historians have also uncovered examples of people mixing the "new" therapies and techniques with traditional ones. Similar to the marketplace for veterinary practitioners, the globalized therapeutic marketplace offered a broad menu of choices that were widely reported and often available even in remote areas.

Ancient centers of Ayurvedic and Tibetan medicine extended from southern India to what is now Mongolia, and these were also centers of production for high-quality sheep and horses during the eighteenth century. Many trading routes crossed this vast area, as did religious pilgrimage routes, and knowledge traveled with the caravans. Knowledge about animal husbandry and healing for elephants, camels, and cattle was the most important in places that used or venerated those animals. The special place of cattle as sacred animals in some parts of South Asia meant that sanctuaries for healing sick and injured animals were widespread by the eighteenth century. Elephants had their own traditional healers (*kaviraj*), especially in the more rural areas. The *kaviraj*, which are still an active group of healers today, practiced traditional medicine using medicinal plants, and they were kept busy treating elephants in remote villages and the countryside. Cattle and elephants were also treated with a type of homeopathic medicine. The treatments were small doses of medication that, at normal doses, would cause the same symptoms from which the animal suffered. For example, if an animal had diarrhea, small doses of a laxative or purgative would be given to prompt the animal's system to react against the diarrhea. These are only a few examples of the complex traditional healing practices, which not only dealt with more minor complaints but also addressed complex conditions such as pneumonia, diabetes, and tumors.

The rich medical ideas and practices of South Asia continued to circulate to Europe in the late eighteenth and early nineteenth centuries, especially with the activities of the imperialist British East India Company (EIC). EIC goals focused on the extraction of wealth from South Asia. In parts of what is now the nation of India, a ruthless British colonial military regime, which depended on controlling large numbers of animals, was an active occupying power by 1800. British veterinarians began to arrive in India in 1799. Paramount to the EIC's success was the acquisition of horses, which were used for military purposes. Efforts to send horses from the West to EIC outposts in India were extremely expensive and often unsuccessful (the horses died on the long journey). Moreover, what some viewed as the greatest horse pasture in the world lay to the north: the steppe lands of Central Asia, the western part home to the famed Akhal-Teke "golden horses," reputed to be fast as the wind and able to run without food or water for days. By 1800, over 100,000 horses (most of them considerably lower quality than Akhal-Tekes) were being brought to markets of the Hindu Kush, stimulating the EIC to consider breeding their own horses locally.

From their base in Bengal, EIC officers founded a stud farm for horse breeding at Pusa and brought the British veterinarian William Moorcroft (1767–1825) to run it in 1807. After his graduation in Lyon, Moorcroft had worked briefly as professor at the London veterinary college, but soon returned to his lucrative equine practice. He constructed a colossal apparatus to make horseshoes, but this enterprise failed; so Moorcroft decided to follow his passion for adventure travel and go work for the EIC in India. He brought the French veterinary educational model to Bengal, and although no school was founded, there is evidence that local people employed at the stud farm learned a great deal from Moorcroft. In turn, Moorcroft immersed himself in Bengali culture, learning languages and marrying a local woman; but he disappointed the EIC because on two major expeditions he failed to find reliable sources of the best Central Asian horses for the British stud farm. Most important for veterinary medicine, he sent copious notes about medicinal plants and local knowledge (and even a flock of Tibetan sheep) back to England during these travels. Moorcroft was an important conduit for animals, plants, and ideas from South-Central Asia that traveled to Britain, and he probably brought European veterinary ideas to northern India as well. While there is little evidence that Moorcroft's findings greatly influenced early British veterinary medicine, he is a good example of the ways in which veterinary knowledge circulated around the world with individuals as well as institutions.

Of course, this knowledge exchange was not new, particularly in China, which harbored Jesuit missionaries, diplomats, and other conduits of European ideas since at least the Mongol khanates of the thirteenth century. In the mid-1800s, European visitors to Chinese territory found local animal healers who combined traditional botanical remedies with practices the Europeans knew well: firing (cautery of external lesions), drenching with purgatives, and bleeding. For example, Scottish veterinary surgeon George Fleming (1833–1901) published his notes from a trip on horseback beyond the Great Wall in 1863, after he participated in the British invasions of China. Remembering that Fleming's point of view was very imperialist, we nonetheless learn quite a bit about local veterinary *chang-ta* (farriers), who used stocks and the nose-twitch to restrain animals, just as in Britain. Fleming compared the Chinese hoof-knife to that used by French *maréchaux-ferrants*.

Fleming then described the *Yi-ma* or horse-doctor, who traveled between the larger rural towns (see Chapter 2, Fig. 2.4). The *Yi-ma* informed the British visitor about the principles of *yin* and *yang* and referred him to a text on "Chinese Veterinary Medicine." The *Yi-ma* was a well-respected professional whose work included the use of medicinal herbs and drenches and other practices (bleeding, cautery) familiar to Europeans. Fleming recounted the *Yi-ma*'s instructions about feeling the pulses, and how he had understood the animal's body in terms of *qi* and its movements, especially in the internal organs. The *Yi-ma* applied plasters to the affected areas and manipulated body parts in accordance with his understanding of these bodily flows of energy. By explaining this system of understanding the body in some detail, Fleming transferred this knowledge to his readers in Britain. Perhaps just as important, Fleming's writing showed his surprise at finding a system of veterinary healing that made a certain sense to a European and aspects of which were very similar to European practice. Regarding horseshoeing, for example, Fleming noted that the Chinese practices of affixing a light metal plate to the horse's hoof more closely resembled the practices of Europe than of neighboring Japan, where horses' feet were protected by woven-straw sandals. Clearly, horseshoeing and healing knowledge from around the world had been circulating for years, including in the isolated rural regions of northern China.

Veterinary knowledge exchange, therefore, was not new during the late 1700s and early 1800s. As in previous historical eras, trade and war spread veterinary knowledge. Nor was the use of animal healing as a tool of imperialism and colonialism new, but the 1800s saw the rapid expansion of European colonial regimes (and the French veterinary meme) onto other continents, notably Africa. For example, the colonial French veterinary presence in northern Africa began in the summer of 1830 with the invasion of Algeria. According to veterinary historian Diana K. Davis, the veterinary regime developed there (later expanded to include Tunisia and Morocco) was crucial to successful French settler colonialism. In contrast to the situation in British in India, veterinarians in northern Africa were expected to manage livestock production and pastures (not just horse diseases). French ideas and practices clashed with well-established local regimes of animal husbandry and the marketplace for animal healing, especially in the steppe areas populated by nomadic pastoralists. To maintain control, French colonizers utilized strict regulations that applied to animals as well as local people. The aims of controlling animal disease, supplying military animals, regulating pasture use, and regulating the food supply fit closely with (and greatly assisted) the goals of controlling rebellious local populations – and the French veterinary meme provided the expertise.

Another conduit of veterinary knowledge exchange took place in a part of the vast Ottoman empire, in Egypt. In 1798, the French dictator Napoleon led an expedition to, and military occupation of, Egypt. Although short lived, this incursion included French military veterinarians whose ideas and practices came from their training back in France. In Cairo and into the countryside, exchanges of animals and knowledge began to spread along with the army. Scientists, including the eminent zoologist Étienne Geoffroy Saint-Hilaire, also took knowledge of Egyptian animals back to Europe. In terms of the domesticated animal economy, the French ideal was based on bureaucratic control that extended into remote areas in occupied Egypt. This pattern seems to have survived after the French left in 1801. The eventual new Egyptian leader, the government of Mehmet 'Ali, ushered in dramatic changes in human–animal relationships during the late 1700s–early 1800s based on the French veterinary regime and animal management model. As Alan Mikhail has shown, the institutions of the new Egyptian State increasingly took charge of regulating and providing care for animals. Mehmet 'Ali actively cultivated the French "veterinary meme" by employing two French veterinarians from the Alfort school in 1827 to investigate an outbreak of disease in rice-field draft animals. One of these, Pierre Nicolas Hamont, began training Egyptian students; this was the beginning of the first French-style veterinary school in the Ottoman empire. Financed by Mehmet 'Ali's treasury, the growing school began in Rosetta, moved to Abu Za'abel, near Cairo, in 1831, and, finally, to Shubra in 1837.

This Egyptian School of Veterinary Medicine exemplified the goals of early French-style institutions (controlling disease in economically valuable livestock and keeping animals healthy for the military), but it also illustrates the important point that the French "veterinary meme" was deliberately used by government officials in other nations and not merely imposed upon them. European colonialism often used French-style veterinary medicine as one of the key tools for controlling subjugated regions. Competing powers, including nations allied with the mighty Ottoman empire, cleverly adapted European ideas and techniques to suit their own economic and military purposes. The Islamic medical and veterinary traditions of the *madrassas* were still very important, and, just as in Western Europe, a vibrant veterinary marketplace included large numbers of folk healers (sacred and empirical) as well as the educated elites. The French-style schools added another, government-sanctioned, group of practitioners to the Egyptian veterinary marketplace: during the 1830s, between 50 and 100 students were enrolled in the School of Veterinary Medicine. As we will see, even more military personnel were trained in the French veterinary meme to maintain the health of cavalry horses. These formal, bureaucratic efforts to manage Egypt's animals reflected the government's concentration on safeguarding the economic and military wealth of its animals. A wealthy nation depended on healthy animals, and alert government officials tested many different ideas and practices, including foreign ones.

Imagine that you are an Egyptian veterinary student in 1840. What would you study, and where would you work after graduation? Until 1846, veterinary and medical students studied together during the first year. They focused on learning comparative anatomy, especially the skeleton and muscles, and also the basic sciences such as botany, chemistry, and physics. After that, veterinary and medical students separated and began more species-specific studies of anatomy, physiology, pathology, and simple surgeries. The third and fourth years of veterinary school included more clinical experience and courses in medicine, disease pathology, and surgery. This curriculum probably looks familiar to veterinary students today. The Egyptian School took full advantage of the French "veterinary meme" and the fact that French was the common language of European veterinary medicine in those days: the veterinary students were required to take courses in the French language during all four years.

Upon graduation, veterinary students were assigned professional positions throughout Egypt. Most were sent to agricultural areas, where they functioned as veterinary public health officials as well as treating individual animals. Veterinarians were empowered to enforce government regulations about clean water, proper feeding, and not working animals during the hottest weather. The veterinarian also treated horses, camels, or buffalo that were sick, injured, or suffering from parasites. If he suspected a contagious disease, the veterinarian could force the slaughter and burning of sick animals' bodies and prevent livestock owners from moving animals from one place to another. Certain diseases were reportable to the agriculture ministry in Cairo, and veterinarians could declare and enforce quarantines. Although the Egyptian School of Veterinary Medicine was closed by Mehemet 'Ali's successor, 'Abbas, in 1849, this regulatory structure remained to control one of Egypt's most economically and militarily valuable resources: its domesticated animals.

Notably, this Egyptian veterinary regime included a focus on comparative medicine and an assumption that animal diseases could also afflict humans. Because they studied anatomy alongside medical students, Egyptian veterinarians understood the similarities between human and animal bodies right away during the first year of veterinary education. These scientific studies reinforced generally held beliefs that some diseases were contagious and could infect humans as well as animals; and that the pollution generated from a sick animal's body could make an exposed person sick. This was a kind of miasmatic theory that assumed that sick or dead animal bodies (and blood) produced poisonous vapors, especially in the case of febrile or purulent illnesses. If such an animal was dying, the practice of *wa'da* dictated that it be buried alive to avoid exposing the person slaughtering it to the tainted blood, vapors, and bodily excretions. After sick animals' bodies were buried (dead or alive), workers poured ammonia or shoveled lime over the slaughter or burial sites, according to State regulations, to prevent healthy animals or people from exposure. All of these measures reflected the assumption that the organic boundary between human bodies and animal bodies was porous to the malevolent influences of disease, and that preventive measures worked for both livestock and people.

Conclusions

From this very brief survey of two centuries, we can conclude that:

1. In Europe, the enlightenment (1700s) stimulated the development of formal veterinary education, especially in France. Concern about epizootics and the existence of the military riding school as a model also contributed to the establishment of the first French schools. A vibrant print culture, the growth of medical knowledge, and royal (later republican) governmental sponsorship enabled formal veterinary education to grow quickly in France. The rationale for these French-style veterinary schools began with the growth of natural history, science, and medicine; but the schools' purpose slowly became more practical, driven by economics and the needs of the nation-state.
2. The French veterinary meme quickly spread abroad, due to other European nations' interest in developing their own schools; French imperialism; and the concerns of national leaders in other parts of the world about epizootics.
3. During the 1700s, animal diseases such as cattle plague/*peste bovine*/ rinderpest threatened agricultural production. Some government officials (in France and other locations) believed that veterinary schools should focus on understanding and responding to these livestock diseases. This goal contrasted with the next point:
4. Horses, donkeys, and mules were crucial to military units and in warfare. Keeping horses healthy required professional healers, including horse-doctors, farriers, and shoeing-smiths. This was another argument in favor of establishing veterinary schools. Balancing the curriculum between these two goals – the needs of agriculture and the needs of them military – was a source of tension for almost all veterinary schools.
5. Veterinary school graduates had to compete in the veterinary marketplace, against unschooled horse-doctors, farriers, cow-leeches and other folk practitioners, and many other types of professional healers. Animal owners had many choices. The establishment of formal veterinary schools did not end the activities of other healers or the availability of "do-it-yourself" veterinary care booklets used by farmers and animal owners.
6. Military veterinary medicine, often combined with imperialism, became even more important during the 1800s. For example, the states of the Ottoman empire established a corps of army veterinarians, as did the Napoleonic army.

7. The establishment of veterinary education was just one step in the different phases of the long professionalization process of veterinary medicine.

Question/Activity: Find examples of how veterinarians and other animal healers were trained in your home country, 1700–1850. What was the veterinary marketplace? When were formal veterinary schools established in your country? Finally, we have seen the importance of horsepower in armies around the world during the 1700s–1800s. How did the use of horses in warfare change over time?

---

4   Veterinary Institutions and Animal Plagues, 1800–1900

Introduction

In the early 1800s, students of veterinary medicine in the recently established European-style schools varied quite a bit. Many had some basic education; but their major qualification was hands-on experience with animals, particularly horses. These were working-class or middle-class people – the sons of farmers, shoeing-smiths, or village farriers. They were already familiar with what we call the "veterinary marketplace" (the array of mostly unlicensed veterinary practitioners from which animal owners could choose, from botanical healers to castrators and dentists). A much smaller group of veterinary students had had the benefit of more formal education and better social connections. These students, along with the most talented and ambitious of the farmers' and farriers' sons, became the leaders in the effort to professionalize veterinary medicine and veterinary research during the nineteenth century.

The mid-1800s was an exciting time to be a veterinary student because scientific knowledge was being created rapidly. In Europe, the fields of zoology and natural history had been revolutionized by such thinkers as the Frenchmen Buffon and Lamarck; the British Owen, Chambers, and Darwin; the Germans Haeckel and Weisman; and the Swiss Rütimeyer. Embryology and cell theory (Schleiden, Schwann, and Virchow) laid the foundations for understanding comparative anatomy and development. Together, these developing fields of thought and experiment supported the notion that natural laws underlay the study of animals in health and disease, just like the laws of physics or chemistry. This fast-developing corpus of knowledge was the basis for "scientific" studies of healthy and diseased animals, in the European tradition that eventually spread around much of the world. This new veterinary regime was shaped by the problems of rapidly growing, industrializing, and colonizing nation-states.

Between 1800 and 1900, the circulations of systems, goods, ideas, people, animals, and diseases transformed much of the world. The ability to move live animals on an international scale was made possible by the development of railroads and steamships from the 1850s onward. Railroads and steamships

134

moved quickly; therefore, even sick animals could reach new regions before dying and transmit diseases to indigenous animals. Observations and ideas about these animal diseases moved in multiple directions. As we will see, animal experts in regions of Africa and Asia influenced European knowledge about animals and healing, just as European veterinary knowledge and institutions were brought to India, Java, and South Africa. But this knowledge exchange took place against a background of violence due to wars and colonial imperialism, destruction of natural resources, and the destruction caused by animal diseases (such as rinderpest) brought by Europeans to Africa, East Asia, and India. Rinderpest, which killed about 90 percent of the cattle it infected, devastated entire societies and cultures. This particular legacy of imperialism persisted for a long time: for example, rinderpest was largely eradicated in Europe in the nineteenth century, but it remained endemic in Africa until 2011. In Africa, rinderpest was devastating not only to livestock and the environment, but also to peoples such as the Maasai, vaShona, Bahima, and Zulu, whose societies and cultures were based on owning livestock. These world-changing events, as well as the need to increase and secure the food supply of the growing world population, shaped the development of the veterinary sciences, veterinary medicine, and government regulation of animal health and disease.

Understanding and Controlling Animal Plagues and Zoonoses in the Nineteenth Century

During the nineteenth and early twentieth centuries, the need to understand and control continuing outbreaks of epizootic and zoonotic diseases stimulated innovations in organized veterinary medicine that continue in some form today. An important step was the establishment of veterinary institutions: schools, (state) veterinary services, serum production and research institutes, meat and milk inspection services, and field stations. The nineteenth century also witnessed the formation of national veterinary professional associations and international veterinary congresses. Both were aimed not only at better controlling animal plagues and zoonoses, but also at obtaining veterinary legislation including state-sponsored animal disease control (the Cattle Acts on notification and stamping-out, for example); meat inspection acts; and legitimizing veterinary medicine as a state-sanctioned profession. It was in the late nineteenth century that the veterinary school graduate began to have an advantage in the veterinary marketplace, as other animal healers and practitioners were gradually outlawed (a process that took decades). In many parts of the world (but not all), the state licensing of animal healers contributed to the normalization of a particular model of animal healer: educated by an approved veterinary school, licensed by the state, and charged with enforcing the state's dictates and laws.

In this chapter we examine major outbreaks of epizootic and zoonotic diseases in the nineteenth century, how these diseases spread around the world (especially by European imperialism and colonialism), and the societal and veterinary response to them. Growing industrial cities consumed ever-larger amounts of meat, milk and other animal products. Food hygiene developed along with sanitation and public health in the cities, but its authority extended into the countryside where animals were born and raised. These regulations depended on scientists' ability to judge food as "healthy" or "safe," both in the abattoir and in the laboratory. Laboratories that were attached to the newly established veterinary institutes played a major role in understanding and controlling animal and zoonotic diseases. There, methods from the natural sciences (physics, chemistry, biology, statistics) were applied alongside laboratory animal science (animal models) to develop new tools such as preventive vaccines and therapeutic serums. These tools promised to ensure a supply of safe foods of animal origin and healthy horses for services in agriculture, transport, and the armies. The new institutes and laboratories, in turn, depended on the impression that veterinary medicine was becoming "scientific" and that some of its leaders were allies with (human) public health officials in the framework of the so-called sanitary movement. Veterinary research work also connected veterinary medicine with human medicine through the study of "comparative" pathology, physiology, and medicine. These comparative studies were based on shared ideas about disease etiology (causation), transmission, and pathophysiology between physicians, veterinarians, and natural historians (early biologists).

In the middle of the nineteenth century, the scientists who worked within veterinary and medical institutions developed the basis of disease causation theories (germ theories) still used today. Especially in the Global South, veterinary investigators moved beyond the germ theories to elucidate the ecology of vector-borne diseases such as Texas cattle fever, East Coast fever, and equine encephalitis. Veterinary parasitologists studied macroparasites (such as *Ascaris*) and microparasites (such as *Trichinae*), linking parasitology and disease ecology with germ theories. Some young veterinarians learned these methods at veterinary schools, which were increasingly becoming associated with universities and national professional associations. The knowledge, vaccines, and other "products" of microbiology began to convince farmers of the added value of trained veterinarians over other healers – but only very slowly. By 1900, trained veterinarians were also better equipped with diagnostic tools such as auscultation, thermometry, microscopy, and culturing microbial organisms by letting them reproduce in predetermined culture medium under controlled laboratory conditions. While theories, knowledge, and new tools were available, they were also expensive – and their widespread use depended on the economic value of veterinarians' animal patients.

Veterinarians and Food Production

Most people think that veterinarians are only active as "animal doctors." However, the scope of professional activities is much broader, including, for example, veterinary food hygiene. Today in some countries about 10 percent of the profession finds employment in the public health sector with the main task of controlling zoonotic diseases and guaranteeing a safe food supply. When and how did veterinarians get involved with public health and food hygiene? We will show that the formation of laboratories, where research was conducted to support food inspection with scientific knowledge, played a crucial role in why veterinarians obtained (legal) responsibilities in the food supply chain and could include public health in their professional domain.

From the early nineteenth century onward, a gradual transition from a traditional rural society to a modern bureaucratic state occurred in many parts of the world. This process of modernization was accompanied by characteristic changes including rapid human population growth, urbanization, industrialization, economic growth, and a gradual rise in the standard of living. Colonialism continued to extract natural resources and bring wealth to Europeans, while spreading European livestock production methods around the world. Due to a higher disposable income of the working class in industrialized countries like Great Britain, Belgium, France, and Germany, a shift in food consumption patterns took place: Europeans expanded their consumption of foods such as milk, meat, and other products from animals. At the same time, the developing laboratory sciences supported an increase of meat and dairy consumption.

Many physiologists, chemists, and physicians stressed the importance of a high intake of animal protein; additionally, meat and dairy consumption were traditionally important to many cultures. Especially between the 1850s and early 1900s, knowledge about the chemical composition of foods and nutrient requirements (of humans and non-human animals) increased. Laboratory research based on the unit of energy, the calorie, and emphasis on proteins meant that many scientists considered foods of animal origin to be more nutritious than vegetable foods. Most European authorities, especially, claimed that a population deprived of animal protein would become weak and produce only moderately strong and productive laborers and soldiers. Reflecting imperial biases, British economists attributed the seemingly effortless manner in which Britain controlled its Indian empire to the high meat consumption of the "British Beefeaters" (in the nineteenth century Britain had the highest per capita meat consumption in Europe) as compared with the vegetarian diet of the Indians. In addition, technologists argued that European nations with a high meat consumption generated the most successful colonists and that the future belonged to the "flesh-eating nations." Such notions help explain why scientists, politicians, economists, and military authorities attached such great importance to a high meat consumption.

As a result, dairy and meat production increased worldwide overall due to expanded animal feed production, innovations in cattle breeding, and organized campaigns against livestock diseases. In addition, the nineteenth century witnessed a rapid expansion of the domestic and international meat trade. Of course, some regions still suffered from famines and meat shortages. Egypt, for example, experienced widespread weather events, crop failures, and animal losses between the 1780s and 1820s. Government officials and the army seized livestock and the scanty meat supplies, leaving the populace without sufficient food. But in other parts of the world, both crop and livestock farming dramatically increased, especially in sparsely populated colonial territories and countries such as Argentina, Uruguay, the United States, New Zealand, and Australia. Although the new regimes based on cattle and sheep production in these areas often had negative effects on the local land and peoples, farmers could increase profits. Newly developed transportation possibilities (steamships and cooling technology) meant that animals and meat could be exported to help meet the demand in the fast-growing cities.

The increase in meat and dairy consumption and concerns about the quality of these commodities facilitated the entry of the veterinary profession into food hygiene during the 1800s. Veterinary leaders in several nations saw the opportunity to bring aspects of public health under the purview of organized veterinary medicine. This did not happen quickly; it took time and effort for veterinarians to assume control over food inspection and regulation, and this process played out differently in different nations. The development of scientific veterinary medicine in the second half of the nineteenth century was supported by the growing need for veterinary expertise in safeguarding the food production chain, from the growth of livestock farming and meat and milk production to the expanding demand from consumers. Veterinarians argued that they were uniquely qualified to carry out the two essential factors for effective meat inspection: mandatory inspection of meat for sale and centralized slaughtering in municipal or public abattoirs on the outskirts of towns. Likewise, milk production could be regulated by linking veterinary inspection of cow byres, the fresh milk produced by them, and the urban regulations necessary to ensure that milk was not adulterated and did not carry diseases. These would be developments of late nineteenth-century municipal, state, and national governments.

From the consumer's point of view, the quantity and quality of meat and dairy destined for the working class in the second half of the nineteenth century left much to be desired. Historians have shown that, in the cities, dairies and slaughterhouses were often "filthy" and their products adulterated with false ingredients. Home slaughtering was common in the countryside, and barter in food between villagers relied on trusting the farmer who produced the food. But the chain between producer and consumer became much longer and convoluted for citizens during the development of a large-scale domestic and international meat trade. Urban consumers had few guarantees that they were purchasing healthy or pure milk and meat. One rare example of a regulatory institution was the pre-revolutionary French guild system, in which retired butchers were sworn in as municipal meat inspectors. But state regulatory power and interference were limited due to the prevailing liberal economies prevalent in most industrializing nations.

In most cities, butchers slaughtered animals in small, privately owned butcheries. Population growth and urbanization went hand in hand with an extended network of such butcheries where slaughtering often took place under unhygienic conditions. In London in the 1870s, it was estimated there were 1,100 operational slaughterhouses scattered around the metropolis. Cheap meat and sausages were sold in these butcheries, shops, and markets. Meat from knacker's yards was marketed or processed into pies and sausages and sold to the poor. Old, worn-out, and even dead horses were collected and processed by knackers, after which the meat was sold as "smoked beef." Cats were sold as rabbits and dogs as mutton. Milk cows were fed the rancid waste products from distilleries and breweries, sickening them and tainting the milk. Bovine tuberculosis affected as many as 80 percent of animals in major cities in the United States, Latin America, India, Russia, and Europe.

Almost inevitably, calamities followed. Numerous outbreaks of "summer diarrhea," scarlet fever, diphtheria, typhoid fever, and undulant fever (brucellosis) in children and adults were traced to tainted milk. Infected and spoiled meat caused trichinosis (a microscopic parasite) and meat poisonings in hundreds of people, killing dozens of them every year. Consequently, local and national authorities were confronted with complaints about the filth and nuisance of dairies and butcheries as well as the poor quality of the food offered. The regular outbreaks of meat-borne diseases alarmed the authorities and demonstrated the need for meat hygiene control. Improvement of the urban environment, the meat trade, and meat and milk inspection regulations became regular issues in local and national politics in the mid- to late nineteenth century. Apparently radical measures were needed.

These concerns were not altogether new. Inspired by the intellectual developments of the Enlightenment, the Paris Council for Public Hygiene had created a set of municipal regulations for meat inspection at the end of the eighteenth century. However, active interference by a state bureaucracy was needed to achieve real progress. Following the French example, health boards were established in most larger towns in Western Europe around 1850. Within these boards the so-called hygienists, a group of progressive physicians, engineers, physicists, chemists, lawyers, civil servants, and veterinarians played a predominant role. Due to the veterinarian's knowledge of food hygiene, they participated in these health boards from the beginning. The great accomplishment of the members was to turn public health into a social and political issue. In the United States similar groups, known as the "sanitarians," also tried to improve sanitary provisions, such as garbage disposal, sewage system, drinking water, hospitals, food inspection, abattoirs, and animal rendering. By means of professionalization and a scientific approach to public health care, including research in laboratories, such sanitary measures were gradually realized in the course of the nineteenth century. Federal regulations about the domestic meat supply, however, were not enacted until public scandals erupted in the first decade of the 1900s.

As for public abattoirs (slaughterhouses), Napoleonic France was the European leader. Until well into the nineteenth century the Parisian abattoirs (built 1810–1814) were regarded as exemplary. There and elsewhere in Europe, butchers were forced to slaughter their livestock centralized in municipal slaughterhouses or public abattoirs under mandatory veterinary inspection. However, this was only accomplished after long debates in local politics between a faction of hygienists with demands for adequate meat inspection, allied with animal protectionists and citizens with nuisance complaints on the one hand, and a coalition of butchers and meat traders whose independence was threatened on the other hand. Due to the prevailing liberal doctrine of free trade and restriction of state interference, at first economic interests and the objections of the butchers outweighed the public health arguments. Authorities believed that meat inspection was best left to the private sector, and that consumers were their own best food inspectors. By the turn of the century, however, socialist ideas and interference by local and national authorities in commercial life tipped the balance in favor of public slaughterhouses. The establishments of slaughterhouses were further promoted by the enactment of meat inspection acts in various countries that obliged local authorities to establish a meat inspection service and to impose hygienic requirements concerning private slaughter places and butcher's shops. Many private butcheries could not meet the new hygiene standards, leading many cities to build abattoirs in order to institute an adequate meat inspection service. Most of these acts stated that inspection should be carried out by veterinarians. This also applied to slaughterhouse directors, thus creating many job opportunities for the profession.

In meat-exporting countries the situation was different. A large-scale meat industry with centralized slaughtering in huge commercial slaughterhouses developed from the 1850s onward, first in the United States and later in South America, Australia, and New Zealand. These large private slaughterhouses proved more cost-efficient than public abattoirs and were quicker to incorporate new technology. Cincinnati ("Porkopolis") became the early center for meat packaging. Chicago took the lead in 1865. Stimulated by the Civil

War, the large-scale "corn-hog cycle" for fattening pigs, and an expansive network of railways, Chicago became the city having the world's largest meat-packing industry, including meat canning. There the meat industry started a vertical integration by taking over farming and transports and succeeding in expanding consumer tastes to include by-products such as bacon and lard on a large scale. One commercial meat packer boasted that his company had found markets for almost all parts of a slaughtered pig: "we sell everything but the squeal." Also, large technological innovations that revolutionized mass production in the meat industry, namely, division of labor and the disassembly line (conveyor belt), were developed in Chicago. In 1883 not less than 5 million pigs, 2 million bovines, 750,000 sheep, and 30,000 calves were slaughtered there. However, the working conditions of labor were very poor, which, together with published meat scandals and fraud, eventually led to the federal Meat Inspection Act in the United States in 1907.

These developments took place amidst growing industrialization and inequality between the world's richer and poorer peoples. During this period, increasing global imports and exports of live animals and products of animal origin led to increasing political and economic conflicts in some places. In East Asia, China battled European aggression aimed at forcing open borders and open markets (for European benefit). At the end of the 1800s, empires weakened as colonies rebelled; and battles over international trade and power in the early 1900s led up to World War I. In addition to food destined for the fast-growing civilian populations, the need for feeding armies increased due to growing international tensions in colonial territories, declining empires, and among European nations. Veterinary care was also required for the horsepower wars directly preceding World War I, such as the Franco-Prussian War (1870–1871), Spanish-American War (1898), Anglo-Boer War (1899–1902), the Russo-Japanese War (1904–1905), and the Balkan Wars (1912–1913).

Modern veterinary medicine formed during the late 1800s: its system of formal education; alliance with the bureaucratic state; and major scientific breakthroughs. These developments did not happen quickly or easily, however, and they were shaped by the growing animal industries, trade, and military conflicts. Devastating animal disease crises, including the return of the dreaded rinderpest, also influenced veterinary medicine's development. Hitching a ride with European armies and colonizers, rinderpest quickly became a historical force that changed not only veterinary medicine but also societies and cultures around the world.

The Homelands of Rinderpest in Europe

As we know today, rinderpest is caused by a virus, and it can be transmitted by live animals or infected animal products. Rinderpest is extremely contagious to cloven-hoofed animals (cattle, sheep, goats, and wildlife), and it has a long incubation period of up to 21 days. Rinderpest had been the scourge of European cattle since at least the early 1500s (see Chapter 2). Circulations of animals around the Continent and high livestock densities in some places (especially near cities and other large human populations) enabled the disease to flare up repeatedly over the next 400 years. For example, a "plague of horned cattle" hit what is now northern Germany in the 1740s–1750s, and again in the 1770s, killing 70 to 90 percent of the cattle across a wide area. (Due to this high mortality, this plague is likely to have been rinderpest by modern definitions.) In the period 1744–1749, England lost half a million, and the Netherlands 1 million cattle. During the third wave of 1768–1786, again millions of cattle succumbed in Europe, in spite of the fact that Austria, France, and Switzerland followed a cull-and-slaughter policy while compensating victimized farmers. The nineteenth-century global spread of rinderpest ("steppe murrain") probably originated in cattle imported to Europe from areas around the Caspian Sea. These steppe oxen were very resistant to the disease, and they could appear healthy while shedding the virus. Sporadic outbreaks of rinderpest occurred in Europe regularly throughout the early 1800s, as well; but the most devastating epizootic was the "cattle plague" of the 1860s in Europe and the United Kingdom. Between 1865 and 1867, the height of the epizootic, 75 to 90 percent of cattle in some affected areas died despite the efforts of local officials to contain the disease. This was a disaster that demanded the full attention of national governments and gave the young veterinary profession a chance to demonstrate its value – but the correct course of action was often highly contested.

How governments and veterinarians responded to epizootics depended on the larger social and cultural context, as we have seen; and in 1865 several broader changes in European science, print culture, and governance led to greater governmental intervention to prevent rinderpest's spread. In the case of Britain, historian John Fisher has asserted that the "cattle plague" (rinderpest) outbreak in 1865 was the most widely discussed problem of its time. This was probably one reason why veterinary legislation to control cattle movement and rinderpest followed rapidly: The Contagious Diseases (Animals) Acts were expanded in 1869, for example. The British government supported pathologists' investigations into rinderpest and, later, experiments with potential vaccines, in the hope of finding alternatives to shutting down the cattle trade. Unfortunately, in the 1860s–1870s laboratory experiments did not offer any effective solutions to the problem of rinderpest. Veterinary leaders pointed out that the only effective short-term measure was to stop moving cattle domestically and internationally; isolate and slaughter infected animals; and cull animals that may have been exposed to infected ones.

This classic technique for containing the spread of a veterinary disease is called "stamping-out," and it consists of the government forcing animal owners to kill all animals that might have been exposed to the disease and establishing a *cordon sanitaire*, or quarantine. Cattle-owners, reluctant to kill healthy animals and concerned about economic loss, often opposed stamping-out policies. In the Netherlands, the first national Livestock Act dated to 1799 and a government fund was created to pay farmers for culled animals. When rinderpest returned in 1865, the cattle export trade plummeted and veterinarians could not agree on the correct combination of stamping-out, establishing *cordons sanitaire*, or trying other measures such as isolation and treatment. After a year of debate, a newly elected conservative national government mobilized the military to force farmers to surrender their cattle for slaughter as part of a stamping-out campaign. This campaign, against which the farmers fought, stopped the rinderpest outbreak within three months. The 1870 Livestock Act established a national Veterinary Service (although that was also contentious). These examples from European countries responding to the crisis of rinderpest outbreaks reminds us that there was no single correct policy for preventing and controlling rinderpest during this time period.

In the Ottoman empire and what is today the Middle East, rinderpest devastated communities during the late 1800s. For example, the disease broke out in Rison Le Zion and Mikveh Yisreal (present-day Israel, then called Palestine) in 1894–1895. Outbreaks in Palestine were thought to be imported with cattle from Damascus, Egypt, or Turkey – demonstrating the multiple trade routes that connected the outposts of the vast Ottoman empire. Veterinarians from the Veterinary School in Istanbul were sent to try to control these outbreaks; they instituted restrictions on animal movement and attempted treatment and prevention with serum from resistant animals. By the 1890s, laboratory experimental research was beginning to yield some beneficial discoveries for both human and animal diseases: Pasteur's rabies treatment (1885), tuberculin (1891), the diphtheria antitoxin (1895), and serums (sera) against specific diseases (discussed below). However, for most disease outbreaks, the most effective control techniques for epizootics continued to be quarantine, *cordons sanitaire*, and stamping-out. This general pattern continued even as European imperialism spread rinderpest around the world during the nineteenth century.

Rinderpest: The Imperial Disease

Wherever Europeans and their animals traveled, rinderpest traveled with them and unwittingly helped them to invade, explore, and colonize. Animal diseases were one component of the violence and destruction brought by Europeans to

Africa, East Asia, and India. This was an example of what historian Alfred Crosby called "ecological imperialism:" European colonialism depended in part on the introduction of European cattle diseases that devastated the cattle-owning cultures, such as the Maasai, vaShona, Bahima, and Zulu in sub-Saharan Africa. Colonialism was not a monolithic and superior system of Western dominance; rather, it was a process of mutual adaptation, negotiation, and conflict between the Indigenous peoples and the new European arrivals. Veterinary knowledge about rinderpest moved in multiple directions. As we will see, animal experts in regions of Africa and Asia influenced European knowledge about animals and healing, just as European veterinary knowledge and institutions were brought to India, Java, and South Africa.

From Europe, rinderpest spread in Asia in the late 1860s and 1870s, carried by steamships. Once established in Asian ports, rinderpest moved between countries quickly. In 1872–1873 Japan was confronted with an outbreak, which probably was due to imports of live cattle from China. In India, the first of a series of rinderpest outbreaks began in water buffaloes and cattle in 1868. Between 1872 and 1877, the province of Berar alone lost more than 90 percent of its cattle and buffaloes to rinderpest, an estimated 11 million animals. Indigenous cattle owners compared *puschima* (rinderpest) to cholera in humans – highly contagious and often lethal. They attempted to control rinderpest by restricting open grazing, keeping healthy animals away from sick ones, and fumigating cattle shelters by burning aromatic resins. The British colonial government installed the Indian Cattle Plague Commission to investigate the disease and make recommendations for controlling it. As historian Saurabh Mishra has demonstrated, this commission's report included important ideas from Indian cattle owners: the control measures mentioned above; and the belief that a mild infection with the disease would protect the animal if later exposed to virulent *puschima* (the basis for vaccination). In 1871, the Indian Cattle Plague Commission confirmed that the outbreak was similar to the European one and estimated that the disease could kill 200,000 cattle every year in India. Recommendations to control rinderpest and to curb livestock losses included the establishing of veterinary departments and a veterinary school, and eventually an act for the prevention of rinderpest spreading.

In India in 1871, a stamping-out policy was not even mentioned, perhaps due to the question of who would pay for the destroyed animals. This is a particular problem in colonies, where the major goal is to send economic profits back to the colonizing government. If animals simply died of the disease, the government was not responsible for paying the cattle-owners. For small-scale Indian farmers, rinderpest was devastating, contributing to a series of famines that killed millions of Indian people. The enduring spread of rinderpest and its impact on the rural economy, however, became a priority for the colonial government when it began to affect British-owned farms and the colonial government's profits. These experiences with rinderpest stimulated veterinary research, contributing to the establishment of the Imperial Bacteriological Laboratory in Poona in 1889 and the Indian Civil Veterinary Department in 1891. Both worked to develop a vaccine against rinderpest but failed. Two more major famines, 1896–1897 and 1899–1900, affected both humans and cattle as fodder and crops failed. With British colonial policies protecting only the wealthier farmers, untold millions of native cattle died, leaving peasants impoverished and starving.

A similar pattern can be observed in the former colonies of the Dutch East Indies (now Indonesia). From December 1878 onward, severe outbreaks of rinderpest, introduced with cattle from India, occurred on Java, Sumatra, and Borneo. These outbreaks and the resulting food shortages caused tremendous distress among the population. The Civil Veterinary Service, established in Batavia (now Jakarta) in 1853 and consisting of only a few veterinarians, asked for assistance to control the outbreak. Jacobus Laméris (1842–1918) an expert on rinderpest, and a team of eight other veterinarians were sent to the colony to control the disease. The local vets worried that the experts had never seen the local type of buffalo before, and that Dutch methods of disease control and treatment would not work in the local environment. At first, Laméris advised the government to let the disease burn out by simply waiting for the animals to die in great numbers. But stockowners, who would lose a lot of money, demanded a rigorous stamping-out policy. At the end of 1879, about 75,000 buffalo, cattle, sheep, and goats had been slaughtered in Java, at the expense of the colonial government. Government officials then ordered a double north–south bamboo fence to be built. This fence crossed the entire island to separate the rinderpest-free area of Java from the rest of the territory. Military forces conducted surveillance and sealed off infected areas to avoid further spreading of the disease, thus condemning the (mostly poor and Indigenous) cattle-owners who lived there. The disease raged for six years, finally contained in 1884 after a loss of more 223,000 animals and devastation for the peasant cattle-owners.

Along with the draconian military presence, the fences, and the stamping-out campaigns, the colonial government decided to develop a local veterinary workforce and invest in veterinary research. To support the work of the Veterinary Service, "Mantries" (paraveterinary assistants) were trained and appointed from 1880 onward, while Indigenous veterinarians were trained at the Dutch Indian Veterinary School at Buitenzorg on Java, which was established in 1907. This school was attached to the Laboratory for Veterinary Research built in the same year, and these veterinary institutions were examples of the innovative experimental research carried out by veterinary scientists in imperial spaces. We might assume that knowledge about veterinary diseases would travel only in one direction – from the great research centers of Europe out to the peripheral colonies. But this was not the case, as the Dutch Indian Veterinary School and Laboratory for Veterinary Research demonstrates. It is remarkable that the research program and publications on surra, dourine, and Newcastle disease performed in this colonial laboratory surpassed those of the veterinary colleges back in Europe (what is now the Netherlands). The curriculum of the Dutch veterinary school (Utrecht) only began to include tropical diseases in 1912, thirty years behind the Javanese Veterinary School.

Rinderpest did not stop in Europe and Asia; perhaps its worst devastation hit sub-Saharan Africa in the 1890s. This was not the first importation of rinderpest to the African continent, but the earlier outbreaks of the disease were confined to the continent's north. In 1841, Egypt was the first country on the African continent to experience an outbreak of rinderpest. About 75 percent of Egypt's cattle and buffalo herds died after they were infected by cattle imported from Romania (in eastern Europe). This earlier outbreak did not spread throughout the continent for three reasons: first, Indigenous African kingdoms had border checkpoints, reflecting their understanding that diseases were (both spiritually and materially) contagious and Europeans were the source of the problem. For example, in 1859 the King of Ndebeleland ordered that Europeans and their cattle were not allowed into the kingdom until they had been subjected to three months' quarantine and healers' cleansing rituals, which consisted of sprinkling them with medicated solutions. These strict quarantines helped prevent the disease from infecting the rest of the African continent. Major geographical features, such as the Zambezi River, also helped to contain rinderpest since it was difficult to get cattle across them. Finally, until the disease spread to wild animals, the density of animals was low enough in many places to slow rinderpest's progress to the south.

Rinderpest returned with Europeans and their cattle, however, entering eastern Africa in the Eritrean port of Massawa in 1887. The Italian army, keen to subdue and colonize Somalia, probably brought the disease with infected cattle from India, meant to feed the Italian soldiers. This was the beginning of what is still known in sub-Saharan Africa as "The Great Rinderpest Pandemic," a tragedy that changed the history of the entire continent. About 95 percent of Ethiopian cattle died, causing famine and the starvation of one-third of the human population of Eritrea and two-thirds of the Maasai peoples of Tanzania, within two years. It is difficult to imagine the sufferings of these people who, in losing their cattle, had lost not only their food supply but also their culture and way of life. In Tanzania, the Swahili name for this disease was *sadoka*, especially when referring to the epizootic in wild animals. German colonial veterinarians and officials at first did not believe *sadoka* was rinderpest, which enabled them to claim it was an "African" disease that they could ignore.

Within seven years, this disease spread all over sub-Saharan Africa, killing 80 to 90 percent of all domesticated and wild cloven-hoofed ungulates (such as cattle, goats, wild buffaloes, and other wildlife). Therefore, rinderpest was also a modern ecological disaster. Rinderpest swept from the Horn of Africa west to the Atlantic Ocean and south to the Cape of Good Hope. Within human memory, no similar devastating livestock epidemic had ever visited Africa. It is estimated that it killed more than 5.2 million domestic bovines, sheep, goats, and wild populations of buffalo, giraffes, and wildebeest. Attempts to prevent rinderpest from spreading by proclamations, days of prayer, inoculation, isolation, containment, and slaughter of infected livestock all failed. Both European aggression and fighting between African kingdoms interrupted the traditional measures for stopping the disease, such as border checkpoints. Rinderpest destroyed cattle culture, which had been the basis for family relations, transhumance, and political stability in many eastern and southern African kingdoms and regions. It is impossible to exaggerate the rinderpest epizootic's disruption of African societies and cultures that had been built around cattle herds. This disruption, another example of what historian Alfred Crosby has called ecological imperialism, only hastened the violent European takeover of Africans' lands.

Rinderpest reached the Senegal river by 1891, wiping out wild animals in the Rift Valley such as buffalo, waterbuck, impala, eland, wildebeest, giraffe, and even bush-pigs. After rinderpest crossed the Zambesi River in 1896, it was reaching the southernmost part of the entire continent. The British Cape Colony government attempted to stop it by erecting a 1,000-mile-long fence patrolled by soldiers on horseback and disinfecting the people and possessions that crossed into southern Africa – similar to what the King of Ndebeleland had ordered in 1859. Despite these measures, rinderpest marched into the Republic of South Africa, where the colonial Veterinary Officer reported it in the Cape Colony and German Southwest Africa (now Namibia) in 1897. Veterinarians working as government officials attempted stamping-out to try to stop the disease; nevertheless, rinderpest annihilated the south's cattle. Within just ten years, rinderpest had infected an entire continent and changed the lives of most of its people permanently.

As was the case with the Dutch colonial government in Java, the British and German colonial governments and European colonists took action to try to prevent future epizootics. In German Southwest Africa, the colonial govern-ment established a buffer zone or no-man's-land from east to west across the whole country. This zone separated the south, where rinderpest was being stamped out, from the north (location of the Black African tribes and their cattle). Later, a fence known as the "Red Line" was built in the buffer zone and enforced by soldiers (this fence is still present today). In the colonies that would become the Union of South Africa in 1910, the colonial governments expanded the state veterinary services and established veterinary research laboratories. Like their colleagues in Java, veterinary scientists at this colonial laboratory (later the Onderstepoort Veterinary Research Institute, described below) developed new serums, attempted innovative vaccines, and made discoveries about tropical diseases that generated important new scientific knowledge. Rinderpest, a devastating effect of imperialism, thus also transformed knowledge about animal diseases in Africa by motivating European colonial governments to establish veterinary institutions. With no more cattle to kill, the epizootic finally burnt itself out in 1905. But rinderpest remained endemic in eastern Africa, reemerging in Kenya in 1907 (and for decades afterward), and spreading due to raiding and illegal movement of cattle by Europeans and Africans.

Another disease that travelled, contagious bovine pleuropneumonia (CBPP), was probably present in some parts of Central Europe around 1700. CBPP invaded the rest of Europe in the first half of the nineteenth century due to the French Wars and increasing livestock trade. From Western Europe it spread to all continents except South America. Often it was confused with anthrax or rinderpest. It was studied intensively in the laboratories of the newly established veterinary colleges in France, where it was described in detail based on pathological-anatomical abductions. The causative agent of this livestock disease (*Mycoplasma mycoides*) was not identified until late in the nineteenth century. Supporters of the miasma theory did not believe in the contagious nature of this disease and thus disapproved of a system for cull and slaughter. As with cattle plague in the eighteenth century, these vets made attempts to preventively inoculate bovines with setons drenched in saliva or lung fluid from infected animals. Particularly in Belgium, the Netherlands, and France, experiments with inoculation on a larger scale were executed around 1850.

Most influential were the experiments by Louis Willems (1822–1907), a Belgian physician (Fig. 4.1). After training in France, Germany, and the Netherlands, Willems entered a prize contest sponsored by the Académie Royale de Médecine de Belgique and wrote a positive report on containing CBPP. His claims received international attention. Except for Britain, where the Royal Agricultural Society took the initiative, all the major Western European governments ordered their veterinary authorities to test and evaluate the Willems tail inoculation method. In most cases a painful swelling developed, accompanied by fever. Mortality ranged from 1 to 3 percent, while 7 to 9 percent of the animals lost part of their tail. In hindsight, the inoculation with attenuated cultures of mycoplasma must have induced some immunity. However, the results were mediocre, probably because inoculation was being performed on already-infected animals. Therefore, many farmers and veterinarians worried that inoculation would only perpetuate the presence of the causal agent among herds. Their resistance was the main reason why

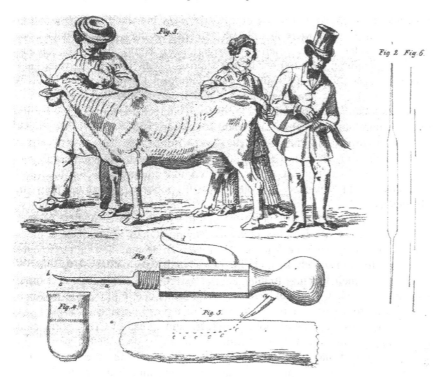

Figure 4.1 Tail inoculation according to Belgian physician Louis Willems
(1822–1907), Cologne, Germany, 1854.
Source: C.Th. Sticker, *Die Lungenseuche des Rindviehs und die dagegen
anzuwendende Impfung* (Köln 1854), attached plate. Courtesy: Library, University of
Veterinary Medicine Hannover, Germany.

inoculation was replaced by the proven measure of stamping-out (slaughter of
all infected animals) in most countries toward the end of the nineteenth
century.

As a veterinary reflex, stamping-out programs had been a consistent feature
of public animal health strategies in Europe and elsewhere for about three
centuries. As a disease control strategy, stamping-out has even survived to the
early twenty-first century for a very simple reason: it works. As critically as it
was approached in the course of time, particularly from an animal protection
point of view, killing diseased animals and those in proximity proved to be the
most cost-effective means of preventing and eradicating infectious livestock
diseases. In the case of CBPP, the emerging national veterinary services could
choose between a strategy of stamping-out or the pre-Pasteurian form of

vaccination (Willems' tail inoculation). Veterinary bureaucracies, particularly on mainland Europe, were anxious to demonstrate their professional value. The choices they made differed from nation to nation, depending on the political economy: the strong national approach with centralized veterinary state supervision versus a liberal economy with local autonomy, where disease control was left to municipal and regional boards. Only the state had the resources to support eradication programs and compensate farmers, the ability to order unpopular slaughter and trade restriction, and the power to punish those who ignored the imposed rules.

Compared to rinderpest, CBPP did not cause as much social, cultural, and demographic disruption. It was considered more a problem for the rural economy. CBPP revealed the difference in public appreciation between physicians and veterinarians around the middle of the nineteenth century. Just as veterinarians had trouble controlling this lung disease, medical doctors stood powerless against cholera outbreaks among humans. Nevertheless, medical doctors maintained their status of learned men despite their failure to cure people suffering from cholera. On the other hand, veterinarians were roundly criticized for their inability to cure lung disease/CBPP, while their economic benefit for a healthy livestock economy was questioned until the 1900s, when they could provide effective preventives or therapies for some diseases.

The rinderpest panzootic (global outbreak) and spread of CBPP stimulated the establishment of veterinary institutions in many parts of the world. By 1900, the United States had taken over the Philippines and other parts of the old Spanish colonial empire, and the Americans inherited the problem of rinderpest epizootics. Rinderpest had entered the Spanish Philippines in 1887, imported by infected animals from Indochina and Hong Kong. Veterinarians from the Spanish army tried to contain the outbreak, with little success. The American invasion in 1898 brought a second wave of rinderpest that was much worse. The American army spread the disease along with the soldiers and their draft animals, and to protect the new colony the U.S. colonial government established a veterinary department in 1899. Sixty civilian American veterinarians, functioning as inspectors of livestock imported through the port of Manila, worked closely with the U.S. Army's Veterinary Corps. But Filipinos continued to fight for independence until 1902, and the U.S. Army's military maneuvers continued to spread rinderpest. In the period 1901–1902 alone, more than 629,000 cattle and water buffaloes were killed by the disease. Spanish and American authorities did not apply a slaughter policy but tried to contain rinderpest by imposing quarantines against imported animals from China and Australia in the harbors. In 1905, the colonial veterinary department was placed under the management of the U.S. Department of Agriculture's Bureau of Animal Industry, making it an arm of the U.S. government rather than a small colonial office. This greatly increased numbers of veterinarians, and two years later the Philippine Veterinary Medical Association was established (1907). Rinderpest stalked the Philippines, causing up to 90 percent of cattle to die at times, until the 1940s.

Around the world, the ruinous effects of rinderpest were part of European colonialism. Where European animals traveled, rinderpest came along; and European science followed it. Increasing numbers of veterinarians associated with the military, colonial governments, and even colonial farmers' associations went to these colonies for employment (and the more ambitious ones, for scientific fame). In this way, rinderpest stimulated the formation of veterinary regimes of control that included regulations, field stations, checkpoints, research laboratories, professional associations, and schools. These veterinarians working in these institutions and in private practices tried to understand and control animal disease problems while legitimizing veterinary medicine as a state-sanctioned and state-supported profession. Their activities, in turn, supported the goals of colonial governments and helped to transform animal husbandry and the land in places like eastern and southern Africa, Southeast Asia, and the Pacific Islands. Rinderpest was an agent of death and destruction to indigenous African and Asian cattle, and to the lifeways of the people who raised them. It also significantly disrupted natural ecosystems by killing wild grazers. As one observer in eastern Africa wrote, rinderpest created landscapes of desolation. As we discuss later in this chapter, these were the landscapes that stimulated some of the most important developments in the veterinary sciences and disease research.

The Disease of Madness: Rabies

Another greatly feared disease was rabies. Rabies, *lyssa*, *hydrophobia* (Latin), *Tollwut* (German), водобоязнь (Russian), kuduz (Turkish), *rage* (French), has been associated with dogs since ancient times. As with other animal diseases, until the 1800s it was primarily diagnosed by observing the symptoms: dogs that appeared "mad," snarling, salivating, jerking, or convulsing, and biting other animals and humans. Once a bitten person or animal became ill, the disease was almost 100 percent fatal. Today tens of thousands of people die from rabies annually, particularly in parts of Africa and Asia and in any place with a high number of unvaccinated dogs. Humans can also be infected by bites from rabid foxes, cats, wolves, monkeys, bats, raccoons, or skunks. The centuries-long circulation of various recipes against bites of infected dogs indicates the regular reemergence of this ancient disease.

Several theories about what caused this disease existed; today, we know that rabies is caused by an RNA virus from the *Lyssavirus* family. You may be surprised to learn where the name "lyssavirus" came from. Since antiquity, the idea persisted that rabies was caused by the *lyssa*, a "worm" that was located under the tongue of all dogs that could cause them to "go mad." (Today we call this anatomical structure the *frenulum*. Look under your tongue: humans have a *frenulum* also.) Cutting out this alleged "worm" in healthy dogs was a standard preventive measure that was practiced until well into the nineteenth century. For a long time, spontaneous generation was taken as the cause of rabies. Other rabies causation theories were summer heat, poisoning, lack of water, bad food or tainted water, incurable canine immorality, and unsatisfied libido. (Some French and German towns even considered establishing "brothels" for city dogs to prevent rabies!) The traditional therapy in humans consisted of cauterization of bite wounds followed by applying various drugs from herbal, mineral, or animal origin. Cattle and other livestock, if bitten by a rabid dog, were bled and the bite wound was cauterized. As we have seen in the case of other diseases, the treatments corresponded to theories about what caused rabies. Infection of livestock and humans represented a societal problem: the financial losses of dead cattle and the great fear among humans of a horrible death were considerable.

Towns and regional governments responded with regulations designed to control the dog population and therefore control rabies. From antiquity onward, laws, decrees, and placards were issued in Europe and Asia, allowing or even encouraging the mass killing of infected or suspected stray dogs to prevent rabies. Many cultures associated rabies with the late summer, the so-called dog days, and an outbreak of rabies usually led to mass killing of dogs in the affected region. This often meant that dogs were chased and stoned, burned, or beaten to death. In ancient Greece and Rome, there were even designated days for the destruction of dogs; *kynophantes* and *dies caniculares*, respectively. In some countries "dog slayers" were appointed to do this job. (These should not be confused with dog butchers, who slaughtered dogs for human consumption or for the preparation of medicine based on dog tissues. Dog meat was consumed in Europe until well into the twentieth century and is still consumed in Asia today.) Of course, some dogs learned to evade their pursuers, often forming groups that may even have helped the virus to spread.

Dogs with owners had a better chance of survival. Although many larger towns and cities charged dog-taxes to limit dog populations, even poorer people quietly kept dogs on chains or leashes or in yards. The muzzle, which prevented the dog from biting, also has a long history around the world. A Japanese regulation of 1695 ordered owners of aggressive dogs to keep them confined and muzzled. Especially during epizootics of rabies, healthy dogs were ordered to be kept confined to avoid contact with infected animals. Any suspected case of rabies usually meant the dog would be killed immediately, or at least isolated from other animals and people. In cities, regions, or countries with formalized public health systems, animal healers were required to notify the officials about suspected cases of rabies. In predominantly Muslim areas, dogs were regarded as unclean animals and forbidden except for a small number of exceptions. Although this was a spiritual law, it also had the effect of controlling rabies.

Despite these efforts, citizens found dogs difficult to control. For 10,000 years, dogs had evolved in association with humans. Dogs were clever, they understood how to live near and evade humans; and they reproduced efficiently. They were small enough to hide and quick enough to run away successfully. People valued their dogs as sources of companionship, work, and food; and they hid them from the dog catchers. Unable to control the canine population, some places, especially islands or isolated areas, chose to completely ban the importation of dogs. For example, compulsory quarantine for all dogs and a ban on importing dogs was proposed in Britain in 1793. In 1897 these measures were adopted to eradicate rabies from the UK, which was successful. Apart from separate Dog Acts and Rabies Acts, this disease was one of the first animal diseases to be included as notifiable in Cattle Acts that were enacted in many countries in the second half of the nineteenth century. Generally, enforcement of veterinary supervision on a national level proved more successful than on a regional or local level.

In 1800, several theories about what caused this disease existed, but one thing was clear: the bite of a rabid animal conveyed the disease. This observation led to the study of rabies in early veterinary schools and research institutes, especially in France. These veterinary institutions usually focused on horse and livestock diseases, but rabies was the exception that brought attention to diseases of dogs (and other smaller animals, such as cats). In 1823, the physiologist François Magendie (1783–1855) inoculated two healthy dogs with saliva from a human victim of rabies. One dog developed rabies and infected other dogs and sheep by biting them. Lyons veterinary school professor Pierre-Victor Galtier (1846–1908) further revealed the etiology of rabies, particularly the role of saliva and nervous tissue in transmission during bites. By 1879, he demonstrated that the disease could be transmitted from dogs to rabbits using injections of blood and saliva. This established an animal model that could be studied in the laboratory. As we will see, the famous microbiologist Louis Pasteur also began studying rabies at about this time, and the work of Pasteur and his colleagues on rabies led to major discoveries in vaccine development. Pasteur and his colleagues developed an effective post-exposure treatment for humans in 1885. Some historians believe that Pasteur used Galtier's ideas without crediting him fairly. Ironically, Galtier accidentally infected himself during experiments with rabies and had to be treated with Pasteur's emergency vaccine. We return to discussing rabies later in this chapter.

Indigenous Healing Regimes around the World Continued to Thrive

Although Western veterinary medicine was introduced in Java in the nineteenth century, local stockowners continued to use traditional medicines. The local population had at least one name for each disease, while livestock keepers seemed to have had an elaborate knowledge of livestock diseases. Some of this knowledge was brought into formal veterinary concepts and practices. There is evidence that Dutch veterinarians occasionally acquired or utilized Indigenous knowledge. For instance, farmers in West Java treated foot and mouth disease with *ayer asem*, derived from tamarind. A mixture of salt and tamarind was applied to the blisters on infected animals. Another example is surra, a disease of equines that was unknown to most Europeans. Based on close observation, Indigenous Javanese animal owners believed that surra was transmitted by flies. Western veterinarians were slow to accept the Javanese experience, until the link between trypanosomiasis and tsetse flies was demonstrated in Africa in 1902.

A clash between Western scientific and local knowledge also occurred in the British-ruled Cape Colony (part of today's South Africa) in the 1870s through 1890s. British vets appointed by the Cape Colony government, with their Western ideas on miasmatic environmental or contagious causes of livestock diseases, were often opposed by European settler farmers (Boers) and Indigenous Khoikhoi shepherds and farmers. In the case of liver flukes in sheep, for instance, farmers were advised to drain their land, which in hindsight could be considered bad for the environment. However, farmers let sheep roam in brackish bushes or administered salt to get rid of internal parasites, as was also done in Australia. The Boers used many home remedies, made from indigenous plants, or ones based on Khoikhoi knowledge. The British colonial vets put efforts into the establishment of an experimental farm in 1880 and the enactment of the Contagious Diseases Act in 1881, which increased their power to control the livestock of the Khoikhoi and Boer farmers. In many places, animal owners did not rely on formal veterinary medicine. Printed sources such as books, recipes and pamphlets remained major sources of knowledge for animal owners that enabled them to treat their own animals. In the United States, for example, two popular books by the physician George Dadd stressed the importance of rational empiricism: *The Modern Horse Doctor* (1854) and *The Modern Cattle Doctor* (1851). The organized veterinary profession viewed Dadd with suspicion because he called into question standard treatments such as bleeding and purging; but his books provided widely used guidelines for veterinary care.

These examples remind us that, although the European-style veterinary regimes were increasing in scope and power around the world, it is important to remember that most animal health care was still provided on an individual basis by folk healers and animal owners. This veterinary marketplace, and the local knowledge that went with it, was well established. It often powerfully contested the developing veterinary regime. Outside of Western Europe, veterinarians were almost always outnumbered by local healers. Additionally, they were usually employed by the European military or local, regional, or national colonial governments – whose major concerns were often epizootics and zoonoses. Therefore, in most settler colonies, animal health care could be loosely divided into two separate realms: individualized, traditional healing and the imported veterinary regime of the colonial government. Although the specifics of these veterinary regimes varied from place to place, all had some combination of regulation and the development of physical institutions, including schools and laboratories. These institutions' goals were to understand and control the most economically serious animal disease problems. In the process, they also legitimized veterinary medicine as a state-sanctioned profession during the nineteenth and early twentieth centuries.

Veterinary Institutions

Schools: Continuing the Imperial Veterinary Education Model

Like the history of medical schools, in veterinary medicine the early centers of education were in France, followed by Scotland. The "Paris school" of clinical (human) medicine, hospital based, had its counterpart in the early schools of Lyon and Alfort and their competitors. Another center of medical education, built up within the Scottish Enlightenment of the late 1700s, encouraged the development of veterinary education in Edinburgh (see Chapter 3). Along with the French, German, and Spanish schools, these nodes of veterinary education launched further expansion of the European-style schools into Asia and the Americas. For example, the German veterinary educational and research traditions were very important in Asia. In Japan after the Meiji Restoration (1868), the first European-style veterinary school was founded in Tokyo in 1876. The Meiji government actively recruited teachers of "Western methods" from Germany, France, and Britain. Between 1900 and 1910, new veterinary departments were founded in at least two universities in China (in Jilin and Guangzhou), based on agricultural animal husbandry and the need to control epizootics. In the 1920s and 1930s, the Chinese government selected students to be sent to Europe and the United States for veterinary training. Returning to China, veterinarians such as Luo Qingsheng (罗清生) (Nanjing Agricultural University) founded veterinary departments or schools using the Western curriculum.

In Edinburgh, William Dick's school and a competitor, the school headed by John Gamgee (1831–1894), trained the next generation of young leaders who transported the formal educational model to North America during the 1860s–1880s. Andrew Smith (1834–1910), who graduated in 1861, was recruited to Toronto (Canada) to found what became the Ontario Veterinary College (1862), the first permanent school in North America. He was joined by fellow Edinburgh graduate Duncan McEachran (1841–1924), who established the Montréal Veterinary College (1866) in French-speaking Quebec, Canada. McEachran's school was very progressive. With a three-year curriculum based on the latest in comparative pathology and medicine, the school was home to one of the great leaders of modern medicine, William Osler. Back in Edinburgh, a classmate of Andrew Smith, James Law (1838–1921), was hired by Cornell University in 1868 to establish the first school of veterinary medicine in the United States. At Cornell, Law trained the scientists and veterinarians who established the research and meat inspection programs at the U.S. Bureau of Animal Industry. The Edinburgh educational model was not the only one transferred to North America, however. The U.S. veterinary profession was also shaped by the Parisian veterinarian Alexandre Liautard (1835–1918), trained at Alfort and Toulouse, who ran veterinary schools in New York City beginning in the 1860s. Liautard edited a popular journal and was highly influential. Other early veterinary leaders included Heinrich J. Detmers (1835–1906), educated at the Royal Veterinary Colleges in Hannover and Berlin, Germany. Detmers immigrated to the United States and taught veterinary sciences/medicine at several state universities in the 1870s and 1880s: Iowa, home to the first state (public) university veterinary school in the United States; and the veterinary faculties of Kansas, Missouri, and Illinois. Finally, Detmers moved to the School of Veterinary Science at the Ohio State University in the 1880s, where he established the first bacteriology course in an American veterinary curriculum and served as director of this School. Through Detmers and his students, the German model was very influential in the U.S. state (public) universities.

In south Asia, the British imperial regime (the Raj) brought veterinarians to India and what is now Pakistan. These were mostly graduates of the Royal Veterinary College, London, and they included the talented researcher Griffith Evans (1835–1935), who had also acquired a medical degree while posted with the military in Canada. Sent to India in 1877, Evans researched animal disease problems and eventually discovered the trypanosome that caused the disease *surra* in horses and camels (both important animals for military transport). Veterinary education in British India has a fascinating history: as early as 1821, military veterinary surgeon J.T. Hodgson trained Indians to be veterinary assistants to the corps of Indian cavalry. In 1862, the army veterinary department opened a school at Poona that concentrated on equine health care. The first permanent veterinary school that addressed a broader range of animal health problems was the Punjab Veterinary College established in Lahore (1881–1882). The Bengal Veterinary College began accepting local students for a three-year course in 1896, and its students were expected to address problems with cattle diseases. By 1900, new veterinary colleges had been founded in Calcutta, Bombay, and Madras, and post-graduate training was available for field veterinarians at the Imperial Institute of Veterinary Research. The Indian veterinary regime was hierarchical, from the more elite "veterinary assistants" at the top to the most-humble "low caste" veterinarians in local towns and cities. Although this structure has evolved quite a bit since then, the robust system of formal veterinary education continues in India today.

The French-Spanish model, based on the national veterinary school at Madrid, also spread rapidly with imperialism and the development of new nations in Central and South America in the second half of the nineteenth century. Schools were established at Llavallol, Argentina (1883); Santiago, Chile (1898); Lima, Peru (1902); Montevideo, Uruguay (1905); and Havana, Cuba (1907), and Rio de Janeiro, Brazil (1913). These schools adapted European knowledge to the political and agricultural needs of their locations, and governments could hire European-trained veterinarians from several countries. For example, the founders of the School of Veterinary Medicine established in Havana, Cuba, had been trained in Madrid, Córdoba, and Zaragoza, Spain (Francisco Etchegoyen Montané and Francisco del Rio Ferrer); Toulouse, France (Julio Brower Etchecopar); and New York, USA (Honoré Laine). The Chilean government imported Julio Besnard from Toulouse, and several other French-trained veterinarians were engaged to oversee national meat inspection, the president's horse guard (Daniel Monfallet), and the development of bacteriology laboratories. Besnard even established a Zoological Garden in which scientists could study comparative anatomy and physiology, and animal diseases such as foot and mouth disease and anthrax in numerous species. In 1905, a military veterinary school replaced the old cavalry school, and this school's curriculum was heavily influenced by the German model. Another interesting example is the establishment of the veterinary school at Montevideo, Uruguay. In this case, the government enticed Daniel Elmer Salmon (from the U.S. Bureau of Animal Industry) to come to Uruguay and establish the school. Therefore, this school was based on the model at Cornell University in New York, USA (as was the school established in Manila, the Philippines, by U.S. military veterinarians in 1910). These complex networks of veterinarians, and the further spread of European-style veterinary regimes, deserve more study by veterinary historians – especially in terms of how local circumstances both constrained and shaped the imported European institutions.

In the European-colonized regions during the late 1800s, only a few graduate veterinarians had relocated permanently, and these formed the elite of the new veterinary regimes. They almost always carried very heavy duties and held multiple offices. Andrew Smith, for example, ran the Toronto/Ontario Veterinary School for over forty years, helped establish the Ontario Veterinary Association, pushed for national legislation to forbid non-graduates from practicing animal healing, served as the Dominion stock inspector, and military veterinary surgeon, and worked on commissions to address recurrent epizootics. In his spare time, Smith studied and passed the examination to become a member of the (British) Royal College of Veterinary Surgeons. Even after the turn of the twentieth century this remained true. In the United States, Leonard Pearson (1868–1909) served as the Dean of the University of Pennsylvania Veterinary School, developed and oversaw a model bovine tuberculosis eradication plan, was the Pennsylvania State Veterinarian, served as an officer of multiple veterinary associations, and declined an offer to become Chief of the U.S. Bureau of Animal Industry. Pearson died at a young age of "overwork" (archival letters hint at suicide), a major loss to American veterinary medicine. By 1900, there were still only 8,000 graduate veterinarians in the United States to care for tens of millions of animals spread over a vast territory, carry out state and federal meat inspection, conduct research, and run disease eradication campaigns. Until enough home-grown veterinary leaders could be trained, the early veterinary elite suffered with heavy workloads. They also had a great deal of influence over the shape of the developing veterinary regimes in the Americas and places such as Japan, the Philippines, and Australia.

Australia's veterinary schools developed mainly from the Edinburgh model of veterinary education. Graham Mitchell (graduate of the Dick Veterinary School in Edinburgh) and, later, William Tyson Kendall (graduate of the Royal College of Veterinary Surgeons, London) emigrated to Melbourne. They worked hard to start a veterinary school in the 1870s–1880s; in 1908 it had become part of the University of Melbourne. Another Edinburgh graduate, James Douglas Stewart, campaigned for and designed a new veterinary school associated with the University of Sydney. With two locations, urban Sydney and more rural Camden, this school's curriculum encompassed both equine medicine and the control of livestock diseases. As Dean of this school, Stewart was remarkable for sponsoring native New Zealanders and women as students at this school (at a time when women and minority groups were mostly excluded from veterinary education).

Veterinary schools benefited from many of the scientific discoveries of the 1800s, beginning with the application of antisepsis and anesthesia in surgery. Antisepsis traces its history to early notions of cleanliness when manipulating animal and human bodies. However, antisepsis only became well established in human and animal surgery after the work of English surgeon Joseph Lister (1827–1912), who famously developed carbolic acid solutions to spray on wounds and the surrounding areas and protective dressings to maintain cleanliness. Although these methods significantly increased survival rates, especially with thoracic and abdominal surgery, veterinarians were slower to adopt them overall (compared with physicians). Isolating superficial wounds from dirt was difficult, especially in the case of livestock. Anesthesia was similarly slow to become standard practice in veterinary practice, in part due to the expense of ether and chloroform for such large animals, and because animals could simply be physically restrained with ropes. For humans, anesthesia was used from the 1840s onward in dentistry, surgery, and childbirth.

But for veterinary medicine, the major problem remained the recurring outbreaks of livestock diseases, which stimulated the formation of various veterinary institutions with attached laboratories where research was conducted to better understand the underlying principles of health and disease in both animals and humans. To this goal often laboratory animals were used as a model, next to the application of physics and chemistry, the two major natural sciences influencing and enforcing (veterinary) medicine.

Laboratories: Colonial and National

The establishment of colonial and national laboratories was an important development for veterinary knowledge. Most of these laboratories were freestanding institutions, but some were connected to the newly founded veterinary schools. There, research was conducted on questions related to the transmission of livestock diseases. At the beginning of the nineteenth century, this included mainly rinderpest and sheep pox, while attention was drawn to contagious pleuropneumonia and bovine tuberculosis somewhat later. Research on veterinary topics took place in all kinds of labs around the world. National examples include the Pasteur Institute in Paris, the Robert Koch Institute in Berlin, and the Istanbul-based *Bakteriyolojijâne-i Baytâri* (Veterinary Bacteriology Laboratory) headed by Adil Mustafa Sehzadebasi. There were also municipal bacteriological labs, (military) hospitals, (bio) chemical institutes, bacteriology, vaccinology, and serum institutes, colonial or tropical institutes, and general hygiene and public health-care institutes. Additionally, laboratory methods were used to test drinking water supplies, meat from slaughterhouses, commercial products, and in the pharmaceutical industry. The boundaries between human and animal medicine were not as sharply divided then as they are today: scientists from various disciplines worked closely together on comparative medicine.

In tropical areas of the world, medical laboratories often conducted research on veterinary topics. Almost all used experimental animals. In 1888, a medical research laboratory was established on Java in the former Dutch East Indies. One of the research officers was physician Christiaan Eijkman (1858–1930), who studied polyneuritis in fowl. He noticed that the symptoms of *beriberi* in chickens used in his laboratory disappeared when these were fed with unpolished instead of polished rice. Eventually this led to the discovery of the etiology of human *beriberi* (thiamine/vitamin B-1 deficiency) and contributed to a general understanding of vitamins in nutrition (for humans and animals). Eijkman himself at first was convinced that *beriberi* was caused by a bacterium, but his assistant, animal physiologist Gerrit Grijns (1865–1944), convinced him that thiamine present in rice membrane played a crucial role. Polish biochemist Kazimierz Funk (1884–1967) shortened the term "vital amine" to create the word "vitamin." In 1929 Eijkman received the Nobel Prize for his work on vitamin B. In this same laboratory in 1890, physician Joost van Eecke (1860–1895) diagnosed hemorrhagic septicemia in buffaloes, a disease which was until then considered a form of rinderpest by Dutch vets. Some veterinarians worked in these medical research teams. Other vets performed research at the Pathological Laboratory of the Deli Land Cultivation Company at Medan and investigated trypanosomiasis, piroplasmosis, and rinderpest. There, a disease called *farcin du boeuf* (tropical actinomycosis) was first diagnosed in cattle suffering from chronic skin abscesses.

Perhaps the most well-known and influential international network of disease research institutes was the Pasteur Institutes. Based in Paris, where scientists were initially trained before being sent around the world, the network included laboratories that had been established in places such as today's Vietnam (Southeast Asia); Algeria, Tunisia, and Morocco in northern Africa; Madagascar; St. Petersburg, Russia; and Tehran, Iran. Each of these institutes was a unique blend influenced by the local disease problems, the scientific interests and personality of the institute's director, and the standard Pasteurian techniques and approaches. Historians have approached the international network of Pasteur institutes from the perspective of human medicine. However, just like the parent Institut Pasteur in Paris, all these institutes had a broad view of the interesting and necessary disease problems that should be studied, and they often carried out important research on animal diseases such as rabies. Comparative medicine was an integral part of the Pasteurian approach.

National governments began supporting animal disease laboratories, often associated with meat and food inspection efforts, during the second half of the nineteenth century. One example was the Bureau of Animal Industry (BAI), established in the United States in 1884 to address the twin problems of trichinosis in pork and contagious bovine pleuropneumonia (CBPP). Its first director was Daniel Elmer Salmon (1850–1914, Fig. 4.2), who studied at Cornell (USA) and the Alfort veterinary school (France). Salmon established the first major microbiological laboratory in the United States at the BAI,

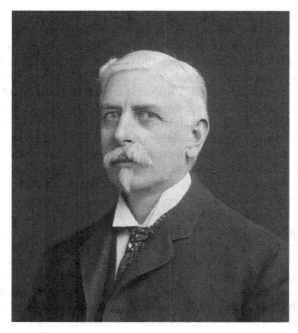

Figure 4.2 Daniel Elmer Salmon (1850–1914), the first American who was granted a DVM degree (from Cornell in 1876) in the United States. First director of the Bureau of Animal Industry, U.S. Department of Agriculture. The bacterial genus *Salmonella* was named in his honor.
Source: Public domain, Library of Congress (USA).

choosing research problems that could be easily justified to farmers and government officials. Annual reports always included calculations of the estimated numbers of animals saved and their economic worth as well as the BAI scientists' technical research. Some of this research, notably the Texas cattle fever experiments of the 1890s, transformed the scientific understanding of causation and transmission for both animal and human diseases. The Texas cattle fever experiments established the roles of insect vectors in transmitting diseases and served as an important stimulus to research on many animal and human diseases (including yellow fever and malaria). The BAI also developed important strategies designed to eradicate animal diseases across vast, sparsely settled and relatively unregulated territory (a very different situation from Europe).

CBPP, a disease that long plagued cattle in Europe, had spread during the 1850s–1860s to places such as the United States and Australia (where it became enzootic). It spread easily because the incubation time is 3 to 7 weeks and outbreaks follow a slow course. The morbidity rate is 10 percent, while mortality is about 50 percent. Twenty-five percent of recovered cattle remain carriers for a very long time. By the end of the nineteenth century, the etiology of this disease was elucidated by the French veterinarians Emile Roux (1853–1933) and Edmond Nocard (1850–1903). CBPP had puzzled veterinary researchers: it was caused by *Mycoplasma*, a bacterium that was difficult to culture in the laboratory; and it was difficult to control because it had a long incubation period (during which the animals often did not show symptoms). CBPP was highly contagious in animals being shipped or housed in close quarters. In 1879, the United States experienced an outbreak so severe that the British government blocked U.S. cattle exports to the UK and Canada. The BAI developed a federally coordinated area-eradication strategy, based on dividing the country up into different levels of infection and corresponding restrictions on cattle movement. While experiments on finding an effective vaccine against the disease failed, the specific area-eradication strategy successfully eliminated the disease from the United States by 1892. (This strategy was a model for some other nations' modern disease eradication programs and, a century later, for the successful global elimination of smallpox in humans.)

Drawing on the rapidly increasing knowledge of blood-borne immunity, scientists used a comparative medicine approach to develop tools to fight diseases in the late 1800s. Next to the pioneering work of Russian scientist Ilya Ilich Metchnikov (1845–1916), German physician Emil von Behring (1854–1917) was renowned as a pioneer in serum therapy and discoverer of diphtheria and tetanus antitoxin. He worked closely together with German physician and chemist Paul Ehrlich (1854–1915), the founder of modern chemotherapy. Observations of animals that survived an illness led to the identification of substances in the blood that could transfer resistance to the disease to another animal (or even humans). Scientists also quickly learned that large animals, particularly horses, could serve as "factories" to generate blood sera that provided resistance to diseases such as diphtheria. In 1895, the development of diphtheria antitoxin in horses was the first major *serotherapy*. Veterinary and medical microbiologists, including von Behring and Shibasaburo Kitasato (1853–1931), injected horses with toxins and small amounts of infectious material. Later, they harvested the horses' blood sera; and although they did not yet understand exactly what factors supplied the protection, they knew that purified sera injected into victims of diphtheria, cholera, tetanus, and other infections saved many lives. These early "biologicals," as the animal-manufactured treatments were called, promised future discoveries to help control the ravages of infectious diseases in animals and humans.

Development of Veterinary Pharmacology in Laboratories

This brings us to the beginning of veterinary pharmacology. Until the end of the eighteenth century, handbooks and manuscripts dealing with drugs (*materia medica*) usually contained uncritical descriptions of therapeutic effects in patients. The first two more critical handbooks on veterinary drugs were both published in 1840 by the French veterinarian Henri M.O. Delafond (1805–1861) and German veterinarian Carl Hertwig (1798–1881). The first half of the nineteenth century witnessed experiments in laboratories in attempts to find explanations for these observed effects. Experimental techniques were aimed at investigating the physiological and chemical modes of action of substances on laboratory animals, and an effective protection against poisoning. An important part of research was dedicated to the isolation of active substances from medicinal herbs. Morphine, emetine, strychnine, colchicine, and quinine were extracted and isolated and the pharmaceutical industry started to produce these commercially.

Pharmacokinetic research by French researchers François Magendie (1783–1855) and his successor Claude Bernard (1813–1878) followed during the nineteenth century. Their interest in the structure and synthesis of drugs was aimed at understanding the relation between structure and operation. The first synthesized drug was the anesthetic chloral hydrate in 1832 and employed since 1869. In 1875, aspirin was first used in therapy. Salicylic acid was extracted from willow bark. For ages the antipyretic operation of this bark was known. More synthetic drugs followed that were listed in handbooks. From the 1870s onward, the pharmaceutical industry started to produce and market synthetic agents. From then on veterinarians had synthetic antipyretic, anti-infective, laxative, anesthetic, and emetic drugs at their proposal. Legislation to control the release of new veterinary drugs became effective from the turn of the century. In the United States, for example, the Pure Food and Drugs Act was established in 1906.

These newly developed drugs as well as new surgery equipment and techniques were first tested on laboratory animals. During the nineteenth century their number increased rapidly, causing public criticism, particularly when vivisection was applied (as we discuss later in this chapter). Research projects dealing with animal breeding (crossbreeding) and testing animal fodder to increase growth and production were performed at experimental farms, attached to veterinary and agricultural colleges and institutes. Vaccine and serum production (previously mentioned) were particularly important reasons to establish veterinary laboratories. Medical and veterinary acts to control contagious diseases were adopted in many countries in the last quarter of the nineteenth century. These acts usually included provisions for traditional measures such as quarantines, but they also established medical and veterinary services for surveillance and institutes and laboratories to produce vaccines and chemotherapeutics for human and animal diseases. Since serotherapies for human diseases were mostly produced in horses, veterinary institutions were logical places to do this work. These institutions were excellent examples of the comparative medicine approach, as first articulated by Rudolf Virchow. Major producers of veterinary serotherapies and biologicals included the State Serum Institute in Vienna (established 1893), the Danish State Serum Institute (1902) located on the island of Amager in Copenhagen, and the National Serum Institute established in Rotterdam in 1904.

Laboratories: Food Hygiene

Another important topic was the transmission of zoonotic diseases, directly from animals to humans (glanders, anthrax), or indirectly via consumption of food of animal origin (meat, milk, eggs). Initially, research findings in vet school laboratories formed a major impediment to the introduction of meat inspection. Namely, it was shown that meat from animals that had died from rinderpest was not harmful to humans. More and more cases where meat from diseased animals was consumed without any detriment to human health were described. This led to the one-sided conviction that all meat from livestock suffering from different diseases posed no threat to human health. If only such meat was heated long enough, no danger could occur. However, from 1850 onward the standing of meat inspection as a veterinary discipline increased when the scientific background of several diseases in humans related to consumption of food of animal origin were discovered one after the other. This was another example of comparative medicine. For example, Dutch and German researchers worked together in the 1890s on bacteriological meat research in the Hygiene Institute in Amsterdam, later Institute for Tropical Hygiene. In cooperation with the local slaughterhouse laboratory, these scientists discovered and described thermostable toxin-forming bacteria as the causes of food poisonings, as well as the development of standard procedures for such research.

Around 1850 scientists became aware of the problem of drug residues in meat and milk. There was a long tradition of giving animals substances to obtain therapeutic, prophylactic, or growth-promoting effects. Apart from treatments such as injections, the majority of drugs were administered as additives to feed or drinking water. The potential danger of veterinary drug residues present in foods of animal origin was recognized when scientists warned against the excessive use of mercury (sublimate), lead, creosote, arsenic, and strychnine in veterinary practice. Nonetheless, in the 1850s and 1860s, animal drug manufacturers were quite successful in advertising and marketing and were generally not hindered by restrictive legislation. The Spanish physician and chemist Mateo Orfila (1787–1853) is considered the father of toxicology and forensic medicine. He studied the toxicological properties of various herbs, drugs, and poisons and the speed of uptake in various tissues of the body, particularly in dogs. For food-producing animals,

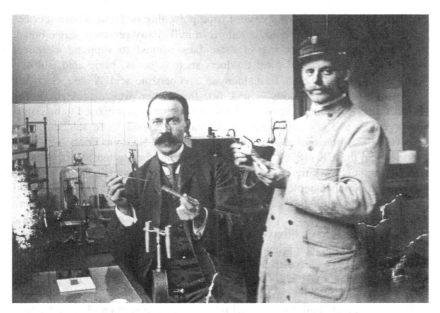

Figure 4.3 Bacteriological meat research at the Amsterdam abattoir
laboratory in 1900 by veterinarian Dirk van der Sluijs (1849–1923)
and his assistant.
Courtesy: Collection Veterinary Medicine, Utrecht University Museum, 0285-151480.

research on applied dose, toxicity level, and withdrawal periods before slaughter was conducted from 1890 onward.

In the second half of the nineteenth century, many municipalities as well as food-producing companies established independent laboratories where research was conducted to support food inspection with scientific knowledge (Fig. 4.3). This was due to changes in the food industry and food supply, distrust concerning industrially produced food, as well as to an increasing number of adulterations in the (international) meat and dairy trade. In addition, foreign markets demanded (veterinary) surveillance to guarantee quality standards of imported meat and dairy. Labs were designated where quality control of these products was performed according to laws regulating the inspection of domestic foods as well as food import and export. Research included the search for safe and effective preservation methods, developing chemical, physical, histological, and microbiological methods for quality and safety control of livestock and food of animal origin. Around 1850, the bourgeoisie in larger cities could go to a pharmacist to have their food inspected. A few decades later, food inspection services were established with labs where the broader public could go to in case of food poisoning or fraud. These services were mainly occupied with adulterations in milk, dairy products, eggs, bread, and drugs. Chemists working in these labs wanted to suppress chemical preservatives in meat and meat products such as borax, boric acid, sulfites, sulfuric acid, salicylic acid, formaldehyde, and benzoic acid. A plea was made to return to "natural foods." In 1900, the matter was discussed at the International Hygiene Congress in Paris, in which it was proposed to ban most preservatives and colorants. Later congresses showed more tolerance and admitted small portions of salt, nitrites, and sugar. National Food Acts were made law in the UK (1875), Germany (1879), and the United States (1906).

Veterinarians working in laboratories established at municipal abattoirs and large commercial slaughterhouses were mainly occupied with microbiological research and investigating cases of meat poisoning. Around 1850 there were the findings in the field of parasitology that enabled control against parasitic nematodes (see below). From 1880 onward, meat hygiene research obtained a more scientific character when bacteriological research carried out in slaughterhouse laboratories accelerated. The pioneering work of Pasteur and Koch, and other microbiologists like Auguste Chauveau (1827–1917), Otto Bollinger (1843–1909), August Gärtner (1848–1934), Emile van Ermenghem (1851–1932), and Daniel Salmon with their discoveries in the field of bacteriology, was decisive for the further development of meat inspection. They focused on diseases such as bovine tuberculosis, trichinosis, and several others. The etiology of meat poisonings was mapped after the isolation of several meat-borne pathogens such as *Salmonella* spp., *Clostridium botulinus*, and *Mycobacterium tuberculosis bovis*. Around 1890 it became clear that meat poisonings could be caused by postmortem growth of thermostable, toxin-forming bacteria in meat. Such findings influenced the canning industry, which adjusted pasteurization and sterilization procedures.

Veterinarians extended the science of meat inspection, while the practical execution of meat inspection is equal to the pathological anatomy of livestock. The most widely used, translated, and reprinted handbook on meat inspection (Berlin, 1892) was published by the German professor Robert von Ostertag (1864–1940), who had studied human and veterinary medicine. He was also editor of the *Zeitschrift für Fleisch- und Milchhygiene* [*Journal for Meat- and Milk Hygiene*], which was published from 1890 onward. Until the 1960s, the guidelines and regulations on meat inspection were based on this handbook. Inspection involved ante- and postmortem inspection of each animal by a qualified veterinarian, by pathological and anatomical examination, and by bacteriological tests in doubtful cases. Based on this, meat was stamped and declared sound, conditionally sound, or unfit for human consumption. Slaughterhouse labs also played an important role in animal disease control, since they provided statistics on the occurrence of various livestock diseases.

Veterinary Associations and International Cooperation

During the second half of the nineteenth century, traditional empirical meat inspection was transformed into an applied veterinary science, and this grew along with veterinary associations. Research findings on food safety were published in handbooks and specific scientific journals, while theoretical and practical food inspection became part of the veterinary curriculum. The efforts of veterinarians to establish veterinary public health and to elevate the scientific prestige of the profession were strongly supported by national veterinary associations. Veterinary associations were very keen on obtaining legal protection of the title "veterinarian" by which the competition of other animal healers could be eliminated: "the battle against empiricism," in their rhetoric. Often it was a slow process before such legislation was granted. Governments feared unemployment among unlicensed healers, who often still outnumbered the formally educated vets. Moreover, many animal owners (and officials) believed the work of unlicensed healers to be effective and important in maintaining animal health. Indeed, not all empiricists can simply be dismissed as quacks. Many of them were very skilled and as effective as the educated, licensed veterinarians. But change was coming: many professions were organizing at this time in European countries, and veterinarians seized the chance to push for restrictive licensing that required formal education. The Netherlands passed a law defining "veterinarian" as an educated, licensed individual in 1874. In Britain, the Veterinary Surgeons Act was adopted in 1881, which made it illegal for unqualified individuals to use the title of "veterinary surgeon." However, these acts were symbolic because many empiricists continued their practice in both countries.

Veterinary associations recognized the potential job opportunities in food inspection services and slaughterhouses, and a possible broadening of the legal basis of the profession. In Romania, for example, members of the Society of Veterinary Medicine (founded 1871) pledged to work together on food hygiene, contagious diseases, and forensic medicine in the service of the nation and the well-being of all its people and animals. Not only would the livestock economy be enhanced, but as well protecting the food supply gave veterinarians a strong role in the public health. Legislation and food inspection requirements also helped elevate veterinarians to nationally prominent roles. Cattle Acts or Contagious Disease (Animal) Acts were established in Austria (1844), India (Tamil Nadu, 1866), the Netherlands (1870), Switzerland (1872), Prussia (1875), England (1878), Canada (1879), France (1881), Germany (1886), the United States (1903), and Australia (Quarantine Act, 1908). Under these acts, State Veterinary Services were established in various countries. In this way, a large sector of (human) public health was entrusted to vets. This can be considered a very important step in the scientific and societal recognition of the veterinary profession.

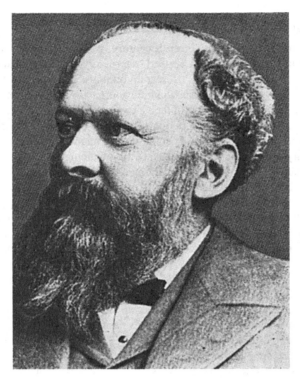

Figure 4.4 British veterinarian and inventor John Gamgee (1831–1894). He initiated the first international congress for veterinarians in 1863 in Hamburg. *Source:* Reinhard Froehner, *Kulturgeschichte der Tierheilkunde: ein Handbuch für Tierärzte und Studierende. Band 2: Geschichte des Veterinärwesens im Ausland* (Konstanz: Terra, 1952) 110.

It was the remarkable veterinarian and inventor John Gamgee (1831–1894, Fig. 4.4), son of a Scottish vet, who took the initiative to organize the first International Veterinary Congress in Hamburg, Germany, in 1863. This was well before the first international medical congress was held (London 1881). About 100 participants from 10 European countries mainly discussed measures such as quarantine length and isolation. Delegates framed their concerns as a European defense against dangerous Asian diseases. The second and third congresses held in Vienna (1865) and Zurich (1867), respectively, also dealt with stamping-out and inoculation strategies against CBPP and rinderpest, as well as the usefulness of trade and cattle movement restrictions. Although these were primarily veterinary-technical debates, they prepared the basis of national and international legislation on controlling livestock diseases. John

Gamgee was also founder of a second veterinary school in Edinburgh. He visited mainland Europe and noted that European standards of veterinary care were much better than in Britain. For example, he reported that only 8 percent of horses in Paris were lame, compared to the high figure of 42 percent in Britain. After studying rinderpest, Gamgee was a convinced follower of the germ theory. He routinely used the rectal thermometer and established that fever as a feature of rinderpest. As an inventor, Gamgee was also involved in the development of refrigeration technology and the frozen meat trade. Considering the problems with contagious livestock diseases and meat poisonings, in 1872 he made a plea for ending the harsh and inefficient live cattle trade. Instead, he argued, transporting and selling inspected meat from animals killed near where they lived would stop the spread of diseases among live animals.

An important step in livestock disease control was taken during an international conference hosted by the Austrian government in 1871 in Vienna. The recommendations listed in the final report "Principles for an International Regulation for the Extinction of the Cattle Plague" received wide international attention and supported the eradication of this disease in many countries in Europe. The necessity of organized veterinary action, including an early warning system for reporting an outbreak to neighboring nations by fast communication (telegraph), was stressed, next to government compensation of farmers for slaughtered animals. These recommendations proved to work well during the last outbreak of rinderpest in Britain in 1877, caused by a shipment of infected animals from Hamburg. As soon as the German veterinary officials had noticed that this livestock was infected, they warned their British colleagues, who could limit the outbreak by immediate action.

After a break of 13 years due to the Franco-Prussian War, four more international veterinary congresses were held in the nineteenth century. During the 7th congress in Baden-Baden (Germany) in 1899, the name was changed from International Veterinary Congress into World Veterinary Congress. This better reflected the delegates: over 1,000 participants from 39 countries, of which 16 delegations came from countries outside Europe. A Permanent Committee responsible for the organization of the congresses was established during the 8th meeting in Budapest in 1906. These efforts grew into an internationally influential organization, which by 1959 had adopted the name World Veterinary Association (WVA). Since 1955, this organization has established official relations with the global Food and Agriculture Organization (FAO) and World Health Organization (WHO). From the first meetings in 1863, the WVA was designed to gain international cooperation regarding animal diseases spreading globally and it had grown into the only non-governmental organization (NGO) representing the veterinary profession globally.

The second half of the nineteenth century witnessed the rise of various international congresses, which also had veterinary topics on the agenda. The French government organized the first International Sanitary Conferences in 1851. The main aim was to standardize international quarantine regulations against the spread of cholera, plague, and yellow fever. Up to 1938, in total 14 of these conferences took place, and they would play a major role in the formation of the World Health Organization in 1948. International Congresses on Hygiene and Demography were held in Europe from 1877 onward. Veterinary issues such as animal food, zoonotic diseases, and sanitary provisions were part of the programs. Between 1899 and 1912, five International Congresses on Tuberculosis were held in which scientists exchanged information about the relationship between bovine and human tuberculosis. The first International Congress on Tropical Diseases, which included veterinary topics, was held in 1913.

These institutions – regulation, laboratories, schools, associations, and international organizations – owed their existence to several social factors such as European imperialism, industrialization, and the threats to those factors posed by animal diseases. The historical spread of veterinary educational institutions also provided training grounds for the professionals who asserted their authority over animal health and disease, thus promising governments and other patrons the economic benefits of preserving livestock and the social benefits of helping to preserve human health. However, these promises depended on making veterinary medicine "scientific" and allying its leaders with (human) public health and medicine through comparative pathology and medicine. Next, we turn to the major intellectual and practical scientific developments during the nineteenth century that enabled veterinarians not only to compete in the veterinary marketplace but also to participate in regulating human and animal bodies and the global animal economy.

The Growth of European Sciences and the Growth of Veterinary Medicine

Historians have written volumes about the developments of the life sciences and the medical sciences during the nineteenth century. We consider these developments only as they helped shape veterinary regimes, according to these themes: how these sciences emerged from comparisons between human and animal bodies; how veterinary practices and disease-control procedures interacted with developing ideas about disease and society; and how scientific disciplines developed from the veterinary point of view. Although many of the names and achievements, such as those of Louis Pasteur and Robert Koch, will be familiar, we will focus on veterinary ideas, research, and practices. This focus is valuable in part because it changes the stories that have been carefully crafted by supporters of different heroes and national traditions, bringing a richer and more sophisticated understanding of these complex events. From the establishment of microbiology and bacteriology to comparative pathology and "one medicine," veterinary problems and veterinary scientists were important co-creators of modern medicine and public health as we know them today. In turn, the promises of "scientific" solutions to long-standing animal disease problems supported the growth and expansion of professional, state-supported veterinary medicine.

Outbreaks of animal disease were commercial crises, not only bankrupting farmers and drovers but also interrupting international credit cycles and threatening the financial and political solvency of governments. Outbreaks of contagious animal diseases led to quarantines and prohibitions against moving animals domestically and between countries. One rational and very practical and efficient measure based on this theory was quarantine, derived from the Italian word *quaranta*, meaning "forty." Physicians had learned that isolating diseased people from healthy people for an (incubation) period of at least 40 days prevented contagious diseases from spreading. This was applied to arriving ships in the harbor of Venice to avoid outbreaks of bubonic plague; and similar principles could be applied to animal diseases. This was very controversial in capitalist societies because government restrictions impeded the free market. Both materially and metaphorically, a serious epizootic was a serious threat to prosperity and, potentially, to political power and social stability. The stakes were high and the pressure on veterinary leaders was enormous. These factors shaped both the development of the veterinary sciences and the veterinary response to disease outbreaks during the nineteenth century.

New Approaches to an Old Question: What Caused Animal Diseases?

Between 1850 and the 1890s, European veterinary medicine experienced wide-ranging changes in ideas about etiology (theories about what caused animal diseases). In the 1850s, veterinarians could choose between several types of disease causation theories: environmental (including the effects of climate, miasmas, and toxins); contagionist (including zymotic theories); and anti-contagionist (such as the humoral theories and the hereditary theories). These categories or types of causation theories are somewhat artificial. Often, veterinarians explained the causes of individual diseases using ideas from *more than one* of these types of theories. For example, German anatomist/pathologist Friedrich G.J. (Jacob) Henle (1809–1885) classified sheep pox, anthrax, and rinderpest as miasmatic diseases that could later develop to be contagious in larger groups of animals. The eminent British veterinarian John

Gamgee stated in 1866 that cattle plague (rinderpest) was caused by a type of dangerous poison originating in the body of the sick animal after being spread by contagion. While the disease was not strictly caused by environmental conditions, Gamgee believed it was native to a particular place, climate, and environment: the interior steppe of Russia. Nonetheless, over time, environmental causation theories were joined and slowly overtaken by contagionist theories, especially germ theories. In the 1890s, both these types of etiological explanation were joined by another theory that implicated the broader ecologies of insect-borne diseases. A good example of this ecological theory (mentioned above) is the work of Theobald Smith, Fred Kilborne, and Cooper Curtice on the disease Texas cattle fever in the southern United States. They observed the development of a microorganism in blood-sucking insects that transmitted it to cattle, causing the disease. In summary, the general trends in prevalent etiological theories in veterinary medicine changed as follows: from a mixture of broad humoral, contagionist and environmental theories; narrowing increasingly to more reductionist germ theories; with the addition of ecological, vector-borne disease theories of germ transmission in the 1890s.

How did the competition between these multiple theories affect veterinary activities in controlling and treating animal diseases? There is no single answer. Often, veterinary practitioners selected treatments that combined these theories, for example, recommending both improved diet and bloodletting for a sick animal, combined with isolation in case the illness was contagious. Diseases that affected a single animal looked different from an outbreak in most of the herd, but even then, multiple causes could be at work: maybe the animals ate the same toxic plants, or maybe an unhealthy miasma affected them. One thing is certain: germ theories did not immediately or completely replace the other causation theories. No "revolution" suddenly replaced older ideas with newer ones. In veterinary medicine, we see a broad variety of ideas and responses continuing throughout the late 1800s and early 1900s. New ideas were often slowly accepted. Veterinarians with different training and backgrounds, working in different places and situations, used the ideas that seemed most effective to them at the time. Moreover, individual veterinarians often had a great deal of influence on local laws and regulations. At the level of municipalities and regions, we can trace changes in veterinary policies over time that reflect trends in disease causation theories.

Veterinary medicine in South Africa, 1850–1900, provides an excellent example. Cattle diseases such as pleuropneumonia and rinderpest, and sheep diseases such as heartwater and *lamsiekte*, stimulated the Cape Colony (British South Africa) government to establish the formal position of Veterinary Surgeon in 1876. The first person to hold this office, William Branford, trained in London and then served as an instructor at the Royal Edinburgh (Dick) Veterinary College for seven years. Branford, reflecting the knowledge of the 1860s and mid-1870s, believed that the unique attributes of the environment around Cape Town caused the diseases afflicting animals there. Branford was not an anti-contagionist; he recognized some diseases as transmissible from sick to healthy animals. However, he understood the Cape environment to be the most important determinant of whether signs of a disease would appear in an animal. His recommendations for preventing diseases in cattle and sheep relied on carefully regulating animals' seasonal diets, housing, and work regimes. The next person to serve as Cape Colony Veterinary Surgeon, Edinburgh graduate Duncan Hutcheon, succeeded Branford in 1880. Hutcheon advocated the germ theories that were rapidly developing in Europe. However, Hutcheon first had to acquire knowledge about the influences of South African environment and geography on animal diseases, which he then combined with germ ideas. (Hutcheon had many difficulties at first persuading Afrikaner farmers to accept germ ideas.) Around 1900, Hutcheon, the Swiss-trained veterinarian Arnold Theiler, and other veterinary scientists increasingly focused *beyond* the germ theories to explain the etiology and transmission of African animal diseases. They realized that direct transmission of bacteria from one animal to another (the major premise of germ theories) could not explain or control common diseases such as heartwater, nagana (trypanosomiasis), redwater, and East Coast fever. To understand these diseases, South African veterinarians combined Indigenous African expertise with new ideas emerging from America: they suspected that insects, such as ticks and mosquitoes, spread these diseases. Controlling the environment, cleaning up "germs," and fighting insect-borne diseases all guided veterinary research and practice in South Africa after 1900.

One other crucial theory about disease causation remained important throughout this time period: the toxin theory. Toxins were compounds that poisoned the body, and animals could get sick by directly inhaling or eating toxic substances. Jotello Festiri Soga (1865–1906) made important discoveries about the role of toxic plants in causing diseases in grazing livestock during the 1890s (see Fig. 4.5). Soga, whose father was Xhosa African and whose mother was Scottish European, was the first South African to qualify as a veterinarian (he graduated from the Royal (Dick) Veterinary College in Scotland). In 1889, he became the first Black official in the Cape Colony civil service. Here we see another interesting combination of Indigenous Africans' knowledge, collected by Soga, and the practices of European experimental science. For example, Soga investigated a disease called *nenta* in the Khoikhoi language of local herdsmen (Afrikaner farmers called this disease *krimpsiekte*). *Nenta* affected all breeds of sheep and goats, causing lameness and paralysis. Soga's colleague and boss, Duncan Hutcheon, had tried and failed to find a microorganism that caused this disease.

After talking with Indigenous African herdsmen, Soga surmised that the animals were being poisoned by eating a toxic plant also called *nenta* by the

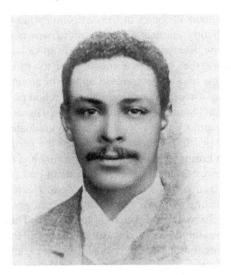

Figure 4.5 Portrait of Jotello Festiri Soga (1865–1906), first South African to graduate from a veterinary school and first Black South African employed by the Cape Colony civil service. Soga combined Xhosa knowledge with European science to elucidate the role of toxic plants in causing diseases in grazing livestock during the 1890s.
Source: Public domain.

herdsmen. He experimentally fed this plant to some goats and reproduced the disease. Thus, Soga proved that the plant called "(klip)nenta" (*Tylecodon ventricosus*) caused the disease *nenta/krimpsiekte* and he recommended eradicating this plant where livestock grazed. He also researched the medicinal properties of many South African plants and today is known as the father of ethnobotany in South African veterinary medicine. Sadly, Soga suffered from racial discrimination, and despite his education and research contributions, he never held a permanent position in the government veterinary services. Historians' recent attention to Black veterinarians has led us to rediscover Soga's major research on plants in veterinary medicine, and this reminds us of how important the toxin theory of disease causation still is today (although histories of disease seldom mention it).

Parasitology

It was in Italy that the basis for microbiology was laid by physician Francesco Redi (1626–1697), a pupil of Galilei. In 1684 he described 108 parasitic species and looked for specific causes of a disease. With his observation that maggots cannot develop from rotting meat, unless flies laid eggs on it, he challenged the prevailing idea of spontaneous generation. His pupil Giovanni Cosimo Bonomo (1663–1696) made a remarkable observation on scabies, a mite infection of the skin that was (and still is) widespread, particularly among poor people living under bad hygienic circumstances. Before Bonomo described it, mites were not considered to be a cause of the disease. It was attributed to humoral factors such as abundant melancholic humor, corrupt blood, or pungent ferment caused by internal ailment. The drawings made by Bonomo in 1687 prove that he did actually study the mite as a causative agent of scabies, observing a tiny worm which reproduced in the human skin. (Under the microscope he had seen an adult mite laying eggs and the turtle-like larvae that hatched.) As an effective therapy, he recommended treating the skin with a sulfur ointment. Macroparasites, such as large tapeworms, could also be observed with the naked eye. By the middle of the nineteenth century, the complete life cycles of a number of parasitic diseases in humans and animals, including ones with a zoonotic character, were elucidated with the aid of microscopes.

A well-known example of a fatal parasitic disease which caused considerable losses among infected sheep or bovine herds in winters was liver-rot. It was long known that this disease was due to the presence of large numbers of parasites in the liver of affected sheep, the so-called liver-fluke or *Fasciola hepatica*. These parasites live in aquatic mud snail species in wet or flooded pastures and thus invaded grazing sheep. The life cycle of sheep liver fluke was experimentally discovered in the period 1881–1883, independently by German zoologist Rudolph Leuckart (1822–1898) and Algernon Thomas (1857–1937), a New Zealand biologist. A major finding in the cycle of pathogenic nematodes was made in 1852 by German physician Friedrich Küchenmeister (1821–1891). Then he published his theory that bladder-worms (cysticerci) are juvenile tapeworms, originating from eggs of these tapeworms. He later proved this by an experiment in which he fed pork containing cysticerci of *Taenia solium* to prisoners awaiting execution. After they had died, he recovered the developing and adult tapeworms in their intestines. It was clear that cysticercosis was caused by the ingestion of the eggs of *Taenia solium*.

Next to his work on liver fluke, Leuckart is also remembered for his work in tapeworms. In 1861 he showed that the bladder-worm *Cysticercus inermis*, found in the masseter muscles of bovines, developed into the long tapeworm *Taenia saginata* in humans. Leuckart also proved that *Taenia saginata* only occurs in cattle (and humans), and *Taenia solium* only in swine (and humans). Another risk was infection with *Taenia echinococcus*, a small tapeworm occurring in dogs, but for which humans are intermediate hosts. Dogs get infected by sheep; eggs from this tapeworm can develop to bladder-worms in the human liver, brain, and lungs. Infection in humans often occurred where many sheep and dogs lived in close contact, such as in Iceland or the Basque country in northern Spain. There, but also elsewhere, slaughter waste of sheep slaughterhouses was fed to working dogs who in turn infected humans. To break this cycle, dogs were banned from slaughterhouse premises. By the results of parasitological research meat inspectors were able to conduct preventive control. Systematic examination of each slaughter animal involving the incision of certain organs and tissues revealed the presence of worms or bladder-worms. The occurrence of these parasites declined during the nineteenth century.

An important parasite that played a significant role in the development of meat inspection is the small roundworm *Trichinella spiralis*. Although known to zoologists, *Trichinella* was not considered harmful until research around 1860 showed that humans could become severely infected. Trichinae predominantly occurs in the intestinal tract of rats and pigs. The larvae encapsulate in their muscle tissue. Humans get infected by consuming raw pork, which could lead to 6 to 30 percent mortality by encapsulation and buildup of trichinae in the heart or diaphragm. In 1835, the first-year medical student James Paget first observed the larval stage of the nematode *Trichinella spiralis* while witnessing an autopsy in a London hospital. He took special interest in the presentation of muscle with white speckles, described as a "sandy diaphragm." However, the credit went to his professor, anatomist Richard Owen, who named the parasite and published a report. However, Owen did not realize that the worm in human muscle was a larval form. Further steps in *Trichinella* research were taken in Germany. The adult worms were described by Rudolf Virchow in 1859. Pathologist Friedrich A. von Zenker (1825–1898) confirmed this observation in 1860 and recognized the clinical significance of the infection, concluding that humans became infected by eating raw pork. Leuckart was the first to document the life cycle of *Trichinella spiralis* both in swine and humans. Von Zenker and Leuckart stressed the public health danger of trichinosis in the 1860s and supported Rudolf Virchow's campaign to create meat inspection laws in Germany.

Due to the consumption of raw ham and sausage, serious outbreaks of trichinella had occurred in Germany, involving hundreds of victims. Between 1860 and 1890, Europe witnessed 90 outbreaks of trichinosis. This was also due to the import of huge quantities of bacon and pork in refrigerated vessels from the United States from 1876 onward. In 1879 the meat from almost 5 million pigs was exported to Europe from the United States, and 8 percent of it turned out to be infected with *Trichinella*. During the nineteenth century, meat inspection was instituted at first mainly on a local level. Particularly in countries with a high consumption of raw pork, federal or national meat inspection included laboratories testing for *Trichinella*.

Germany began banning importation of infected meat, forcing exporting nations (such as the United States) to develop their own meat inspection programs to control animal infections transmissible to humans. Understanding diseases as the result of infection with macroparasites or microparasites (including bacteria) developed in the context of changing ideas about disease causation.

Environmental Theories of Disease Causation

Environmental theories can be summarized in this phrase: the belief that unhealthy environments lead to sick animals (and people). The unpleasant odors of rotting vegetation, trash heaps, and sewers (and even graveyards) were thought to contain particles that caused diseases in people or animals. Disease-causing bad air (*miasmas*) was especially dangerous during climate conditions (heat, wind) that allowed the miasmas to spread widely, causing illness in groups or populations of animals and people. This standard theory of miasmas explained epidemics for centuries. In addition, people often thought that unfamiliar environments produced sickness in animals brought from other places, for example, from the Global North to the Global South or vice versa. This belief played a very important role in imperialism and settler colonialism, because horses and food-producing animals were essential components of both. Especially during the European invasions of areas in the Global South during the nineteenth century, an understanding of how to keep European animals alive and well was critical to imperial success.

During the eighteenth and nineteenth centuries, questions about acclimatization and improvement took on deep sociocultural meaning in the context of European colonialism. Peoples whose lands had been invaded, plundered, and colonized were often characterized as primitive, unimproved, or barbaric, and so were their animals. The ability to "civilize" such animals and peoples depended on the ability to change them according to European expectations. Animal breeding and inheritance were thought to be governed by a combination of heredity and environment. Ongoing ecological imperialism meant that Europeans brought their breeds of domesticated animals with them: horses, cattle, sheep. In new climates and environments, European breeds of animals often did not survive well at first. As we have seen, the specter of diseases hung heavily over circulations of animals between regions and continents. European colonizers complained that each place, from South Africa to Australia to Vietnam, seemed to have its own suite of diseases fatal to European animals.

Europeans believed that animals native to a particular area could survive because they were used to its atmosphere, while "foreign" animals died when brought to the same place. This theory was mainly based on heredity and the notion that different "races" of animals lived naturally in the climate/environment best for them. However, if "foreign" animals survived for a year, they were thought to be "seasoned" or "acclimatized": their bodies had managed to change enough to fit the new environment. To accomplish this, animals needed to be cared for properly, with good stables, clean water, nutritious food, and limited work (especially during very hot days). People who did not follow these careful instructions could expect their animals' health to decline. Another way to create an acclimatized animal population was to interbreed imported animals with the indigenous herds. Native animals, although viewed by Europeans as unproductive and inferior, were interbred with European breeds in the hope that a carefully controlled infusion of native blood would help European animals acclimatize. The resultant offspring often survived more readily in the new environment, reinforcing a hereditary theory about animals' adaptation to new environments.

Environmental theories never entirely disappeared because they explained so many observations about the survival of animals in different environments. Environmental theories were also easily expanded to encompass the idea that parasites and insects caused or spread diseases. A general understanding of how the "seeds of disease" could be present in the atmosphere or air existed at least since the days of the Veronese physician Girolamo Fracastoro (1478–1553). Fracastoro wrote that sick people (or animals) could transmit these "seeds" (*contagium vivum*) by direct contact to people (or animals) around them or by breathing the "seeds" into the air, where they multiplied and spread. Healthy animals could then become infected from the atmosphere. This theory easily accommodated the idea of "germs" spreading through the air, which developed 300 years later. Combined with the power of new technologies, such as the microscope, environmental theories helped to explain the diseases encountered by peoples raising animals in many places, from the warm equatorial regions to the cooler, drier north.

Contagionism and Anti-Contagionism

As we have emphasized in veterinary history, ideas and theories changed slowly over time, and the nineteenth-century debate over the theory of "contagionism" is an excellent example. Some historians of (human) medicine made this debate into a battle between two sides: those scientists who advocated contagion as a cause of disease (contagionists) and those were against it (anti-contagionists). The anti-contagionists were often viewed by these historians as "backward," while the contagionists were portrayed as "progressive" because their ideas led toward our thinking today. But this is historically inaccurate, especially for the case of veterinary medicine, in which we see a spectrum or range of ideas over time (more recent medical histories also take this position). For centuries, people had observed that a healthy animal (or person) could acquire an illness from a sick one; contagionism was not new. But most classical theories of disease causation, from the Ayurvedic to Chinese traditional to Greek humoral theories, defined disease as a functional disorder in the body of the animal. Because these theories were so ancient and widespread, it was difficult for most veterinarians, physicians, and scientists to abandon them. For example, the French veterinary professor Philibert Chabert (1737–1814) believed that the equine disease glanders occurred due to individual predisposition, inadequate feeding, and poor working and housing conditions. Later, a professor named Dupuy at the same veterinary school (Alfort) compared glanders to human tuberculosis, which physicians considered to be a hereditary disease of families rather than a strictly contagious one. (This belief about tuberculosis continued, in some form, into the 1900s.) At the same time, both Chabert and Dupuy acknowledged that glanders spread rapidly in a stable. For the case of glanders, Chabert and Dupuy combined environmental, hereditary, and contagious theories. It was very common for veterinary and medical investigators to use combinations of causation theories to explain diseases.

The leading scientists of the time (1830s–1850s) knew that the body was complex. Illness could occur without any evidence of something foreign entering the body. Whether the body responded with a fever, or pustules, or diarrhea, these symptoms arose from organs and tissues that had their own roles and activities within the body's metabolism – and these activities were causes of "disease" (the lack of normal function). To many scientists, the idea that tiny, unseen particles alone caused disease seemed unrealistic and too simple. In other words, the idea that disease could only be caused by an infectious particle was reductionist – this idea *reduced* the complexity of diseases to one simple thing. But diseases were not simple to veterinarians and physicians; and what they observed was sometimes not completely explained by the reductionist theory of contagion developing in Europe after 1850.

Many anti-contagionists, including the eminent German physician Rudolf Virchow, focused on the complex disease processes within the body. As we described in Chapter 2, Virchow contributed to cell theory and created a new way of classifying and thinking about diseases as pathologies of individual organs. Virchow was the world's expert on animal tissues and how those tissues changed with disease. His explanation for the cause of glanders illustrates the complexity of his thinking. In 1863, Virchow wrote that glanders was transmitted when a horse inhaled some type of irritating agent that stimulated the body to form a granuloma that exuded pus – the distinctive sign of this disease. Aspects of anti-contagionism remained important throughout the late 1800s, bolstered in part by the observation that strict *cordons sanitaires* did not always prevent the spread the most dread diseases. In nineteenth-century veterinary medicine, this point was driven home by the experience of rinderpest. Many scientists fell somewhere in the middle as "contingent contagionists" (those who believed in contagion under certain conditions), and common observation of animal epizootics supported this view.

Contagionists believed that disease could only be passed from one animal to another due to the transfer of a material substance. With their interest in animal diseases and their ability to experiment on animals, veterinarians were early leaders in contagionist research. For example, in 1664 Jacques de Solleysel succeeded in experimentally passing glanders from an infected horse to a healthy one. He wrote that a "venom" transmitted glanders. A century later, the director of the veterinary school at Lyon (France), Claude Bourgelat, confirmed that glanders was directly transmitted to humans when several Lyon veterinary students died of it after being exposed to infected horses and cadavers. The Danish veterinarian Erik Viborg (1759–1822) speculated that a "poison" contained in the pus exuded from the noses of glanderous horses spread the disease. In 1802, Viborg also demonstrated that lymph from the swollen glands of horses with another disease, strangles (*Streptococcus equi*), transmitted that disease to healthy young horses. The French veterinary schools were vibrant centers of research on infectious animal diseases such as glanders, strangles, rinderpest, and sheep pox. They also investigated diseases passed to humans, such as tuberculosis, glanders, and anthrax. Contagionist beliefs were common among the Maasai and Zulu cattle-herders of sub-Saharan Africa, as well. They believed that wildlife, such as wildebeest, impala, and eland, served as reservoirs for diseases that spread to their cattle herds and killed their animals.

By the 1860s, European contagionists were also becoming reductionists: they believed that particles caused diseases to pass from one animal to another. They did not know what these particles were because they could not see them or observe their actions. Especially in the case of diseases caused (as we know today) by viruses, researchers could only trace tissue damage – the footprints of the contagious particles in the animal's body. Jean-Baptiste Auguste Chauveau (1827–1917), professor at the Lyon (France) veterinary school, conducted some of the most important early work on animal and human diseases such as smallpox, anthrax, tuberculosis, and sheep pox (although he is relatively unknown compared to Pasteur and Koch). Chauveau's sheep pox experiments demonstrated the existence of contagious particles in 1868–1869, when he was able to diffuse and filter them out of "virulent liquid" from the pustules of infected sheep. Although Chauveau could not see the particles under the microscope, he believed that they were there because his filtrate caused pox when injected into healthy sheep. This research influenced physicians and scientists, such as the British physiologist John Burdon Sanderson.

Sanderson wrote that he learned Chauveau's techniques while visiting the Lyon veterinary school in 1869 – and he immediately replaced his own "inferior" laboratory methods with those of Chauveau.

By 1870, many contagionists suspected that the infectious particles were living things, not just inert crystals or chemical compounds. The theory of *contagium vivum/contagium animatum*, as declared by Burdon Sanderson, stated that disease was sparked by living particles that had invaded the tissues of the sick animal or person. What sort of life did these particles possess? And what explained their ability to transform from an inactive state to causing tissue damage and the signs of disease? Living things that lived on animals' tissues – these ideas reflected both an understanding of parasitology and agricultural ideas about how seeds grew in the soil. Zoologists and physicians compared the *contagion vivum* to a tiny insect or parasitic "animalcule" – clear references to parasitology. Veterinarians were quite familiar with the problems of internal and external parasites, which multiplied in/on animals' bodies. Too many parasites could cause illness or death in the host animal; by analogy, if the infectious particles were living and reproducing, they too could cause disease in this way. As historian Michael Worboys has shown, among British scientists the agricultural metaphor of "seeds" that germinated in the proper soil also made sense. For disease, the seeds or "germs" literally propagated in animal bodies, but only if the conditions were correct within the body. This explained many problems for contagionists in the late 1800s, for example, why certain diseases affected certain species, and why some animals exposed to the same materials got sick and others did not.

Germ Theories and the Development of Microbiology and Bacteriology

Although microscopes had been used by natural historians before the mid-nineteenth century, technological advances and falling prices made these tools much more widely available by 1850 and increased the resolution with which people could observe insects, parasites, and other microorganisms. Not surprisingly, the rod-shaped *Bacillus anthracis*, one of the biggest bacteria (length 8 microns), was the first pathogen for which the microstructure was identified. It took decades before mechanical innovations in microscopy, such as compound, polarizing, and phase-contrast microscopes and immersion oil, enabled the identification of smaller bacteria. Within this context, the microscope became the symbol of medical and veterinary progress in the nineteenth century, as did the stethoscope around the neck of medical and veterinary doctors.

In the mid-1800s, scientists in Europe had developed several "germ theories" that linked organisms visible under the microscope with diseases of animals and humans. (Similar theories had been proposed much earlier, by

Fracastoro in 1546, for example, but did not catch on at the time.) Many others studied the tiny organisms, known today as *bacteria*, devoting their careers to "discovering," naming, and classifying bacteria. Some bacterial species are named after a person, for instance *Salmonella* spp., after the American microbiologist Daniel Salmon. Others are named after the shape of the organism such as *Campylobacter* spp. (*kampulos* [Greek], meaning "curved") or the location where the bacterium occurs (*Escherichia coli*, which lives in the colon). *E. coli* is also named after the discoverer, the German physician Theodor Escherich. Although most bacterial species are not pathogenic for animals or humans, these scientists were most interested in the pathogens. They classified bacteria using criteria including shape, size, and position of the bacterial cell; its reaction to chemical dyes; its morphology and activity (flagella, for example); and whether it could transform into spores. Three basic shapes of bacteria were observed: spherical (*coccus*), rod-shaped (*bacillus*), or curved rod shape (comma or spiral form). One of the most commonly used classifications today is based on the microorganisms' reactions to chemical dyes, Gram staining, a color reaction developed by the Dane Hans Christian Gram (1853–1938). Different structures of the bacterial cell walls react differently to the dyes/stains, dividing bacteria into the categories of Gram positive (taking up purple stain) or Gram negative (taking up pink/red stain).

The development of histological techniques from around 1780 onward included microtomes, fixation, and embedding techniques and staining methods to differentiate between various tissues and cells. These techniques stimulated research on the concept of tissues and cells and particularly lesions therein. The same is true for cytology and blood research. Classical methods in bacteriology included culturing methods with various media, in vitro experiments with flasks, test tubes, Petri dishes, centrifuges, and incubators. Louis Pasteur, for instance, cultured bacteria in liquid media during his research on alcohol and lactic acid fermentation. He thus proved that spontaneous generation of microorganisms did not occur. He also showed that avoiding food spoilage by means of heating (later called pasteurization or sterilization), a technique used in canning, was based on killing bacteria. Robert Koch introduced solid media (gelatin, agar) and aniline coloring agents to stain bacteria to better visualize and classify these. Developments in chemical methods enabled the determination of the chemical composition of foods (protein, carbohydrates, fat), which initiated the discourse on healthy food for humans and animals alike.

For the next several decades, the specifics of exactly how these microorganisms caused disease were open to investigation and debate, and scientists around the world joined their European counterparts in the race to discover various "germs" and how they affected animals' bodies. At this time (1850–1900), European institutes were the centers of scientific training; but most veterinarians could not afford to study there. This was certainly true for those from the Americas, which were (in the words of one U.S. veterinarian in the 1880s) a scientific backwater at the time. The few elite veterinarians who had trained in Europe were especially keen to use the new laboratory techniques to solve disease problems. As we will see, they used the exciting new techniques of bacteriology/microbiology to hunt for the microbes that caused disease, which sometimes succeeded and other times led to premature assertions. It was not uncommon for a disease later determined to be caused by plant toxicity or viruses to be wrongly attributed to bacteria at first. Like other scientific theories, germ theories were not *one* unified theory; nor were these ideas understood and deployed the same way everywhere. Ideas about germs and disease traveled and changed somewhat as they moved around the world, and different people understood them and used them in different ways.

Veterinary disease problems are excellent examples of the complex ways in which germ ideas and practices were deployed. During outbreaks of rinderpest in Britain in 1865 and India in 1869, British veterinarians were well aware of the new germ ideas, and many were also contagionists. But they were practical, too. The benefits of inoculation against rinderpest were still uncertain in the 1860s. (This pre-Pasteurian form of inoculation existed but was not reliably effective.) Led by the Gamgee, British veterinarians advocated a system of isolation and stamping-out the disease by killing all cattle in infected herds. This made sense based on long experience with the disease and the high level of government concern. But the germ theories promised even more, according to its supporters: tests to detect the disease (without injuring the animal) and vaccines to prevent it from spreading to healthy animals. The promise of prevention was particularly appealing to agricultural leaders and government officials since it would potentially save a great of money. It was in the realm of agricultural chemistry that some of the most famous discoveries about animal diseases would be made.

Louis Pasteur (1822–1895), considered to be the father of microbiology, was a French chemist who began his research career studying the diseases of wine grapes for the French government. Pasteur and his colleagues were skilled with microscopes and with techniques borrowed from agricultural chemistry, and they carried out a series of elegant experiments that called into question the ancient doctrine of spontaneous generation (life could generate from anything). Studying microorganisms in flasks of broth led Pasteur to imagine the processes of disease developing in the body as a kind of "fermentation," a process that could be interrupted or controlled. Working with the physiologist Claude Bernard, Pasteur focused on fermentation in fluids such as milk and urine. He invented a process ("pasteurization") that could stop the fermentation and kill the "diseases" of wine, beer, and milk. He then wondered if diseases in animals worked in a similar way and spent five years studying silkworm diseases. These experiences prepared him to begin studying veterinary diseases in the 1870s. As we will see, Pasteur was well connected and well read; and he was very good at what we today would call "science communication" and "public relations." Pasteur also stood on the shoulders of several French physicians and veterinarians and employed some extremely talented people in his laboratory (such as Charles Chamberland). Much has been written about Pasteur, so we will refocus the Pasteurian story from the veterinary point of view.

Pasteur was not the only researcher working on animal diseases in the 1870s; another major figure is veterinarian Jean Joseph Henri Toussaint (1847–1890), an 1869 graduate of the Lyon veterinary school. In 1876, Toussaint took up a professorship at the Toulouse veterinary school, where he taught anatomy, physiology, and zoology. But his passion was the rapidly developing field of microbiology. He began by analyzing blood, urine, and tissue samples of animals dying of sepsis and other diseases, and (like other researchers at that time) saw bacteria under the lens of his microscope. Beginning work on chicken cholera, an epidemic disease of poultry, he found large numbers of bacteria that he thought caused the disease. Toussaint sent Pasteur some cultures, and Pasteur famously (as a result of a coincidence) inoculated healthy chickens with old cultures. The chickens not only survived but did not die when they were later inoculated with large amounts of live, virulent cultures. Pasteur concluded that this was a way to create a vaccine: by exposing the cultures to oxygen for a time, they became weakened and could then be safely used in healthy animals. Meanwhile, Toussaint began trying to weaken the cultures of the bacteria that he found in animals that had died of anthrax.

Rabies was the disease that made Pasteur internationally famous. In the 1880s, Pasteur's laboratory began inoculating rabies-infected material from sick animals directly into the brains of dogs and rabbits, reasoning that the "canine madness" developed there. When experimental animals died, the scientists removed the brain and spinal cord tissue. By drying and preparing these tissues, Pasteur's laboratory created a crude vaccine that could protect rabies-exposed dogs by inoculating them with successively more virulent material. Today we understand this effect as stimulating the immune system to fight the virus; but at that time Pasteur did not know exactly how it worked. This was still true when he undertook his most risky experiment in 1885: inoculating a human, a 9-year-old boy who had been badly bitten by a rabid dog. Pasteur used his series of inoculations, and the boy recovered. Pasteur became famous, and his laboratory began mass-producing the rabies inoculation material. This method was not perfect, however: it caused some serious side effects; some scientists feared that it could actually cause the disease; and many laypeople were opposed to putting foreign "putrid" material into their bodies. (There were even anti-vaccination groups.) As we have seen, new ideas and procedures take time to become widely accepted. However, Pasteur's fame for saving the lives of rabies victims was rewarded when the French government paid to establish a new, state-of-the-art microbiological laboratory, the Institut Pasteur in Paris. There, scientists conducted research on both veterinary and human medical disease problems, including rabies, anthrax, silkworm diseases, and cholera in chickens. It was an early center of comparative medical research and the pride of France.

Pasteur had a German competitor, however, in the physician Robert Koch (1843–1920). Reflecting the political enmity between their two countries, the advocates of Pasteur and Koch waged bitter battles over who was the greatest microbiologist/bacteriologist. From the veterinary point of view, the approaches and practices of Pasteurians and Koch's followers were different and complementary. Pasteur founded *microbiology*, the study of microorganisms such as bacteria, fungi, and protozoans; Koch founded *bacteriology*, which was more narrowly focused on bacteria. (We can think of *bacteriology* as a subdivision of *microbiology*.) While Pasteur's chemical manipulations created vaccines and other tools, Koch systematically developed the techniques of culturing, staining, and manipulating bacteria. Most of these tools and techniques eventually became important in veterinary practice, and many are still used today (including the pink and purple stains, eosin and hematoxylin). Koch was mentored by Rudolf Virchow and the German anatomist/pathologist Friedrich G.J. Henle, who wrote the influential treatise *Von den Miasmen und Kontagien und von den miasmatisch-kontagiösen Krankheiten (On the Miasmas and Contagions and Miasmatic-contagious Diseases)* that stimulated the discourse on germ theories. Henle is remembered for drawing up the fundamental rules for the clear definition of disease-causing microbes, the so-called microbiological postulates. In 1884 his postulates were refined by Robert Koch and Friedrich Löffler, based on their research on the etiology of cholera and tuberculosis. These postulates were published by Koch in 1890 as a fundamental basis for proving a microorganism caused a disease. (See textbox.)

The Henle-Koch Postulates (Robert Koch, Friedrich Löffler, and Friedrich G.J. (Jacob) Henle)
    First used by Koch to establish the etiologies of cholera and tuberculosis; published 1890.
    For a microorganism to cause a disease:

1. The microorganism must be present in large numbers in animals with signs of the specific disease. The microorganism must not be present in healthy animals.
2. The microorganism must be isolated from sick animals and grown in pure culture.
3. When inoculated with the microorganism, healthy animals must become ill with the same disease.
4. A pure culture of the microorganisms must then be isolated from these sick animals; it must be identical to the microorganism isolated from the original sick animal.

In the 1870s, Koch was working as a country physician when cattle in the area began to die of anthrax. Koch knew this disease could infect multiple species (including humans). As we described in Chapter 2, anthrax was a common and deadly disease that several scientists had been studying for decades. In 1849, Koch's countryman F.A.A. Pollender observed little solid rod-shaped bodies (*stabförmiger Köperchen*) in the blood of an infected cow under his microscope (he published his findings in 1855). Another German, Christian Joseph Fuchs (1801–1871), later a professor at the Karlsruhe veterinary school, had noticed many granulated threads in the blood of a cow with anthrax in 1842. In the late 1840s, French physician P.F.O. Rayer and his student, Casimir Davaine, also found small, elongated bodies present in anthrax-infected blood and tissues obtained from the Montmartre (Paris) abattoir. They were able to infect healthy sheep by injecting blood from sick animals, and they published their results (setting off a battle with the Germans about who was "first" to identify the causative microorganisms).

Working with the most sophisticated microscope of the time, with a Zeiss oil-immersion lens, Koch observed numerous rod-shaped microorganisms in the blood of dying animals. With his more sophisticated microscope, he was able to see the microorganisms much more clearly than his predecessors had; and he found it in both sheep and cattle. Koch knew anthrax was a zoonotic disease. (Remarkably, Koch kept cultures and infected experimental animals in his house, but he and his wife did not become ill.) Veterinarian Friedrich Brauell (1807–1882) in Tartu, Estonia, was the first to demonstrate anthrax bacilli in human blood in 1856. The blood originated from his veterinary assistant, who had contracted anthrax from dissecting an infected sheep and then died of the disease. This tragic accident enabled Brauell to connect human anthrax with the disease in sheep, and he suspected the bacilli were the factor that transmitted the disease. In 1860, Henri M.O. Delafond (1805–1861), director of the veterinary school of Alfort, France, succeeded in culturing anthrax rods in small jars. However, he could not decide whether these were the cause or result of the disease. Delafond performed thorough research on anthrax cadavers, and he introduced the use of rabbits as test animals.

Building on all this work, Koch was able to infect experimental animals and he figured out how to grow the microorganisms in the aqueous humor from cow's eyes (obtained at the local slaughterhouse) by 1875. He was even able to watch the microorganisms, named *Bacillus anthracis*, form spores when exposed to the air. He suspected that the rod-shaped bacilli, in their normal life's activities, caused damage to the host animal's body and thus signs of the disease. However, a question remained: did the rod-shaped microorganisms *themselves* cause the tissue damage and signs of the disease, or did the damage result from some other "poison" from the sick animal's blood? Koch ruled out poison or toxicity by transferring the rod-shaped bacilli into fresh aqueous humor up to 20 times; in this process, any poison or other chemical would have been washed away. After 20 transfers, the bacilli still caused the disease when injected into healthy experimental animals. The microorganism kept multiplying even as it traveled from one animal or culture to the next, thus establishing a chain of infection. Koch demonstrated his findings to other scientists and managed to persuade them of his theory. In 1876, Koch published his famous paper, "The Etiology of Anthrax Based on the Developmental Cycle of *Bacillus anthracis*," which established a definite linkage between the presence and life cycle of a microorganism and the tissue damage and signs of the disease in host animals.

This represented a major change in understanding diseases. Diseases could be understood as generalized phenomena, such as *fevers*. They could also be specific to organs, such as *nephritis* (kidney disease). Germ theories of disease causation made diseases *specific* to a particular microorganism. Koch believed that an animal with anthrax must have *Bacillus anthracis* in its body. Otherwise, it did not have true anthrax. Many people, including many other scientists, did not believe this at first. However, Koch's research, particularly observing the *Bacillus anthracis* life cycle, explained many aspects of anthrax that had puzzled observers for centuries. The disease seemed to reappear in "cursed fields" for years. Koch explained this by showing that the *Bacillus* spores survived harsh conditions for long periods of time. When animals grazed on the same pasture in later years, the spores were still there – sitting and waiting for the next host animals. Activated by the warm, moist, and mainly anaerobic conditions inside the body, the *Bacillus* emerged from its spore-shell and began to multiply. Rapid multiplication explained how quickly the disease could kill an infected animal. Koch's careful and detailed experiments, and a public presentation, persuaded many scientists that the living, multiplying *Bacillus* and not a blood-borne chemical poison caused the disease, but not everyone agreed. In France, Jean Joseph Henri Toussaint and Louis Pasteur, working separately to test the microorganism-contagion theory, conducted further experiments that supported Koch's conclusions and began to test possible vaccines to stimulate immunity to pathogens.

Toussaint, professor of anatomy and physiology at the Toulouse veterinary school, had been a pupil of French veterinary pathologist Auguste Chauveau. Both were interested in how animals developed immunity to pathogens. In 1880, Toussaint achieved promising results by applying low concentrations of phenolic acid and heat to anthrax microorganisms (*Bacillus anthracis*), thus creating an inactivated anti-anthrax vaccine. Toussaint double-vaccinated about twenty sheep in a successful trial conducted at a farm belonging to the Alfort veterinary school. Hearing reports of Toussaint's success, Louis Pasteur and his colleagues began experiments using Toussaint's method. In 1881,

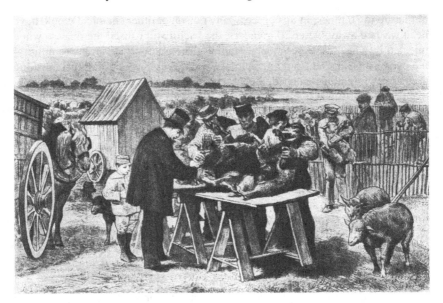

Figure 4.6 Louis Pasteur's vaccination against anthrax during a trial in Pouilly-le-Fort on May 31, 1881.
Source: L' Illustration, November 3, 1881.

Pasteur was challenged to make a public demonstration of an anti-anthrax vaccination at a farm in the commune of Pouilly-le-Fort, France (Fig. 4.6). Groups of sheep were vaccinated with either Pasteur's secret vaccine or placebo; then challenged with anthrax infection. This public experiment was an international sensation in the newspapers, and the pressure on Pasteur and his colleagues was intense to prove the value of germ theories and vaccines. Fortunately for them, the vaccinated sheep survived – a successful trial of the Pasteurian anti-anthrax vaccine. Although Pasteur received the credit for creating the successful anti-anthrax vaccine, historians later discovered that he and his colleagues had in fact used *Toussaint*'s method – without Toussaint's knowledge, and without giving Toussaint proper credit for his discovery. From his provincial and junior position, Toussaint was unable to battle Pasteur for priority; and, suffering from a severe neurological illness, he died at a young age. Overall, the anthrax vaccine story gives us some insight into scientists' "race for fame" during the late nineteenth century. It also demonstrates how scientists from different disciplines (veterinarians, chemists, physicians, etc.) worked on similar research topics, an important basis for comparative pathology and "one medicine."

Comparative Pathology and "One Medicine"

The phrase "one medicine" (OM) was created by German physician Rudolf Virchow, whom we introduced in the discussion about pathology in Chapter 2. However, the similarities between animal and human disease had already been noticed. Based on autopsies and feedback from the pathology dissection table to the clinic, these scholars were convinced that the cause of disease lay in abnormalities in organs (lesions), abnormal tissues, and cells, as described by Giovanni Batista Morgagni (1672–1771), Pierre Louis (1787–1872), Xavier Bichat (1771–1802), and Rudolph Virchow. The Paris hospital also stimulated the development and use of diagnostic tools such as the stethoscope from René Laennec (1781–1826), the percussion hammer, the ophthalmoscope, and the fever thermometer. Between 1850 and 1900, comparative pathology and OM formed the network of scientific relationships and research methods in which the various European theories of disease causation were investigated. Comparative pathology and OM developed from the combined influences of Darwinian evolutionary ideas, observations about animal and human bodies and diseases, and the developing laboratory sciences.

The British natural historian Charles Darwin (1809–1882) was a wealthy gentleman farmer who bred and raised animals such as fancy pigeons. Popular animal breeding influenced Darwin's publication, *On the Origin of Species* (1859), which was a public sensation. In this study, Darwin laid out a theory of biological evolution for all life on the earth. According to this theory, all species should arise and develop through a process of natural selection of inherited variations by which the individual's ability to survive is increased. Certain variations would then increase in animal populations over many generations. *Origin* synthesized several existing lines of European thought about the development of life on earth over long periods of time, using practical examples (such as breeding cattle) to provide evidence for its conclusions. *Origin*'s conclusions transformed the human–animal relationship, animal breeding, and ideas about animals' susceptibility to injury and disease. Most famously, supporters of Darwinian evolution directly linked the ancestry of humans and non-human animals. This sparked intense controversy in some societies, based on the theological belief that a deity created humans separately from all other animals. Anatomists had, for centuries, noticed homologies (similarities) between human and animal bodies. For scientific veterinary medicine, human–animal homologies supported the idea of "one medicine" and the use of animals as experimental proxies for humans. Human and animal bodies could be similarly studied as susceptible to certain diseases, in need of acclimatization when moving to different regions, and subject to "improvement" through controlled heredity or breeding.

Observations about human and animal health and disease confirmed this theoretical relationship, particularly with comparative anatomy (see Chapter 1) and comparative pathology. Comparative pathology is the study of abnormalities caused by disease in animal and human bodies. Because they could freely perform postmortem examinations, the more elite veterinarians were experienced and skilled pathologists. In the late 1800s, pathologists added histological and microscopic examinations of tissues to their postmortem observations, thus expanding pathology to include the rapidly developing laboratory sciences. Many of the diseases studied by pathologists were zoonoses, so it made sense for physicians and veterinarians to work together. Also, animal diseases provided proxies, or models, for human diseases. Finally, epizootics were expensive and devastating, and governments relied on scientists from multiple disciplines to address them. Sometimes the investigators themselves became "test subjects." For example, in the 1880s–1890s it became clear that glanders is caused by infection with a bacterium (*B. mallei*). Knowing that glanders was a potentially fatal zoonosis, Latvian veterinarian Kristaps Helmanis (1848–1892) in St. Petersburg (Russia) and Oto Kalniņš (1856–1891) in Tartu (Estonia) worked hard to develop a specific and sensitive diagnostic, the "mallein test" for horses and other equids. Tragically, Kalniņš and some of Helmanis' co-workers died after becoming infected with *B. mallei*, thus proving this bacillus' zoonotic infection capabilities.

Helmanis was a leader in establishing both a Pasteur Institute and studies on zoonotic diseases at the Institute for Experimental Medicine in St. Petersburg (IEM). This outstanding multifield biological research center brought together interdisciplinary teams of scientists who made many contributions to knowledge about infectious diseases in both humans and animals. In many other places, however, the problem for veterinarians was that physicians often attempted to exclude them from scientific investigations. Also, highly trained veterinarians were busy controlling disease outbreaks and had less time to do basic research. There were only 20 or 30 trained veterinary pathologists working around the world in the late 1800s. Many had low-level positions with little money or support; and technologies such as the microtome, mounting media and coverslips for microscope slides, were crude and expensive. Nonetheless, veterinary comparative pathologists worked long hours to collect information from postmortems, microscopic observations, and animal experiments.

Using comparative pathology techniques, veterinary and medical researchers sought to understand the entire course of a disease within the body – human and animal. This was especially true in French veterinary research, where Auguste Chauveau, Henri Bouley, and other veterinary leaders studied human and animal pox viruses (vaccinia, variola, cowpox, and sheep pox) and Jean Joseph Henri Toussaint became the second scientist (after Koch) to successfully cultivate a pathogen (chicken cholera). The research of Chauveau and others was based in the French veterinary schools, and this model spread to other nations. Early veterinary education in Romania in the 1850s, for example, was established by General Dr Carol Davila (1828–1884) and taught by him and the surgeon Vasile Lucaci (1806–1890) in the Bucharest medical school until the Higher School of Veterinary Medicine was founded in the 1880s. In the Western Hemisphere, several veterinary schools were established on the model of comparative medicine. By the late nineteenth century, this included the Montréal Veterinary College and related professional associations (Québec, Canada); the School of Veterinary Medicine at the University of Pennsylvania (Philadelphia, USA); and the (now defunct) New York College of Veterinary Surgeons and Comparative Medicine and Columbia Veterinary College and School of Veterinary Medicine (New York City, USA). Here, veterinarians such as Duncan McEachran (1841–1924) and physicians including William Osler (1849–1919) led the development of veterinary comparative medicine in full partnership. This emphasis in veterinary education trained generations of North American veterinarians to see themselves and their work as contributions to "one medicine," including finding the causes of diseases.

Researchers worked hard to find bacteria and other microorganisms that caused the major animal diseases, but some diseases yielded their secrets more quickly than others. Bovine tuberculosis is an excellent example. The famous Robert Koch figured out how to stain and culture *Mycobacterium tuberculosis*, an acid-fast bacterium that he and others established as the causative organism of human tuberculosis. For 25 years, microbe hunters (including Koch) used comparative medicine techniques to try to understand the relationship between bovine and human tuberculosis. Koch developed tuberculin, which he thought might be a treatment for human tuberculosis; but unfortunately, tuberculin did not help sick patients. Instead, it became a testing tool – for both humans and animals (cattle). Veterinarians visiting Koch's laboratory carried tuberculin back home with them; this included the American Leonard Pearson (1868–1908), who conducted the first tuberculin testing on cattle in the Western Hemisphere in 1892. Between 1895 and 1902, researchers in the United States and Europe debated whether tuberculosis in animals was a different disease from that in humans. Koch famously declared that these were two different diseases; and the American bacteriologist Theobald Smith (1859–1934) separated *M. tuberculosis bovis* from *M. tuberculosis* in 1898. However, veterinarians and other scientists were correct in asserting that bovine tuberculosis (*M. tb. bovis*) was transmissible to humans, where it caused serious infections in children (Pott's disease of the spine, for example).

Comparative medicine and developments in laboratory research slowly changed veterinary education, training, and status over the next century. From around 1850 onward, the status of professional scientists began to grow.

As a result of the strong growth of scientific knowledge, the gap between laymen and scholars increased. By 1900, scientifically trained experts had obtained higher prestige, particularly after scientific breakthroughs. The position and functioning of universities also changed. Universities were mainly the sites of classical education until the 1850s. Then a professionalization and scientization process began, in which research financed by governments or scientific foundations began to be more important within universities. University graduates were no longer financially dependent on an audience of interested laymen, from which they distinguished themselves and who were excluded more and more. Graduates also organized themselves into professional associations for engineers, physicists, chemists, physicians, veterinarians, and many others.

How did these technological and intellectual developments affect physicians and veterinarians' practices? They benefited not only from the feedback from pathological findings to the clinic, but also from the use of newly developed diagnostic tools such as the stethoscope (auscultation). This was part of the systematic way of examining and diagnosing patients by inspection, palpation, percussion, and auscultation. In addition, the new knowledge on microbiology was also applied in the clinic where disinfection, aseptic surgery, became the standard. In 1867, English physician Joseph Lister (1827–1912) successfully introduced spraying phenol to sterilize surgical instruments and to clean infected wounds. Instead of wood, leather, bone, horn, and ivory, human and veterinary medical instrument manufacturing companies designed equipment of metal and glass that could be easily sterilized. Next to sterile surgery and obstetrics, which decreased mortality significantly, the introduction of general anesthesia, applied first in 1846 with diethyl ether, and local anesthesia with cocaine since 1884, had dramatically changed standard surgical practices in both human and veterinary medicine by 1900.

The development of prophylactic vaccines and treatments instigated a breakthrough in the acknowledgement of medical and veterinary progress after 1900. This process would continue into the twentieth century (Chapter 5), and it owed its success in part to the growing value of the basic sciences in informing medical and veterinary practice (Table 4.1).

As with physicians, veterinarians could increasingly rely on the tools generated by scientific investigations: cultivation of bacteria, diagnostic tests, sera, and vaccines. But this process was slow, and sometimes these new tools and products did not change basic veterinary practices very much. Veterinarians still controlled livestock epizootics using the time-tested *cordons sanitaires* and slaughtering sick or exposed animals, and they treated illnesses, lameness, and injuries in horses with the old techniques of drenching, cauterizing, and suturing. Even after they were developed, specialized medications and treatments sometimes remained too expensive for use in larger animals in the early twentieth century. However, veterinarians increasingly began caring for

Table 4.1. *Milestones in microbiology and therapy*

MILESTONES IN MICROBIAL STUDIES AND THERAPY, 1840–1880

General theories of disease causation, the development of scientific disciplines, and technologies as they influenced Western veterinary medicine

1   C. 1840 THEORIES

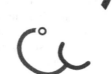

- Imbalance of *qi, prana* or humors
- Miasma theory
- *Contagium vivum*
- Spiritual or divine causes
- Technologies: stethoscope, compound microscope

2   C. 1850 PARASITOLOGY

- Technologies: dissection, compound microscope, microtome
- Tapeworms, roundworms (Paget, Owen, Leuckart, Von Zenker)
- *Trichina*, pathologies of tissues, cellular theory (Virchow)

3   C. 1880 MICROBIOLOGY / BACTERIOLOGY

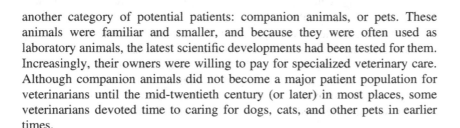

- Technologies: oil immersion microscopes, vaccines, antisepsis techniques, culturing & staining
- Microscopic "animalcules" and microorganisms
- Anthrax (Davaine, Koch, Toussaint, Pasteur)
- Tuberculosis (bovine, human) (Koch)

another category of potential patients: companion animals, or pets. These animals were familiar and smaller, and because they were often used as laboratory animals, the latest scientific developments had been tested for them. Increasingly, their owners were willing to pay for specialized veterinary care. Although companion animals did not become a major patient population for veterinarians until the mid-twentieth century (or later) in most places, some veterinarians devoted time to caring for dogs, cats, and other pets in earlier times.

Pets and Pet Keeping

Dogs, cats, and other small animals had lived alongside humans for thousands of years. These animals assisted with hunting and security, with herding domesticated animals, and with controlling rodents that infested humans' food supplies. They also provided companionship and, in some cultures, were worshipped or accompanied humans to the afterlife. Historians have found clues in documents, paintings, archaeological artifacts, and other sources that indicate how highly different groups of people valued animals for emotional, cultural, and religious reasons. It is reasonable to assume that animal healers provided services for these animals, which were often well cared for and well fed. With the eighteenth-century formation of the veterinary profession, however, there is not much evidence that they spent much time treating companion animals. Companion animals kept by very wealthy people were the obvious exceptions. By the late nineteenth century, veterinary practices and schools in urban areas increasingly treated the illnesses and injuries of dogs and other pet animals. Of course, these animals' proximity to humans also exposed people to zoonotic diseases, such as rabies and parasitic worms transmitted by infected dogs; these problems were research topics for veterinarians and other scientists.

Dogs, cats, birds, and other small animals were also the main victims of animal experiments conducted from the sixteenth century onward (the period covered by this book). Anatomists such as Gasparo Aselli and William Harvey sought to understand the functions of the living animal body, and they established *vivisection* (dissecting a living animal) as a crucial practice for physiology research. By the time the first modern veterinary schools were founded in France, questions about the very nature of life and how animals' bodies functioned were worked out using experiments that we find cruel today (remembering that anesthesia was not available or widely used until the end of the 1800s). Inherent in this experimental model was the assumption that animal bodies' functions were analogous to those of humans, and that knowledge about animal physiology informed that of humans. Although anatomists and physiologists defended vivisection as the only way to unravel the body's mysteries, their critics developed and published anti-vivisection arguments by the 1700s. Along with multiple entries about horses and other domesticated animals, Diderot and D'Alembert's famous *Encyclopédie* (see Chapter 3) included medical articles written by vitalists against experimentation on living animals. Not only were such experiments cruel to the animals, but they also failed to yield good results due to the trauma on the animal's body.

By the mid-1800s, love for companion animals combined with concerns about the cruelty of many animals' lives stimulated wealthy Britons to form popular societies devoted to protecting animals. They drew on the earlier writings of Jeremy Bentham (see Chapter 2), John Lawrence, and others who argued that animals could suffer and therefore had a right to be protected in civilized societies. This philosophical idea was the basis for parliamentary legislation, from the 1822 Martin's Act onward, which provided limited protection to domesticated animals. Initially, British animal protection groups focused on the most visible signs of animal cruelty: overwork and abuse of the horses that did the hard work of transporting people and goods. In India, where bullocks did this work, colonial British authorities formed societies for the prevention of cruelty to animals in the 1860s. Bengali members of these societies argued that ancient Vedic principles called for treating animals kindly. Concern about the welfare of working horses expanded into other groups that advocated vegetarianism and opposed animal experimentation.

In Western Europe and the United States, the growing urban middle class often adopted cats and dogs as domestic companions. After a long history of adoration and affection on the one hand and demonization and killing as a result of superstition and disease (rabies) on the other hand, these animals were becoming accepted members of middle-class households. Cat and dog pedigree associations were established, organizing dog shows and exhibitions with prizes. Pets were depicted as iconic and aesthetic subjects by artists in newspapers, books, and art exhibits. Authors and artists portrayed companion animals as emblems of civilized morality and economic success. At the same time, the rise of companion animals led to a paradox of exploitation and affection for the different kinds of animals that reflected how people valued them. Due to urbanization, livestock disappeared from urban citizens' experiences, especially in wealthy countries. Urban officials created laws that banned pigs, cattle, and other animals. Urban citizens no longer saw slaughterhouses and other reminders of the short and often brutal lives led by livestock, and horses were beginning to disappear from cities. Increasingly, urban citizens' main exposure to animals was seeing dogs, cats, and other companion animals. Kindness to these animals covered up the harsh reality of other animals' lives. This difference between the emotional treatment of small animals in cities and the commercial approach toward livestock in the countryside only intensified during the next century.

In Britain, its colonies, European nations, and the United States, the gospel of animal protection increasingly centered on dogs at the end of the nineteenth century. Popular dog stories and dog "heroes" encouraged ordinary people to view dogs as special – the "best friends" of humans who deserved the best care. Unfortunately, many dogs suffered homelessness or ill treatment. The worst fate for dogs was to become a subject of medical experimentation by medical or veterinary students. Dogs had been used for vivisection for centuries. But with the increasing popularity of pet ownership in many European nations, animal protection advocates increasingly argued that medics' cruelty to dogs led to cruel treatment of humans. Many anti-vivisectionists believed that the serotherapies, vaccines, and other products of medical research were immoral and tainted because they were tested and produced by animals' suffering. The crude serotherapies, they argued, introduced foreign material into peoples' bodies even as the development of these biologicals required cruel experiments on laboratory and experimental animals. Medical researchers responded to these criticisms by arguing that the lives of a few animals could save those of many humans, and that modern medical science was essential to "civilized" society. Veterinarians could not make the same argument, but as we will see in the next chapter, they too justified animal experimentation in terms of humanitarianism and institutionalized the practice of using animal bodies for experiments and demonstrations.

This had some unintended consequences. European Enlightenment principles of the eighteenth and nineteenth centuries encouraged the recognition of suffering, both animal and human, and social principles that would maximize happiness and humanitarianism. By establishing similarities between humans and animal bodies, natural philosophers contributed to concerns about animal suffering and its effects on humans. Conducting public or semi-public demonstrations about animal physiology, such as suffocating birds and small animals in Robert Boyle's air-pump apparatus, inadvertently brought their own observational and experimental methods under broader scrutiny. Was vivisection justifiable? Even Albrecht von Haller found his animal experiments to be gruesome, and he questioned whether they were justified on moral grounds. It is important to remember, also, that these new ideas were seldom accepted right away – especially if they contradicted long-standing medical practices, since most experimenters were philosophers or physicians.

In the United States, animal protection associations maintained veterinary hospitals in large cities that treated horses and pet animals. The most famous was New York's Society for the Prevention of Cruelty to Animals "hospital for dumb animals," which provided veterinary care for 15,000 dogs, 4,000 cats, and 2,000 horses each year by 1910. These hospitals promoted the idea of medical care for pet animals, and pet owner's affection for their animals encouraged them to seek and pay for veterinary care. Veterinarians in large European and American cities established private hospitals for pets (which also provided boarding) in the early 1900s (Fig. 4.7). Some were lavish, with a home-like atmosphere complete with women attendants to care for and play with the animals. Still, most veterinarians in private practice cared for a few dogs and cats in the context of a general practice located in an office or a day clinic. To treat pet animals, veterinarians needed to change the way they viewed their patients. Horses, cattle, and other animals were economically valuable. Dogs and cats were not; but their value lay with the "sentiment" attached to them by their owners. Unlike the rough men working with livestock, these animals' owners were often women and children. They expected

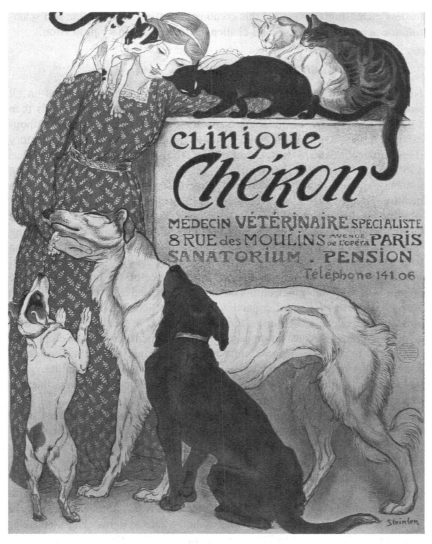

Figure 4.7 Poster of Clinique Chéron in Paris from 1905 in art nouveau style by T.A. Steinlen (1859–1923).
Courtesy: Rijksmuseum Amsterdam RP-P-1968-308, public domain.

kind treatment, clean facilities, and the use of the latest anesthetic and analgesic techniques. By the 1920s, pet owners increasingly expected scientifically trained veterinarians to provide the same services for pets that their owner could expect at a hospital for humans. During the next century, veterinary leaders increasingly leveraged this combination of emotional value and scientific medicine to survive several challenges to the veterinary profession.

The Intensifying Storms of War

Nineteenth-century wars relied heavily on animal power, and armies on all sides expected to sacrifice more horses, oxen, dogs, and other animals than soldiers. Early in the century, the Napoleonic Wars used hundreds of thousands of horses. Military conflicts continued throughout the nineteenth century (Peninsular War, 1807–1814; Crimean War, 1853–1856; American Civil War, 1861–1865; Franco-Prussian War 1870–1871; several colonial wars) requiring a steady stream of war animals and healers or veterinarians to keep them healthy. To specialize in this veterinary field, armies sent students to the early veterinary schools and paid for their education. Some schools, for instance in Germany and Turkey, were mainly established for the purpose of training military veterinarians and their curriculum focused on the problems common to military horses, including horseshoeing. Many nations established formal military veterinary services with veterinary inspectors at home and in the colonies during the nineteenth century. Established in 1880, the British Army's Veterinary School trained veterinary officers in basic first aid of animals, the selection of horses for remounts, and tropical diseases. A new Army Veterinary Department replaced the old regimental system of employing army vets. In other countries, similar military veterinary services were established, in the homeland as well as in their colonies. A corps of military vets developed around the world, although it took a long time before veterinarians reached the higher ranks as officers.

Since the horse was so important for mobility during warfare, army commanders wanted to have enough horses available as a backup, immediately behind the forward moving troops. These horses were kept at temporary stations ("remount depots"), along with hospitals for horses and dogs returning from the battlefield. Army veterinarians inspected the animals before purchasing, maintained the healthy horses, treated injuries and illnesses, and dealt with stray animals and euthanasia. The Napoleonic Wars were excellent early examples of the need for these complex horse care systems. The Peninsular War (1807–1814) was a military conflict between Napoleonic France, which invaded the Iberian Peninsula for control over Spain and Portugal. The British Army joined the fight in support of Spain. In this campaign and all Napoleonic Wars, the horse played a significant role. The newly established veterinary service of the British Army was organized by regiment at that time: horse doctors were recruited directly into cavalry regiments. They saw the problems of trying to maintain replacement horses, care for the injured and recover the stray horses, especially when the army was moving. The British Army developed and began using horse remount depot hospitals during this campaign.

By the mid-1800s, new technologies of war caused new challenges for horses and soldiers alike. During the war between the United States and Mexico (1846–1848), for example, the U.S. Army had added a few veterinarians in addition to the farriers it had hired since 1792. (By 1847, there were only about 15 qualified vets in America, all immigrants from Europe.) During the American Civil War (1861–1865), the Union cavalry counted 284,000 horses; however, only six veterinarians were assigned to the Union Army. Dreadful injuries from exploding shells and repeating rifles caused the deaths of tens of thousands of horses; even more died of glanders, respiratory diseases, and gastrointestinal illnesses. In Europe, the Crimean War (1853–1856) was fought between the Russian empire and a coalition of British, French, and Ottoman troops. The Russians attempted to extend their empire at the expense of the Ottoman empire. In this war, the armies used modern technologies such as explosive naval shells, railways, and telegraphs. However, the Crimean War also quickly became a symbol of logistical, tactical, medical, and veterinary failures. Human and animal losses were enormous. The demand for professional modern nursing care of wounded and diseased soldiers (Florence Nightingale) and horses gained worldwide attention. Again, the veterinary care of sick and injured horses, including proper equipment and medicines during transport by sea, as well as on the battlefield during the severe winters of 1854 and 1855, proved to be wholly inadequate.

The Crimean War was notable for another innovation: canned meat and other food for the soldiers, which varied greatly in quality. In 1855, a million portions of canned meat were supplied to the allied armies in Crimea. Inspecting the armies' food rations eventually became another responsibility for army veterinarians. The use of canned meat in households became common in the second half of the nineteenth century. However, the rising meat-packing industry was also stimulated by the military, which needed food that could easily be transported and preserved for longer periods. Until then, armies were fed with herds of cattle that moved along in the rearguard. Traditionally, people had looked for ways to preserve food and based on empirical experience, and processes like cooling, smoking, salting, and drying had been applied throughout the ages. Large-scale canning techniques promised to feed armies more efficiently, but poor techniques and corruption caused major problems. The U.S. meat-packing industry was mostly unregulated, and profit was the only motive. The cans contained not just meat but were also adulterated with cheap additives such as ground-up cereals and offal. The quality of the canned "meat" was usually very poor, probably due to microbiological spoilage, and it caused food poisoning among the soldiers. Similarly, in

1877 the British Army and Navy stopped the imports of frozen meat from the United States, which was uninspected during transport and spoiled due to lack of proper refrigeration. The problem was so bad during the Spanish–American conflicts (1890s) that soldiers complained that their canned meat had been "embalmed." Some historians assert that more soldiers died from diarrhea, dysentery, and food poisoning than Spanish bullets. The scandal directed public attention in the United States to pure food movements and stimulated the passage of state and federal pure food laws.

These military needs, for food and horses, contributed greatly to the development of modern European-style veterinary regimes during the 1800s. In turn, veterinarians were crucial to military success. As the new century of the 1900s dawned, the world looked ahead with hope but also faced the gathering storms of war.

Conclusions

From this survey of the 1800s, we can conclude that:

1. In the early 1800s, the veterinary marketplace had not changed very much. Veterinarians educated at the new schools competed with farmers, farriers, healers, castrators, dentists, and others for patients. Livestock (especially cattle, sheep, and goats) and equids (especially horses and mules) were the most important veterinary patients in most parts of the world.
2. Fast-developing knowledge about the natural world, including how animal bodies functioned in health and disease, was the basis for "scientific" studies of animals in the European tradition that eventually spread around most of the world. Elite veterinarians contributed to, and incorporated, scientific knowledge into European-style veterinary education.
3. Colonialism, global trade networks, and other circulations of animals around the world led to disease outbreaks (epizootics). Animal experts in Asia, Africa, and Europe attempted to control epizootics using traditional practices: quarantine and slaughter of sick and exposed animals. A major disease that veterinarians attempted to control was rinderpest, which destroyed up to 90 percent of infected animals. Sub-Saharan Africa suffered greatly as both domesticated livestock and wildlife were wiped out by rinderpest, which was imported by Europeans. Rinderpest was an imperial disease.
4. Indigenous healing methods continued to thrive around the world where local people had important knowledge about animal diseases. Healers treated animal diseases and injuries with botanicals and other medications, cautery, and simple surgeries. Indigenous healing regimes were often familiar with concepts such as quarantine and isolation for infectious diseases and associating some diseases with flies and other vectors.

Indigenous knowledge contributed to veterinary knowledge (see the case of *nenta* in South Africa).

5. With an increasing global consumption of animal products (meat, dairy), veterinary leaders began training programs in food hygiene (especially inspection). Veterinarians argued that they were uniquely qualified to conduct inspections of slaughterhouses, dairy facilities, and meat and milk products.

6. With the development of new tools (better microscopes, etc.), veterinary leaders envisioned a "scientific" veterinary medicine (similar to human medicine) from the 1850s onward. Laboratory investigations became increasingly important in food hygiene and veterinary research.

7. Veterinary schools based on the European model were founded in many countries throughout the 1800s. Graduates of these schools established veterinary associations that worked hard to develop laws and regulations that restricted the practice of animal healing and food inspection to graduate veterinarians.

8. The development of germ ideas (especially about disease causation) slowly led to changes in veterinary education, disease control, and food inspection. Other ideas about disease causation included the roles of the environment and insects in spreading disease, the *contagium vivum*, parasitism, and toxins. Veterinarians and animal healers working in different places and situations used the ideas that seemed most effective to them at the time.

9. By working to establish microbiology, comparative pathology, and "one medicine," veterinarians were important co-creators of modern medicine and public health as we know them today. "One medicine" and comparative pathology studied disease in both humans and animals (especially zoonotic diseases). Veterinarians worked alongside physicians and other scientists in interdisciplinary teams. The French veterinary schools, and their daughter schools in Canada and the United States, were centers of the "one medicine" and comparative pathology approach.

10. Most veterinarians worked on horses and livestock, but a few also treated companion (pet) animals. These animals' owners valued them for emotional reasons, and in the West citizens formed associations for the human treatment of dogs and other animals. Pet owners increasingly expected scientifically trained veterinarians to provide the same services for pets that their owner could expect at a hospital for humans.

Question/Activity: What major scientific discoveries or developments occurred in your country or region of the world? Can you connect these scientific developments to epizootics or outbreaks of animal diseases? How were these scientific ideas different from the beliefs of animal owners? When did veterinary practice for companion animals or pets develop in your nation?

5   Veterinary Medicine in War and Peace, 1900–1960

Introduction

By 1900, the major components of modernity had been created: the highly organized, bureaucratic nation-state that regulated people, animals, and environments; large-scale agriculture; industrialization; and new technologies such as electricity, the telegraph, and the internal combustion engine. The first half of the twentieth century (1900–1960) would see an intensification of modernization. As Sigfried Giedion wrote in his book *Mechanization Takes Command* (1948), mechanization in disparate societal sectors was a crucial component of this modernization, and it assumed control of peoples' lives. Examples of innovations he discussed included the assembly line, agricultural production, the slaughterhouse, systems of hygiene and waste management, and kitchen tools. European science was an important driving force that equated modernization with "progress" in solving social problems (such as how to feed the world's rapidly growing human population). Despite implications of "progress," modernization had negative effects: the destruction of local peoples' lifeways, huge increases in burning fossil fuels that damaged the earth's atmosphere, and political, social, and economic instabilities that led to two global wars. In many parts of the world, animal agriculture and animal healing remained local activities, but were increasingly tied to global economies.

For veterinary medicine, the early 1900s saw both a continuation of the previous centuries' themes and new developments and problems. Veterinarians and animal owners around the world were still faced with outbreaks of animal diseases that traveled quickly on ships and railroads. Veterinary institutions, regulations, and regimes continued to develop in many parts of the world, with an increasingly narrow definition of "veterinarian" as a graduate of a European-model veterinary school. Veterinary researchers contributed a great deal of knowledge and evidence to bacteriology as well as in the new sciences of immunology and virology. But veterinary medicine faced important changes due to mechanization and modernization, also. Methods of raising livestock began to intensify, with ever-larger numbers of animals crowded into enclosures and buildings. Public health officials and agricultural leaders often clashed, putting veterinarians in difficult positions. The biggest change, however, was the slow but steady replacement of animal power with that of engines. Horses and oxen used for power, transportation, and traction were valuable animals for whom owners would be willing to pay for veterinary care. Most veterinarians and animal healers focused on these animals, with little attention paid to pets and smaller animals with low economic value. With mechanization, veterinarians lost their most valuable patients. In many places, veterinarians learned to shift between individual clinical care and herd health and preventive medicine.

Veterinarians also participated in, and were shaped by, the great upheavals of the 1900s, especially uprisings and instability in colonized regions, World War I, the global economic depression, World War II, and postwar recovery. Maps of the world's nations quickly became outdated as empires collapsed and new nations arose. The Western European colonial regimes, such as the British in India, weakened or dissolved; and revolutions based on socialism and communism upset old monarchies and capitalist governments (the Russian Revolution and the 1949 Revolution in China, for example). Between the advent of World War I, in 1914, and the end of World War II, in 1945, much of the world lived with war and violence or the equally challenging crises of poverty and famine (that outlasted the wars). For many of the world's people, these were years of crisis. Paradoxically, this time period also increased the pace of scientific and technological developments, especially during the war years.

For veterinary medicine, new therapies and tools, such as antimicrobials and vaccines, greatly increased the ability to control animal diseases and enabled the industrialization of food animal production in the West. In the period 1900–1945, and particularly during the postwar reconstruction, which lasted until 1960, veterinarians oversaw large-scale eradication schemes as a disease-preventive measure. They found new roles as government food inspectors, army veterinarians, and preventive medicine specialists for large herds. These changes were not driven primarily by the new therapies and tools, however, but by changes in the roles of animals in societies. Of course, in most of the world, small-scale animal agriculture and local animal healing practices continued. These practices remained the backbone of human–animal interactions (and survival) for much of the world's population.

The global animal economy began to change during this time period, however: food animal production industrialized, and engines replaced horses in transportation and agriculture. These trends, which began in the United States and Europe, have arguably been the most profound transformation in human–animal relationships since domestication. Under this new regime, food-producing animals lived and died out of sight of the humans who consumed them. Milk appeared in bottles; cheese, yoghurt, ghee, and other milk products could be purchased rather than made at home. Meat, already butchered and cut into pieces, was displayed in a sanitary shop. As animal production industrialized, food prices decreased, and meat consumption increased; these trends continue today. The other major force shaping the global animal economy was the replacement of horses and other animals with mechanized power and transport. To be sure, in many areas of the world, small farmers continued to use donkeys and other draft animals along with machines. Mechanization has spread unevenly. In the West (except for the military), horses became obsolete for most work purposes in society and agriculture by the rise of cars, trucks, and tractors in the first half of the twentieth century, particularly when roads were improved. The equine-oriented veterinary profession in the mechanizing nations had to adapt quickly as their most important patient population disappeared. This was perhaps the greatest challenge the young profession had yet faced.

The Decline of the Horse Economy

Today it is hard to grasp the degree to which economies and broader society depended on horses. In 1720, before industrialization and mechanization began in the West, the number of horses worldwide was estimated at 27 million. Around 1815 this figure had risen to 55 million, while a peak of 110 million horses globally was reached between 1910 and 1920 (Fig. 5.1). European nations (France, Germany) and the UK reached their peak horse populations earlier than North American countries (Canada, United States), reflecting developments in rail and urban transportation. Especially in North America, horses remained important for agricultural use. With its largely agricultural economy, Russia had the largest horse population at the beginning of the twentieth century, estimated at 23 million. However, tremendous losses of the equine population followed due to the Russian Civil War (1917–1922) and both world wars. During the process of collectivization (especially 1929 onward), the horse population dropped from 34 to 16.5 million, contributing to severe famines and poverty in the vast rural areas.

Until the 1920s, horses represented the most important clientele for veterinarians, in society and agriculture as well as for the military, while the veterinary curriculum was built around the horse as model animal. Cattle, pigs, sheep, and poultry had economic value as food producers, but the workhorse had practical value. Veterinarians served livestock owners, but horse owners dominated the marketplace for animal care. Because of these interests, equine medicine had developed the most over the centuries. Veterinarians' focus on infectious diseases, such as glanders, also reveal how horse diseases played a

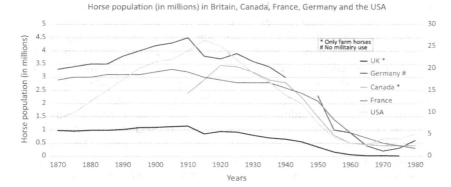

Figure 5.1 Graph showing horse population (in million) in Britain*, Canada*, France, Germany#, and the United States (right y-axis) in the period 1870–1980. (*Only farm horses, #non-military use.)
Sources: Wilfried Brade, 'Die deutsche Reitpferdezucht – aktueller Stand und wirtschaftliche Bedeutung', *Berichte über Landwirtschaft – Zeitschrift für Agrarpolitik und Landwirtschaft* 91 (2013) 1:2; G.K. Crossman, *The Organisational Landscape of the English Horse Industry: A Contrast with Sweden and the Netherlands*, thesis Univ. Exeter 2010) Fig. 2.2; J.P. Digard, *Une histoire du cheval. Art, techniques, société* (Arles: Actes Sud, 2004); Emily R. Kilby, 'The Demographics of the U.S. Equine Population', in: D.J. Salem and A.N. Rowan (Eds.), *The State of the Animals 2007* (Washington, DC: Humane Society Press, 2007), p. 176; F.M.L. Thompson, *Horses in European Economic History. A preliminary Canter* (Reading: British Agricultural History Society, 1983), p. 59. Courtesy: Monique Tersteeg B.Sc. Department of Population Health Sciences, Faculty of Veterinary Medicine, Utrecht University.

significant role in the rise of comparative pathology. In addition, after the discoveries of Charles Darwin and Georg Mendel, much veterinary attention was paid to theories about heredity. Could problems in horses – particularly in their legs, hooves, and lungs – be explained and prevented by knowledge of genetics? Did purebred horses naturally have good legs, lungs, and hooves? Or were hybrids better? Would inferior horses pass this quality on to their offspring? Veterinarians embraced this field and supported pedigree adminis-tration, enrollment in breed associations, and inspection of stallions. Horse breeding was an important tool for veterinarians and horse breeders who increasingly saw themselves as animal engineers.

Animal Engineering

Because horses, mules, oxen, and other draft animals were crucial to industrial and economic activities, scientists and engineers focused on assessing and improving "horsepower." The British engineer James Watt was credited with inventing the term "horsepower," a unit of how much work a horse could perform over time, after studying farm horses and ponies working in coal mines. To increase horses' energy output while keeping maintenance costs low, animal breeders crossed stronger, heavier horses with local animals. Scientists interested in nutrition and efficiency calculated ratios of energy consumed (feeding) to energy output. Veterinary leaders noticed this "scientization" of animal breeding and feeding, and some (such as American Leonard Pearson [1868–1909]) even advocated restructuring veterinary education to produce "animal engineers" along with clinicians. The "animal industry" needed horses that were not only strong and efficient, but also resistant to lameness and injury. This engineering view of draft animals valued them in quantitative terms, like machines; the goal was to maximize power output relative to energy input (and, of course, profit).

Maximizing efficiency in equine bodies meant controlling breeding programs. At this time, several nations around the world maintained state-run horse-breeding farms. Along with private farms, these large establishments supplied horses to governments, armies, urban transportation companies, and agriculture. In Korea, for example, the island of Jeju specialized in producing horses, cared for by specialized *teuri* herders. Ten state-run horse farms and numerous private farms utilized veterinary services and the latest technologies at the end of the 1800s. At this same time, draft-animal breeding during the late Qin dynasty (China) blended traditional Chinese and Mongolian techniques for feeding and breeding, drawing on China's long history of horse breeding. By the end of this dynasty (1911), which was very interested in technology, ideas about increasing the efficiency of horses, cattle, and buffaloes began to appear in government guidelines for running state-owned farms. The famous state stud farms of Europe (France, Germany, Hungary, Austria, Poland, Czech Republic, Spain, etc.) developed horses for cavalry, riding, and sport and employed veterinarians throughout the long nineteenth century. While these specialized breeding farms did not produce most of any nation's working animals, they were testing grounds for applying new ideas about scientific breeding and animal husbandry to the old problem of making an animal a "more efficient machine."

Urban populations of horses and other draft animals peaked at the end of the nineteenth century, just as graduate veterinarians' numbers were rising. In European and American cities, the ratio of horses to humans varied from 1:10 to 1:15, on average. Hundreds of thousands of horses and oxen moved freight and people in the great cities of South and East Asia; and horses walking on treadmills powered urban factories and mills worldwide. Not surprisingly, these horses' heavy workloads meant frequent lameness and breakdowns. In the United States, large urban stables kept veterinarians on retainer (paying them a monthly salary) to treat or (often) shoot lame horses not worth saving. A surprisingly high percentage of European and North American veterinarians earned their living in urban areas, reflecting the large numbers and high value of horses. In the United States in 1900, a horse was worth $50–$60, compared to $30 for a dairy cow, $35 for beef cattle, and $3 for a pig or sheep. Owners were more likely to pay for veterinary care if the animal was valuable. Also, most municipalities employed veterinarians to purchase and supervise the care of the city's horses (used for police, fire-fighting, and hauling). Some cities even had their own horse hospitals, indicating cities' reliance on healthy horses. Veterinary schools' curricula, reflecting this reality, still focused on horses. Most veterinary associations were based in cities.

With their core business and focus on equine medicine, understandably, veterinarians and veterinary authorities feared the consequences of the transition from horsepower to machine power in the urban environment as well as in the countryside. What could this mean for the future of the profession?

After a spectacular drop, then a slow increase beginning in the 1970s, the world's equine population is estimated at 60 million today. However, this latest increase is also due to a major change in the functioning and valuing of most horses: they have become companion animals used in sports and recreation. That change in equine roles only became widespread after the 1950s, however; and only for those wealthy enough to own a horse for leisure purposes. In most of the world, horses were slowly replaced as the major means of transport by motorized vehicles during the first half of the 1900s. The transition from horse to motorized power proceeded unevenly, slowly, but still unavoidably.

Horses had long been cultural and social icons as well as crucial economic resources. This meant that owners' attitudes toward horses, both as living beings and as technologies, influenced how horses maintained or lost economic value and social relevance. Between 1907 and 1917 cars replaced horses as the regular means of transport for people and goods in the United States, for example. About 140,000 cars and 3,000 trucks were registered there in 1907. Long-distance transport of people and goods was made by railroad, and short distances by foot, bicycle, or horse-drawn carriage. Not many people still rode horses. In 1915, the number of cars surpassed the number of nonagricultural horses for the first time. The number of cars processed at assembly lines rose to almost 5 million, and the number of commercial, agricultural, and military vehicles, to almost 400,000 in 1917. The equine population hit its peak in 1917, and by 1930 cars per U.S. citizen had surpassed horses

For urban dwellers horses had become an anachronistic, wasteful, and dangerous minority on the roads. The environment started to play a role as well. In 1908, New York City's 120,000 horses left a pungent 1.3 million liters of urine and 2.6 million kilograms of manure on the streets daily. Pleas were made for a horseless city with clean, odorless streets with transportation by cars, motor bus lines, and electric trams. Unpaved dirty roads were replaced by asphalt, and stables were banned inside larger towns and cities. Another plea for reducing horse work came from the urban animal protection movements. The coming of the motor vehicle would liberate horses and mules from harsh and exhausting servitude. Horses of sport, pleasure, and fashion would have better lives. These humanitarian arguments provide a sense of how progress, technology, and modernity became entangled with humanity, cruelty, and sentimentality in the opening decades of the twentieth century.

Automobiles became popular at the expense of horses as a means of transportation. Not only in urban America but also in larger cities in other countries around the world people rapidly adopted mechanized transportation. However, developments often were slower. For instance, Germany did not become motorized like the United States, Britain, and France until the 1930s. In many countries like India and Australia, railways were built during the colonial period, while the European tradition of horse-powered carriage transportation for passengers, goods, and mail was adopted, but at a much smaller scale, and only for people in high social status. In much of Asia, the majority still used bullock- or oxen-powered transportation, particularly in rural areas, inland waterway systems, bicycles, and the human-powered carts or rickshaws. In North Africa, camel caravans continued to play a role as traditional means of transport, as did horses, donkeys, and mules in Central and South America, next to a slow increase of cars, trucks, trains, and other motorized transport. The means of transport and power that people chose depended on the conditions: the climate, distances, costs, and cultural considerations.

It is important to keep these regional differences in mind when examining the market for veterinary services. For instance, regarding the business for veterinarians, apart from looking at horse populations, it is also important to map out where these animals lived. As historian Philip Teigen has pointed out, many horses lived in urban areas of the United States. By 1910, 14 percent of the total horse population and 6 percent of all mules lived in non-rural areas. Due to the high density of economically valuable urban horses, many veterinarians located their private practice in cities; they also did so because many food animals were kept within towns. Veterinarians in the countryside had to travel long distances to care for animals, which made their practice less profitable (time is money, after all). Not only in cities, but also in the countryside veterinarians were confronted with the process of mechanization. There, the horse was replaced by tractors and trucks. Again, this worried veterinarians in the United States, since 16 million horses were kept on farms against 1.3 million horses performing non-agricultural work in 1930. Moreover, prices of horses had dropped significantly in the 1920s. In Europe, the situation was different. In Britain, for instance, most horses were used outside agriculture, while as many resided in the towns as in the countryside. Nevertheless, the tractor would eventually replace farm horses.

Rural Horses and Tractors

The mechanization of many aspects of agriculture began simultaneously in Britain and the United States. Due to this process, new machines such as combines, cultivators, and milking machines found their way to farms in the twentieth century. Of these, the tractor was one of the most important innovations. In the 1920s it was estimated that one tractor equaled sixteen horses. However, the replacement of horses, particularly heavy draught horses, by tractors in agriculture started later than the rise of cars within urban life. First, the heavy steam tractors were introduced on big farms. These machines proved to be useful for belt work (threshing grain) but slow and impractical for field work. They were also expensive and could be dangerous, so by 1908 gasoline-powered machines were replacing steam-powered ones in North America. However, many North American farmers with small to medium-sized holdings could not afford a tractor or truck until around World War II.

In Europe, Britain was the leading country with mechanization, where about 50,000 tractors were in use in 1939. In total, these represented more traction force (expressed in horsepower) than all agricultural horses at that time. In many other European countries, this transition happened after World War II as part of postwar recovery programs. Many smallholders continued their work using heavy horses as well as tractors until the 1960s and 1970s. Farms represented the last bastion of animal power, owing not only to economics but also in part because replacing horses meant upsetting the entire structure of farm work. Motorization was most profitable on large farms in sparsely populated regions (with a limited labor supply) such as Canada, Argentina, and Australia. By the 1930s, these respective countries became the world's largest exporters of wheat.

As Figure 5.2 shows, the tipping point of horse replacement by tractors occurred in 1944 in the United States and in 1948 in Canada. However, this was a slow process. For several years after acquiring a tractor, many farmers kept one or two horses for particular tasks (cultivating young plants, for example) or because they liked their horses. France also possessed a large agricultural sector, yet the transition to tractors took much longer. The same holds for Germany, which – despite its pioneering role in motor vehicle substitution – had a large unmechanized agricultural sector until after World War II. Germany therefore had a high horse population compared to France and Britain and a rather late transition to tractors. In Australia, despite

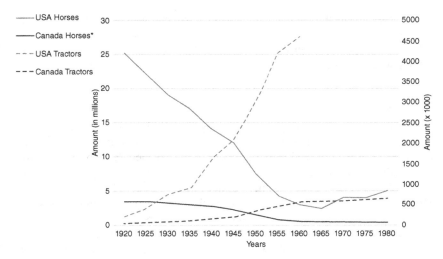

Figure 5.2 Graph showing the tipping point of horses (in millions)
replacement by tractors (× 1000) in Canada and the United States in the
period 1920–1980.
Source: William J. White, "Economic History of Tractors in the United States," EH.Net
Encyclopedia, edited by Robert Whaples. March 26, 2008; Darrin Qualman: www
.darrinqualman.com/high-input-agriculture/canada-tractor-numbers-and-horse-
numbers-historic-1910-to-1980/ Courtesy: Monique Tersteeg B.Sc. Department of
Population Health Sciences, Faculty of Veterinary Medicine, Utrecht University.

mechanization in agriculture, it took the tractor from 1918 to 1950 to completely replace the horse. After the famine of 1921, and due to a loss of horses
during wars, Soviet agricultural authorities wanted to replace horse traction
with tractors. They ordered tens of thousands of tractors, combines, and other
agricultural equipment from the United States. However, industrialization of
Soviet agriculture still proceeded slowly over vast territories, so there was a
continuing need for horses.

Compared with North America, Europe, Australia, and New Zealand, the
transition from horse to motorized power on smallholder farms in Africa, Asia,
and areas of Central and South America happened much later, only partially,
or – in some regions – not at all. Next to horses, oxen and water buffaloes
represented the standard traction power. Oxen, also known as bullocks in
Australia and India, can be regarded as the first "tractors." Usually yoked in
pairs, they can pull more weight and in general are more powerful than horses,
particularly in terms of endurance. Often, they are also used as a source of
power to grind grain or supply irrigation. Depending on circumstances, some
working oxen were shod with two half-moon-shaped irons for each claw.

Unlike horses, oxen cannot balance on three legs; therefore, shoeing was done after throwing the ox to the ground and lashing all four feet to a heavy wooden tripod. The domestic water buffalo (both river and swamp types) is spread over the Indian subcontinent, Southeast Asia, and China. For centuries they have been very suitable for tilling rice fields, and their worldwide population is now estimated at 202 million. Apart from traction, the water buffalo has always been an important source of milk. Their milk is richer in fatty acids and proteins than that of dairy cattle.

In Africa, depending on social, economic, and ecological conditions, the use of animal-powered transport slowly spread from the coastal regions by the activities of traders, settlers, missionaries, and government authorities, who used imported horses, donkeys, and mules. This happened first during the colonial periods in South Africa and Egypt. Except for South Africa, the introduction of animal power in agriculture happened mainly in the twentieth century. In Egypt, Ethiopia, and Sudan, mainly oxen or barren cows are used for traction. After the independence of many African countries, it was assumed that (following the European example) tractors would soon replace animal traction. However, tractor hire schemes for smallholders failed, due to high oil prices and problems with maintaining the machines. Animal traction for tillage and transport on wheels became a major goal of development strategies in many countries in sub-Saharan Africa. There, millions of mules (a cross between a horse and donkey) provide transport and traction. Mules have a better ability to adapt to the harsh conditions of the highlands and drought. Compared to oxen, mules are easier to handle for women, who have been traditionally responsible for transport of water, fuel, and crops. Larger and more prestigious animals (usually bovines) are traditionally handled by men in many cultures.

The collapse of the horse industry in the Western world and the rise of agricultural machines was a gradual transition in most areas. Breeders stopped producing horses in large numbers, while many farmers had their horses slaughtered. Sadly, many unique horse breeds disappeared. In Turkey, for example, the Karacabey Stud was established after independence to develop the Turkish Karacabey breed. Karacabeys were used for riding and light work; but the breed declined dramatically as horses were replaced by motorized vehicles, and today this breed is extinct. In contrast, animal traction in the developing world was only replaced by tractors to a limited extent, while in many places transport and traction by oxen, water buffaloes, donkeys, and mules even increased. The market for veterinary care in those areas remained focused on these important and valuable animals, especially during contagious disease outbreaks.

With the decline of the numbers and economic value of urban and agricultural horse populations in the Western world, veterinarians there faced great challenges for their business and profession. Due to the shrinking market for veterinary services and fears of unemployment, fewer and fewer students enrolled in veterinary schools. The total number of veterinary students in North America fell 75 percent between 1914 and 1924. This was not the case in other countries, where horses and oxen were not so rapidly replaced, the number of government veterinarians and farm animal practitioners had always been bigger, and the need for army veterinarians had steadily grown. Fortunately, veterinarians also provided other crucial services to urban and rural areas, especially milk and meat inspection. Increasingly, as horses disappeared, veterinarians concentrated more on safeguarding the food supply.

Veterinarians: Guardians of the Global Food Supply

Changes in Global Circulations of Animal Products

Veterinarians' responsibilities for meat and milk inspection made the profession vulnerable to political and social controversies, however. In the United States, the federal government's Bureau of Animal Industry (BAI) controlled veterinary meat inspection for domestic use and export. The BAI was the single largest employer of U.S. veterinarians, and the public reputation of American veterinarians depended on the BAI's performance. During the Spanish–American conflict in Cuba (1898), the poor quality of canned and refrigerated meat supplied to the U.S. Army became a national scandal. Army generals complained that the meat smelled "like a dead body" and made soldiers sick. They blamed the huge American meat-packing companies, who then blamed the BAI and its veterinary meat inspectors. Publication of the popular book *The Jungle* (1906) led to the investigation of meat production. Eventually the BAI chief, eminent veterinarian Daniel Elmer Salmon, resigned, although corrupt meat-producing companies and lax governmental oversight were responsible for meat-quality problems. U.S. veterinarians bitterly resented attacks on the integrity of meat inspection and the veterinary profession. They argued that veterinary schools incorporated modern bacteriological training, the profession advocated increased regulation of animal products, and all veterinarians took an oath of integrity and honorable, ethical behavior. This U.S. example demonstrates the politicized nature of food inspection and other veterinary activities, especially in the twentieth century.

The food supply and food patterns changed dramatically due to population growth, industrialization, and urbanization from around 1850 onward, and this process accelerated in the twentieth century. The increasing demand for meat, milk, dairy products, and eggs spurred innovations in agriculture and animal production methods. These innovations included scaling-up, specialization, cooperation, and mechanization in agriculture as well as more extensive and intensive animal husbandry. Economic growth, together with the use of synthetic fertilizers and the resulting surplus of new animal feeds, stimulated the development of mass production in the livestock sector of the Western world over the course of the twentieth century. This so-called modern consumption pattern is characterized by a larger variety of food products, more processed and convenience foods, and a decrease in seasonal influences. Between 1850 and 1930, the annual per capita meat consumption doubled in European nations from about 25 to 50 kilograms. It should be noted that these figures are based on total meat production in a country (that is, carcass weight, minus exports, plus imports) divided by total number of inhabitants. Thus, only about 45 percent of the animal is consumed as food – the balance represents everything from cooling and cooking losses and food left on the plate to inedible materials such as hides and bones

In cooperation with agriculturists, veterinarians contributed to increased animal production through changes in animal husbandry and product processing. With better feeds, livestock selection, crossbreeding, and inspection, the carcass weight of cattle increased by 120 percent between 1800 and 1912. These cattle were smaller and leaner animals, which fattened quickly and could be slaughtered at a much earlier stage. To improve pork production, European pigs were crossed with Chinese breeds. Cheese and butter making moved from farms to collective dairy-processing facilities, private or cooperative steam-powered creameries with boilers and separators. With selective breeding and high-protein feeding, egg production became very profitable. Egg yield increased from about 60 eggs per year per hen (c. 1800) to 135 in 1940. Factory farming of pigs and poultry, and to a lesser extent cattle, changed from a small solitary operation – often a family farm – into a component of the greater production chain from primary production to consumer.

However, it must be stressed that large-scale, capital-intensive farming only gradually replaced peasant farming, and that around the turn of the century, livestock production was still mainly based on smallholder farms. This was true for farmers around the world. As independent farmers or tenants employed by estate holders, most of their products found consumers via local markets. Nevertheless, in addition to that flow of foods of animal origin, the increase in livestock production on larger farms together with modern transport facilities resulted in a growing global trade in live animals and their products. Later, after the development of refrigerated ships, the distant (former) colonies supplied perishables like meat and butter to Europe, to be exchanged for exported European goods and capital. The trading monopoly of the European colonial system made way for an international economy in which European farm products were also exported.

Agricultural historians call the period up to World War I the first of three global "food régimes," or eras, which emerged from European colonialism.

During this first historical era in international agricultural development, colonial governments extended capitalist production relationships to almost every continent. These white "settler" governments and companies sent agricultural exports from sparsely populated countries in Australasia, Africa, and the Americas to Europe, Britain and later North America. Both before and following World War I, the efforts of veterinarians helped transform local agriculture in colonial areas. As historian Diana K. Davis has shown, French veterinarians in the Maghreb (northern Africa) were crucial agents of colonialism. Their activities included facilitating the trade in animals and animal products, research on infectious diseases, and treating sick animals and humans. However, these veterinarians also functioned as spies, advanced troops infiltrating enemy areas, and range managers who helped destroy nomadic peoples' lifeways and alter the natural environment. Serving the French colonial government also served the forcible inclusion of Morocco, Tunisia, and Algeria into the global food régimes of the early to mid-1900s.

Along with livestock production, veterinarians became involved in inspection and quality control of imported and exported livestock and foods of animal origin. National and international associations for professional veterinary food inspection were founded, and meat and milk inspection became important issues for international congresses. Food hygiene was also important for the Office International d'Hygiène Publique (1907) and the Office International des Épizooties (OIE, 1924), both established in Paris. Foreign markets increasingly demanded veterinary surveillance to guarantee quality and safety standards of exported and imported meat. For example, uninspected meat products exported by the United States were rejected by Germany and other nations, whose state-inspected meat-producing industries protested that U.S. meat did not meet German regulatory standards. As discussed in Chapter 4, the BAI was founded in 1884 to provide meat inspection for domestic and export markets, as well as to control outbreaks of bovine pleuropneumonia and other livestock diseases.

For import and export inspection purposes, veterinarians developed quality and safety control as well as legal procedures for certification. In this way, these official veterinarians become key components of the extended food networks, globalization of the agro-food system, and international trade politics. As in the previous centuries, the growth of international trade was regularly hampered by outbreaks of livestock diseases. Sometimes these were caused by smuggling infected cattle (foot and mouth disease) or contaminated products (trichinosis). Regularly this led to trade wars between nations whereby governments banned foreign livestock of products, which in turn was profitable for protecting domestic livestock farming. For instance, in the early 1890s, virtually all livestock from mainland Europe was prohibited from landing in Britain. Animals that were allowed into the country had to be slaughtered at the port of debarkation. The rise in meat imports into Europe made possible by the application of refrigeration meant that meat prices followed cereal prices and declined after 1880. European nations reacted by erecting tariff barriers and other measures, such as declaring the imported meat unsound, to restrict imports. However, as Britain rejected protectionism, her market remained open to meat imports of all kinds until the outbreak of war in 1914.

The two world wars and the economic crisis of the 1930s provided the most severe interruptions to the meat and livestock trade. Both wars seriously reduced purchasing power in Europe, as national expenditure switched from production of food to military needs and the people consumed more grain and less meat. In the early 1920s the international meat and livestock trade was restored quite quickly after the distortion during World War I. World meat imports again remained highly concentrated on Britain. Between 1924 and 1928, the UK bought almost 60 percent of the beef, 94 percent of the mutton, and 72 percent of the pork that entered world trade. In that period, the main exporters were Argentina (61 percent of world beef supplies), New Zealand and Australia (45 percent of world mutton supplies), and smaller European countries such as Denmark and the Netherlands (60 percent of pork and bacon supplies). Because of the expanding market in the United States, the interwar livestock trade was mainly between European countries. The depression of 1929 and the following process of self-sufficiency as part of war preparation had an adverse effect on both the trade in meat and live animals. World War II caused an even greater reduction in international meat and livestock trade than World War I. In 1934–1938, world exports of beef had averaged 661 million tons per year; it fell to 387 million tons in 1948–1952. Beef exports did not recover to the prewar level until 1960. Instead of Britain, the United States became the highest beef importer after World War II, acquiring 30 percent of world imports.

Veterinarians' roles in the care of food-producing animals and sanitary inspection of animal products grew in importance during the first half of the twentieth century, despite the disruptions of war and economic depression. These activities were crucial for the survival of veterinary schools and the veterinary profession. Schools' curricula, many traditionally focused on horses, shifted to training veterinary students to provide care for food-producing animals and scientific assessment of meat and milk. In many nations, federal or national governments sponsored and regulated veterinary education. This was true for most independent nations and also for European-controlled colonial states. Major exceptions included Britain (England and Wales) and the United States, with free-market economies and relatively low levels of governmental oversight. In these countries, both the (human) medical profession and the veterinary profession fiercely opposed oversight, which to them felt like "socialism." Veterinarians wished to regulate their own profession: to write the laws, control the colleges, and determine the cost of their services.

The shift to food-producing animals, however, challenged veterinary autonomy, and this is another example of political influence on the development of veterinary regimes. Surprisingly, in the United States for several years veterinary education was under the control of the federal government's BAI, which was the single largest veterinary employer. Between 1910 and 1930, the BAI employed about 10 percent of all U.S. veterinarians. BAI vets worked on regular salary instead of risking their livelihood in private practice; these were the best jobs. Because they conducted research on livestock and food inspection, BAI vets needed to have excellent training in bacteriology, pathology, and other basic sciences. While not providing any money to the veterinary colleges, the BAI dictated which subjects their students should study, inspected every veterinary college, and tracked every student admitted. The BAI angered veterinary faculties by judging the qualifications of the professors and restricting the number of professors trained at the same school. This detailed, centralized program of standards for veterinary colleges licensed the schools – and eight schools did not pass the test, so their graduates could not apply for BAI jobs or sit for the civil service examinations. Despite veterinary colleges' protests, the U.S. federal government remained in substantial control of the veterinary profession, through the BAI and the military services, until the end of World War II.

All these developments show that veterinarians compensated the partial loss of their activities within the horse economy by entering the market for veterinary services in the area of livestock production, food safety, and public health in the first half of the twentieth century. Veterinary leaders reformed the veterinary curriculum, incorporating more training in basic sciences such as bacteriology and focusing more on livestock and food safety. A few even included a course or two about dogs and other pet animals. Formalized, European veterinary medicine survived by remaking itself into the profession that could turn the tools of bacteriology and other sciences into practical benefits – and fortunately, these sciences expanded rapidly during the twentieth century.

Twentieth-Century Scientific Developments and Disease Outbreaks

Continuing developments in microbiology/bacteriology, immunology, and virology contributed to the success of large-scale veterinary disease eradication schemes during the 1900s through 1960s (Table 5.1). The terrible animal plagues – rinderpest, contagious bovine pleuropneumonia (CBPP) – remained

Table 5.1. *Milestones in microbial studies and therapy, 1880–1960+*

MILESTONES IN MICROBIAL STUDIES AND THERAPY, 1880–1960+

General theories of disease causation, the development of scientific disciplines, and technologies as they influenced Western veterinary medicine

4   C. 1880-1900 IMMUNOLOGY

- Technologies: vaccines of different types, serology, horses as immune serum factories
- Cellular immunity (Metchnikov)
- Humoral immunity (antibodies) (Behring, Kitasato, Ehrlich)

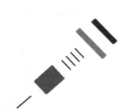

5   C. 1900 VIROLOGY

- Technologies: Filtering apparatus to remove larger bacteria (Chamberland), passaging through laboratory animals
- CBPP (Nocard & Roux)
- African horse sickness (McFadyean)
- Rabies (Frashëri & Remlinger)

6   C. 1900-60 CHEMOTHERAPY

- Biologicals
- Salvarsan & derivatives (1910)
- Penicillin (1929); sulfonamides (1935)
- Streptomycin (1940s); many antibacterials developed
- New vaccines against viral diseases

7   C. 1980-2020 MOLECULAR BIOLOGY

- Technologies: component vaccines, recombinant DNA, PCR, gene therapy
- Prion disease causation theory (BSE, scrapie)
- Rinderpest eradication
- Targeted therapies for cancerous diseases

problems, as did zoonoses such as brucellosis and bovine tuberculosis. Understanding these diseases, and creating vaccines and therapeutics to help control them, depended on expanding knowledge in areas such as thermodynamics, electromagnetism, (an)organic chemistry, atom theory, and radioactivity. Perhaps most crucially, stronger microscopes revealed the astonishing diversity of the microbial world. The stronger the microscope, the more micro-organisms were identified, from parasites, yeasts, fungi, and bacteria to viruses. Viruses were much smaller and could only be visualized using electron microscopes available from the 1930s onward (although their existence was known since the 1890s). Disease control and eradication programs depended on combining traditional strategies (test and slaughter, the *cordon sanitaire*) with the vaccines and other tools being developed from the 1910s onward. An understanding of how and why these tools worked depended on rapidly growing fields such as immunology and virology.

Immunology: The Body's Defenses

Ideas about the body's defenses against diseases were ancient; but a remarkably talented generation of scientists began to work out the actual mechanisms in the late 1800s and early 1900s. There were two types of these mechanisms: the activities of cells (cellular immunity) and the development of antibodies (humoral immunity). Ilya Ilich Metchnikov (1845–1916), a Russian/Ukrainian invertebrate zoologist who supported the Darwin–Wallace theory of evolution, first observed cellular inflammatory reactions in starfish larvae and water fleas in the 1880s. Metchnikov found cells he named "phagocytes": large cells that roamed the body and engulfed foreign microorganisms. In mammals, this cellular response included two different types of cells, the leukocytes and larger macrophages. Metchnikov believed this mechanism explained how the body defended itself against disease-causing organisms. Almost at the same time, however, other scientists found that something else in the blood (not phagocytic cells) could also produce immunity. In 1889, Hans Buchner (1850–1902) showed that cell-free serum killed bacteria, but that heating the serum destroyed this effect. The next year, Emil von Behring (1854–1917) and Shibasaburo Kitasato (1853–1931) worked together in Robert Koch's laboratory to prepare immune sera and antitoxins against tetanus and diphtheria, thus demonstrating humoral immunity. In 1900, Paul Ehrlich (1854–1915) proposed the side-chain theory that explained antibody specificity (the molecular structure was finally elucidated in 1959).

The immune sera were generated in the bodies of horses: after injection with small amounts of toxin, the horse produced antibodies that were protective for other animals and humans. In subsequent decades, horses functioned as living factories within laboratories and medical and veterinary schools and for companies that produced biological products. These immunological discoveries, and the development of mass production in horses, saved uncounted lives (especially children with diphtheria). Realizing the complexity of the immune system, scientists throughout the twentieth century studied serum sickness, allergies, blood type antigens, and many other aspects of the body's defenses. Most of these discoveries were made using farm animals as test subjects. Chickens were used to identify antibody-producing B cells from the bursa of Fabricius, while activation of B cells in lymph nodes was discovered in sheep. Pigs were used in early xenotransplantation studies, including blood transfusions and organ transplantations between species. (Some humans even received transplants of animal organs – including testes and ovaries!)

These discoveries led to advancements in controlling various animal disease problems. Chickens, for example, had been extensively used as laboratory animals and thus their diseases were well studied. The causal bacterium of fowl cholera was detected by microscopy in chicken blood in 1878 by Italian veterinary pathologist Edoardo Perroncito (1847–1936). Two years later, Louis Pasteur succeeded in culturing and attenuating the bacterium, which was later named after him: *Pasteurella multocida*. He also proposed the development of a vaccine, but it was veterinarian Theodor Kitt (1858–1941), professor at the Munich veterinary school, who studied the etiology of *Cholera avium* and who developed a serum immunization method. Later, inactivated agents were developed, providing a longer immunity. All these examples, and many others, reveal the fact that animal diseases were (in some ways) more thoroughly studied than those in humans at the turn of the twentieth century. Moreover, the scientists working on these problems were, from today's viewpoint, remarkably interdisciplinary, including chemists, veterinarians, physicians, microbiologists, and many others. Despite international scientific competition, several worked in multinational groups and scientific ideas and practices circulated around the world due to the increase in published scientific journals and international congresses. These were exciting times for scientists, and perhaps the most exciting new biomedical science was virology.

Virology: The Mysterious Diseases

The development of virology was closely tied to developments in immunology and bacteriology, especially the search for vaccines against common animal diseases. Volumes have been written about the general history of virology, so we will only briefly discuss it here in the context of specific animal diseases. Virology begins with a mystery. Charles Chamberland (1851–1908) was working in Louis Pasteur's laboratory when he developed an unglazed porcelain filter that would trap bacteria in 1884. Disease-infected blood/serum could be filtered, thus removing the bacteria and rendering the filtrate serum noncontagious – *if the disease was caused by bacteria*. However, for some diseases, the filtered serum still caused experimental animals to become sick, proving that some other infectious factor was present. No one could see this mysterious factor, nor could scientists grow it in the laboratory, so this unknown factor was called a "filterable virus." (*Virus*, from the Latin word for "poison," was a general term used for contagious particles.) Ambitious scientists around the world hunted filterable viruses. In Ukraine, Dmitri Iosifovich Ivanovsky (1864–1920) used Chamberland's filter to study tobacco mosaic virus in 1892. The Dutch microbiologist Martinus Willem Beijerinck (1851–1931), also working with tobacco mosaic virus, in 1898 called the mysterious infectious factor *contagium vivum fluidum*.

Filterable viruses remained mysterious until they could be seen with the electron microscope, in the 1930s; but before that, scientists studied them by studying the diseases they caused. Many important animal diseases were determined to be caused by filterable viruses at the century's turn. In 1898, Pasteurian Émile Roux (1853–1933) and veterinarian Edmond Nocard (1850–1903) found that a filterable virus caused CBPP, while veterinarian John McFadyean (1853–1941) determined in 1900 that filterable agents caused African horse sickness. Sheep pox became a filterable virus disease in 1902 with research conducted by French physician Amédée Borrel (1867–1936), who had worked in Metchnikov's lab at the Pasteur Institute in Paris. Borrel compared sheep pox intracellular inclusions with the appearance of cancerous cells (this viral theory of cancer continued to be an important research topic for decades). Borrel also introduced the term "infectious epithelioses" as a category for viral diseases that caused skin lesions (sheep pox, cowpox, etc.) German pathologist Otto Bollinger (1843–1909) declared fowl pox to be a viral disease, finding viral inclusion bodies or "Bollinger bodies" in infected cells. The Albanian microbiologist Rifat-Bey Frashëri, French physician Paul Remlinger (1871–1964), and their assistant Hamdi Effendi in Constantinople (Istanbul), and independently Alfonso di Vestea in Naples, established rabies as caused by a filterable virus in 1903. That same year, pathologist Adelchi Negri (1876–1912) identified the classic cellular lesions of rabies in dog brains: Negri bodies, which are cytoplasmic inclusions in neurons composed of rabies virus proteins and RNA. These were exciting discoveries for research scientists, and, with one exception (yellow fever), all the earliest identified filterable virus diseases in mammals were veterinary ones.

Even rinderpest (the dreaded global cattle killer) and foot and mouth disease (FMD) took on new identities as viral diseases. Despite the low mortality (2 to 5 percent), FMD represented the most economically severe animal plague after the rinderpest, because animals would not gain weight or produce milk. Infected animals could not be easily sold, moved, or exported. In 1897, German physicians Friedrich Löffler (1852–1915) and Paul Frosch

(1860–1928) discovered that a filterable virus agent caused FMD. (FMD was thus the first animal disease determined to be caused by a filterable virus.) Turkish veterinarian Adil-Bey Mustafa (1871–1904) and French microbiologist Maurice Nicolle (1862–1932) used the Chamberland filter to isolate the rinderpest virus from brain tissue and cerebrospinal and intestinal fluid from infected animals. In 1902, they injected healthy cattle with the filtered fluid, and rinderpest developed in all the animals, thus proving the transmission by filterable virus. Dorpat (now Estonia) Veterinary Institute pathologist Eugen Semmer (1843–1906) demonstrated that the serum from a recovered animal had both curative and protective powers. Continuing losses from FMD led the German government to establish a Research Institute on the Island of Riems in 1910, where Löffler and Frosch could experiment safely with this highly contagious disease. In 1922, seven different serotypes of FMD were identified.

These developments of serum-virus methods of immunization against rinderpest became the standard prophylactic procedure and opened the way for the development of several prophylactic vaccines. In the 1920s, British researcher J.T. Edwards of the Imperial Bacteriological Laboratory at Izatnagar (India) discovered that the administration of an attenuated rinderpest (*Morbillivirus*) preparation protected animals from rinderpest for life. In the early 1950s, Dutch veterinarian Herman Salomon Frenkel (1891–1968), director of the State Veterinary Research Institute, had developed an effective vaccine, produced with large-scale *in vitro* virus cultivation. In Germany, veterinarian Otto Waldmann (1885–1955) continued the work of Löffler, and together with Karl Köbe, Waldmann developed an effective vaccine from formalin and heat inactivated FMD virus in 1938 that was widely used in central Europe. The DDR (East Germany) was the first country in the world to introduce an annual vaccination against FMD in 1950.

Other animal diseases whose causation had long eluded scientists "became viral" in the early twentieth century. Several diseases threatened poultry flocks, and avian influenza (fowl plague) was probably the deadliest poultry disease. Italian veterinary researchers Sebastiano Rivolta (1832–1893) and Pietro Delprato (1815–1880) were probably the first to differentiate the clinical and pathological properties between fowl plague (influenza) and another disease, fowl cholera, in 1880. In 1901, Eugenio Centanni (1863–1942) and Ezio Savonuzzi discovered that fowl plague was caused by a filterable virus, and this helped to differentiate it from fowl "cholera." Another poultry disease, Newcastle disease, was also identified as a filterable virus disease during epizootics in 1926 in Britain and the Netherlands. First identified in Indonesia and Newcastle (UK) (although probably present in various places before then), the disease infected both domesticated and wild birds and it remains a severe problem for global poultry production even today.

Classical swine fever (hog cholera) was well described for the first time in 1833 in Ohio (USA) and it spread from North America to other continents. U.S. researchers first believed hog cholera was caused by a cholera bacillus. In 1903, Emile Alexander De Schweinitz (1864–1904) and Marion Dorset (1872–1935) of the Bureau of Animal Industry (BAI) proved that a filterable virus, not a bacillus, caused hog cholera/swine fever. Slovak-Hungarian veterinary pathologist Ferenc Hutyra (1860–1934), working with colleagues in Budapest (Hungary) at the University of Veterinary Medicine, confirmed the Americans' finding that classical swine fever/hog cholera was a filterable virus disease (as did other researchers). BAI researchers, many of whom were veterinarians, continued working on serums developed in hyperimmunized pigs. Copying Pasteur's earlier public anthrax demonstrations, BAI veterinarians carried out serum-inoculation trials observed by meat-packing company personnel and hog farmers, thus launching a pharmaceutical industry so large that some veterinarians specialized only in hog cholera/swine fever prophylaxis.

Another disease, swine influenza, opened a new vista of interspecies infections by viruses. Swine influenza was studied by physician Richard E. Shope (1901–1966), working for Paul Lewis at the U.S. Rockefeller Institute (Princeton). Shope, who had worked on farms as a boy, valued the knowledge he obtained from veterinarians and farmers, and this led him to the problem of swine influenza. Shope and Lewis differentiated a filterable virus from a bacterium present in infected pigs, and Shope proved that the virus caused the disease. Noting that an outbreak of swine influenza raged during the catastrophic human influenza pandemic of 1918–1919, Shope wondered if swine and human influenza were related. In 1933, British virologists Wilson Smith, Patrick P. Laidlaw, and Christopher Andrewes demonstrated that the swine and human viruses were antigenically quite similar, thus opening the question of whether humans could be the source of swine influenza (or vice versa). After sampling human populations, Shope found that adults carried antibodies that cross-reacted with the swine virus. Subsequent research (in the molecular era) has confirmed that influenza viruses are constantly evolving and transferring between animal and human populations, thus making influenza an early example of viral disease with zoonotic origins.

Virological research led to some remarkable advances in vaccine development techniques that circulated between medical and veterinary research groups. For example, in 1905 French veterinarian Henri Carré (1870–1938), who was the director of the Alfort veterinary school's Research Laboratory, identified a filterable virus as the cause of canine distemper. In the 1930s, British medical researchers Patrick P. Laidlaw and G.W. Dunkin found that they could experimentally transmit this virus to another species, ferrets, in the laboratory. Using this experimental system, Laidlaw and Dunkin established the identity of the virus (canine morbillivirus) and created a formalin-inactivated vaccine. They are only the most well-known protagonists in a very active sphere of veterinary research and vaccine development for viral diseases after World War I. For example, in the late 1920s veterinary researchers Raymond Alexander (1899–1965), Petrus du Toit (1888–1967), and Wilhelm Neitz (1906–1979) at the South African Onderstepoort Veterinary Institute, and a competing group at the Kabete veterinary laboratory in Kenya, attacked the problem of African horse sickness using Laidlaw and Dunkin's technique. Although this was not immediately successful, the South Africans next tried Max Theiler's technique of passaging viruses (yellow fever) through mice to create a vaccine. (Theiler, son of Onderstepoort's founding veterinarian Arnold Theiler, was working at the Rockefeller Institute in the United States.) Using this technique, they found that they could decrease the virulence of the target virus without affecting its ability to stimulate the immune system. By the early 1940s, they had developed a vaccine that was widely used in South Africa, Kenya, and elsewhere for thirty years.

Veterinary virology and research on virus-caused animal diseases were one of the pillars on which twentieth-century virology was established. These studies reconfigured disease etiologies, elucidated immunological principles, and contributed to the development of viral cancer biology. At the same time, scientists were discovering the microworlds of trypanosomes, rickettsia, and other causative agents of animal and human diseases. Trypanosome diseases affected humans and many species of domesticated animals across the global South. Working in the Punjab in 1880, veterinarian Griffith Evans (1835–1935) identified the trypanosome species (*T. evansi*) that caused surra, a deadly disease of horses and camels. In 1894, David Bruce (1855–1931) identified *T. brucei* as the cause of sleeping sickness in humans and *nagana* in cattle. Although livestock raisers in endemic areas had long associated these diseases with flies, scientists did not agree that these were vector-borne diseases until around 1900. Moreover, the bacterial diseases had not disappeared. Two of these diseases, brucellosis and bovine tuberculosis, illustrate the importance of zoonotic disease research in the first half of the twentieth century. Both examples also illustrate ways in which political and social context affected the deployment of scientific knowledge, a factor that no doubt contributes to the persistence of brucellosis and bovine tuberculosis in human populations even today.

"Scourges of Man and Animalkind": Brucellosis and Bovine Tuberculosis

One of the infectious diseases that puzzled medical and veterinary bacteriologists around 1900 was brucellosis, also known as "contagious abortion" or

"Bang's disease" in animals and "undulant fever" or "Malta fever" in humans. We now know this disease is caused by bacteria of the genus *Brucella*. It is characterized mainly by abortion, retained placenta, and reduced milk yield in cattle. During the nineteenth century, the contagious nature of this disease was established. The causative bacterium in cattle, *Brucella abortus*, was isolated in 1897 by the Danish scientist L.F. Bernhard Bang (1848–1932), who had studied human and veterinary medicine in Copenhagen. Together with his assistant V. Stribolt, he described the media employed and the cultivation method of *B. abortus*; and the disease was named "Bang's disease" in his honor. Bang is also remembered for his research on smallpox vaccination, for isolating necrosing bacillus in swine, and for drawing up a system for the control of bovine tuberculosis that became a model for many European countries in the early twentieth century. He did not, however, link Bang's disease to Malta fever in humans; that would not happen for another twenty years.

British medical officers recorded a mysterious disease with high fevers in soldiers during the Crimean War (1853–1856) that was probably the first record of this disease in the Western literature. David Bruce (1855–1931), an Australian-born military microbiologist posted to the island of Malta, isolated a bacillus from the spleen of soldiers that had died of Malta fever, which he named *Micrococcus melitensis* in 1893. The Maltese scientist and scholar Themistocles Zammit (1864–1935) isolated the same bacterium in unpasteurized goat's milk and confirmed this as the source of Malta fever among British soldiers in 1905 (to the chagrin of Bruce, who had not found the source). American bacteriologist Alice Catherine Evans (1881–1975, Fig. 5.3), of the U.S. Department of Agriculture, noticed similarities between *B. abortus* and *M. melitensis*, and after testing them extensively argued that this close relationship meant that the bovine *B. abortus* might also sicken humans ingesting it in raw milk. Although severely criticized by both the dairy industry and prominent scientists, Evans' results were confirmed over the next several years and brucellosis was established as a zoonotic infection.

Evans argued that the disease infected humans after ingestion of unpasteurized milk and soft cheeses (primarily from infected goats), insufficiently heated meat from infected animals, or close contact with infected animals' secretions (she even became infected in the laboratory). Along with laboratory workers, veterinarians and slaughterhouse workers became infected. Pasteurization and proper heating of milk and milk products prevented the disease, but for cultural and economic reasons pasteurization was only slowly adopted in many places. From 1910 onward, inactivated and live vaccines against brucellosis for the immunization of young heifers were used with limited success. European research by serological testing in the 1930s showed that many farms were infected, with an abortion rate between 6 and 13 percent.

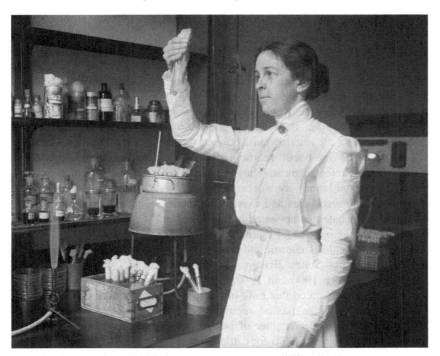

Figure 5.3 Bacteriologist Alice Catherine Evans (1881–1975) working in the U.S. Agricultural Department laboratory c. 1915.
Source: National Photo Company, portrait c. 1915.

After World War II, attenuated *Brucella* strain 19 was introduced as a vaccine. Given to heifers between 3 and 9 months of age, this modified-live vaccine successfully induced immunity in animals prior to breeding. However, it could not eliminate existing high levels of brucellosis in breeding herds, and the most successful way to control the disease was still through old-fashioned test and slaughter. In Europe, the United States, and elsewhere with high levels of brucellosis, culling was the basis for successful eradication. In Europe, some countries used Marshall aid to eradicate Brucellosis as well as bovine tuberculosis in the 1950s; the U.S. eradication program for brucellosis began in 1957.

In the case of bovine tuberculosis, scientific disagreements threatened the early control and eradication programs. Bovine tuberculosis (bTB) and its relationship to human tuberculosis (TB, the leading cause of death worldwide at this time) stimulated bitter debates among scientists from the 1890s to the 1920s. The debates challenged the strict "one germ – one disease" model and forced nations to consider various possible control strategies. The question was: Were bovine and human tuberculosis one disease or two? Robert Koch, who had first identified and cultivated *Mycobacterium tuberculosis*, TB's causative agent, declared in 1901 that *bovine* TB could not be the same disease as human TB. Koch strictly adhered to the "one germ – one disease" model, and the germ that American bacteriologist Theobald Smith had isolated from cattle in 1896 (*Mycobacterium tuberculosis bovis*) was slightly different from Koch's *M. tuberculosis*. Koch advocated ignoring bovine TB, reversing his own previous opinion that nations should try to eradicate it. His critics, including almost all veterinarians, pointed out the fact that humans could be infected with bovine bacilli (particularly children) by drinking contaminated milk or eating infected meat. They detailed examples of bTB contracted by veterinarians and laboratory workers. They argued that horrific cases of children with disfigured faces and twisted backbones could not be ignored. This was a public debate that appeared in all the major U.S., British, and European newspapers, magazines, and journals at the time.

Bovine tuberculosis control and eradication programs were delayed, but in the end the United States, Britain, and European nations instituted anti-bTB campaigns between 1900 and 1960. Pasteurization of milk killed the bacilli, but consumers demanded that milk be "pure" and uncontaminated with bacilli (alive or dead). Cities passed regulations forcing dairy farmers to allow tuberculin testing and slaughter of positive cows. Scientists were unable to develop a vaccine against TB for cattle. However, the bovine bacillus was the basis for a successful human vaccine, BCG, developed by Albert Calmette and Camille Guérin, French Pasteurians working in Africa. A virulent culture of *Mycobacterium tuberculosis bovis*, collected from a cow by the veterinarian E. I. Nocard, was the basis for this vaccine. This research began in the 1910s, but World War I delayed testing vaccine preparations in cattle and other experimental animals. That delay provided more time for the culture to lose virulence yet retain its ability to induce immunity. Could these aged cultures safely vaccinate humans? During the next thirty years, BCG was tested (first in babies) and eventually used around the world as an anti-TB vaccine for humans. Only the Netherlands and the United States do not vaccinate their citizens with BCG. No effective vaccine has been developed for cattle, and bovine tuberculosis still occurs in much of the world today. With the recent discovery of wild animals that can serve as bTB reservoirs (buffaloes, ungulates, and elephants in Africa and Asia; elk and deer in North America; llamas in South America; badgers, squirrels, and possums; otters and seals), global eradication of this disease is unlikely despite the maintenance of national tuberculosis control programs.

Since 1900, veterinarians have been central participants in scientific research and the practical work of testing, surveillance, and slaughtering infected animals to control these and other diseases. In turning to livestock and zoonotic disease control and herd health, the veterinary profession survived the major challenge of motorized vehicles replacing horses. However, there was one unforeseen development which brought many of them back to equine medicine: the care of animals during successive and devastating wars, during which a massive war horse economy developed.

War, Animals, and Veterinary Medicine

Nineteenth-century wars were horse wars. The Crimean War, the Civil War in the United States, the Franco-Prussian war, and the first Boer War (December 1880 until March 1881) in South Africa had clearly shown the importance of mobilizing huge numbers of horses and mules. These animals proved to be as crucial as men. During the U.S. Civil War, the Union Army used not fewer than 800,000 horses, while in total over 1 million would die (one-fifth of the nation's total horse stock). German forces were able to mobilize 1 million horses in a relatively short time during the Franco-Prussian war of 1870–1871. In the first decades of the twentieth century, even greater numbers of military horses, mules, donkeys, camels, oxen, elephants, water buffaloes, dogs, and pigeons participated in warfare, as well as army veterinarians to keep these animals healthy and fit.

Horses and the Boer War 1899–1902 in South Africa

In South Africa, two White populations fought for power amidst the competing interests of their African neighbors. Boers, independent Dutch farmers who wanted to maintain self-rule, lived in their own territory in Free State and Transvaal, where they raised livestock. They were opposed by the colonial British forces advancing inland from the Cape Colony. During the first Boer War, large numbers of British troops were defeated by a much smaller number of Boers in part due to the Boers' good use of their horses and knowledge of the terrain. The British government settled for a peace treaty because a larger-scale war would require the mobilization of more troops, horses, and mules – a very expensive proposition. In 1899, after the discovery of huge gold and diamond deposits, British imperial policy led to the second attempt to annex the Boer republics. The Boers and their African allies fought a British and colonial force that outnumbered them three to one. At first, the Boers conquered three British strongholds; but in 1900 they were finally defeated on the battlefield by the increasing numbers of British and their allies. The Boers kept the war going for two more years, using guerilla tactics to harass the British. To force Boer commandos to surrender, the British troops burned Boer farms, slaughtered their livestock, and imprisoned their wives, children, and African servants in concentration camps where tens of thousands died of hunger.

British prestige was shaken badly by the fact that one the world's most powerful armies could only defeat the minority Boers by applying a scorched earth policy.

The war was also disastrous for horses. The fate of horses employed in the British military was very tragic. The major combat force of the British Army consisted of cavalry and other mounted troops. However, the need for horses in this war was underestimated by the War Office. The mounted infantry was as important as the cavalry, while horses and mules were vital for transporting supplies and artillery. The horse-mounted Boers followed warfare strategies that were first practiced in the American Civil War, employing a mobile combat force that moved too quickly for infantry to engage. Compared to the sturdy, durable and native Boer horses, well adjusted to the local environment, the imported British horses had difficulty in the South African terrain. The number of animals killed in the second Boer War was huge, with many dying of diseases. The British Army even shot stray horses to keep them from falling into Boer hands. About 51,400 mules and more than 400,000 horses lost their lives, of which 326,000 were on the British side.

Veterinary officers working in the British Army Veterinary Department, established in 1881, in hindsight criticized the fact that most of the enormous animal losses did not result from enemy action, but were largely due to disease, starvation, and poor veterinary management by inexperienced mounted troops. British veterinarians criticized top Army leaders for poor decisions. For instance, the veterinary hospitals and remount depots (herds of replacement horses) were all placed on one location, against the advice of the Army Veterinary Department. Inevitably, crowding the horses led to a rapid spread of diseases such as glanders, epizootic lymphangitis and mange. The British went to war in South Africa with dozens of veterinarians, while Arnold Theiler (later director of the Onderstepoort Veterinary Institute) was the only veterinarian conscripted into the Transvaal State Artillery to care for Boer horses. But British horses died in huge numbers and had to be continually replaced with new animals.

With the Boer War, the breeding and international trade of horses became important military and political issues, resulting in the development of a true global warhorse economy. At the center was the British imperial horse economy, with animals imported from other British colonial nations. About 35,000 horses from Australia and 15,000 from Canada were shipped to South Africa. From the time of their arrival at Port Elizabeth, their average life expectancy was only about six weeks. Eventually, the British began replacing their lost horses with more durable African Basuto ponies and Waler horses imported from Australia. The British also imported supplies across the Indian Ocean at huge cost. For example, British mobile veterinary horse hospitals, which each held 300 sick horses, were shipped to South Africa from India. Even the

British veterinarians were mostly imported. About 10 percent of the British veterinary profession, 322 men, served as army veterinarians in South Africa. Britain also purchased large numbers of horses from other nations to import to South Africa. On the European mainland, stud farms (the Haras system) had existed since the eighteenth and nineteenth centuries to control the production of horses for war-based uses (riding horses, troop horses). This continued in the twentieth century, when the Haras system received government support. By 1910, compared to other countries, Germany spent the most government money on breeding stations for army horses and employed veterinarians to care for them. In Britain however, horse breeding was not regulated and was left entirely to private enterprise, due to the liberal economy. This opened opportunities for horse breeders around the world, including Europe and the United States (which supplied more horses than from all the British colonies combined).

New Roles for Horses: The Russo-Japanese War, 1904–1905

Another conflict, fought between Japanese and Russian forces in Manchuria (China), also demonstrated how animals were still important to modern warfare, but, increasingly, in new ways. This was a larger conflict than the Boer Wars, and its trenches, machine guns, and disastrous frontal assaults all foretold the conditions of World War I. This war included Asian and European combatants, and hundreds of thousands of horses, mules, and other animals to support the war effort. Horses served as cavalry mounts, pulled supply and personnel wagons, and moved artillery from place to place. In this war, despite the fearsome reputation of the Russian Cossacks, traditional cavalry attacks began to be less important. The Japanese, with their inferior horses, avoided cavalry attacks as much as possible; the Russians found their traditional mounted combat formations to be useless. Tactics had to change, including abandoning frontal assaults by mounted soldiers armed with swords and other steel weapons. Instead, armed skirmishes, quick incursions, and infantry and artillery support would become the major uses for horses and other animals. The once-proud cavalry officers and troopers often had difficulty accepting these new roles, but their best use was now as scouts for reconnaissance, small surprise attacks, carrying messages, and screening the infantry – tactics learned from the Japanese, who realized the limitations of their horses.

As the value of traditional cavalry waned, however, the value of heavier animals to position cannons and other artillery guns increased. Horses and oxen dragged massive artillery, and the Japanese were at a major disadvantage here, too, because their smaller, lighter horses struggled to pull the heavy gun carriages. Again, compensating for their animals, the Japanese shifted tactics. They began to use their artillery indirectly, during the whole battle, and flexibly, moving it around more. In this way, they kept their enemies guessing and overcame their relative lack of heavy horses. This same strategy would be used during World War I, when millions of horses did the humble work of dragging guns, supplies, and wagons through the mud. Traditional cavalry (reluctantly) became mounted infantry, armed with pistols and rifles. Far from being rendered obsolete, horses and other animals had become crucial support assets, and the proper care and resupply of animals continued to be a military concern.

The experiences during the Boer and Russo-Japanese Wars had a major impact on military tactics leading up to World War I. Military authorities in war departments of World War I's major combatant nations (Austria-Hungary, France, Germany, Russia) learned an important lesson: the horse – as a factor in warfare – had not passed into history, but the roles had changed. Modern technological warfare would require huge amounts of horses and mules, much more than ever before. Veterinary inspection and care in remount depots as well as in veterinary field hospitals was considered indispensable, which meant incorporating veterinarians into twentieth-century military forces (as historians such as Margaret Derry have argued).

Rinderpest Returns: The Balkan Wars, 1912–1913

The Balkans were a group of nations located strategically between the Austro-Hungarian and Ottoman empires. In 1912, war broke out between the four members of the Balkan League (Bulgaria, Greece, Montenegro, and Serbia) and their common enemy, the ruling Ottoman empire. The Balkan "protectorates" were inspired by nationalism and were discontented with the strong centralized policy followed by the Ottoman government after the Young Turk Revolution of 1908. During this so-called First Balkan War (October 1912 to May 1913) the Turkish Army was defeated and lost almost all the remaining European part of the Ottoman empire. In the Second Balkan War (June–August 1913), the former allies Bulgaria, Greece, and Serbia, joined by Romania, fought among themselves for the division of the former Ottoman territories. Bulgaria tried to hold Macedonia, but lost the war against Greece and Serbia, who divided this area between themselves. Albania obtained independence.

As in the previous wars, hundreds of thousands of soldiers and similar numbers of horses and mules were deployed in the Balkan Wars, and tens of thousands lost their lives. Light cavalry remained important in these wars, hitting the flanks of infantry, scouting, foraging, and sabotaging supply lines. Veterinary involvement in both armies increased with the need of maintaining

the health of or treating injured war animals. In addition, veterinary surveillance was required, because, like the Franco-Prussian War of 1870–1871,
troop movements and provisioning during the Balkan Wars caused the spread
of rinderpest in cattle meant to feed the armies. Spreading rapidly in Turkey,
Montenegro, Macedonia, and beyond, rinderpest continued to plague this
region after the war.

The stories of the horrors of the Boer, Russo-Japanese, and Balkan wars
drew more attention to the poor treatment of horses and general cruelty to
animals in various countries. For instance, Our Dumb Friends League, founded
in Britain in 1897, established the "Blue Cross Fund" in 1912 (after the
example of the Red Cross), which started caring and treating wounded and
diseased horses in the Balkan War. Originally, this institution was aimed at
improving the welfare of the many workhorses in London. In 1902 they
succeeded in obtaining a rule that every coach or wagon pulled by horses
carried a bucket with fresh water, thus preventing the spread of glanders via
municipal water troughs. In 1910 the Society for the Prevention of Cruelty to
Animals criticized the selling and transport of sick and worn-out horses to
Belgium and the Netherlands, where they were destined for meat consumption.
Instead, they advocated for worn-out horses to be humanely killed in the UK.
But the fates of horses in wars would also be a major concern for the Blue
Cross and other animal welfare societies.

These Balkan Wars set the stage for the Balkan crisis of August 1914, and
thus served as a stepping-stone to World War I. The Balkan peninsula was
strategically located, and dominance of this area was of political and military
importance for the leading European nations. Around 1910 the two great-
power groupings in Europe, the Triple Alliance (consisting of Germany,
Austria-Hungary, and Italy) and the Triple Entente (a coalition of Britain,
France, and Russia) were evenly balanced. The losing parties in the Balkan
Wars, Bulgaria, and Turkey, chose the side of Germany and the double
monarchy, countries that promised them restitution of the lost territories. In
various ways, the balance of power within Europe was challenged by the
Balkan Wars, and this unstable situation exploded in August 1914.

New Challenges for Veterinary Medicine: World War I (1914–1918)

In 1914, foreign (and colonial) policy within Europe was characterized by a
complicated system of rivalry, alliances, diplomacy entanglements, and
(secret) agreements. The main purpose for all involved nations was the assur-
ance of mutual aid against outside attacks. The spark in the powder keg that
launched World War I was the assassination of the Austrian archduke Franz
Ferdinand by a Serbian nationalist on June 28, 1914. The context of this act

was a conflict between Austria-Hungary and Serbia about control over Albania. War became inevitable, and countries of both the Central Powers (Austria-Hungary and Germany) and Allied Forces (including Britain, France, and Russia) mobilized their armies. On July 28 Austria-Hungary attacked Serbia, and Germany invaded neutral Belgium and northern France. Britain was obliged to defend Belgium and France by treaty and joined the battle on August 4. Because the United States entered the war in April 1917 on the side of the allied force – thereby playing a decisive role in the outcome – and more nations and colonies outside Europe also became involved, the war expanded into a global scale. Ultimately more than 65 million military personnel from 32 nations were mobilized in one of the greatest wars in world history.

On the long and open eastern front of this war, the German and Austrian armies were quite successful and forced the Russians after the communist revolution of October 1917 to a peace treaty in March 1918. On the western front the initial fast advance of the German Army was blocked and turned into a static trench warfare which lasted until November 11, 1918, when the Germans surrendered. This was a global tragedy in which an estimated 8.5 million military personnel and 2.3 million civilians lost their lives. (These losses became even greater with the ensuing influenza pandemic [1918–1919], in which an estimated 40–80 million people died.) The fact that about 8 million equines also died during World War I is less well known.

Horses for Attacking and for Transport

Trenches, barbed wire, poison gas, machine guns, and the introduction of tanks changed the mode of warfare during World War I. However, animals (horses, mules, oxen, camels, pigeons, and dogs) continued to play a significant role. In fact, their role had even increased. In 1870 the horse-to-soldier ratio in the German Army was 1:4; in 1914 this ratio was 1:3. On the eastern front, where trench warfare was less common, cavalry divisions remained important for long reconnaissance rides and artillery traction, as well as for offensive mobile firepower to break through infantry lines. This also applied to horse-mounted troops in the initial stages of the war in the west. After it had turned into a trench war there, armies used horses (and mules) as pack animals mainly for logistical support, such as carrying messengers and ammunition and pulling ambulances and supply wagons, particularly in mud and over rough terrain. In this sense, the loss of a horse was tactically valued higher than the loss of a human soldier, particularly since it became increasingly difficult to replace these animals during the war. Since the role of horses was so crucial, transport of huge quantities of horse fodder to the front by supply train units remained an important logistical challenge.

The roles of war horses were crucial; however, their fate was indeed tragic. Although the company of horses increased morale among soldiers, these strong human–animal relations did not last long, because horses were very vulnerable to machine guns, mortars, artillery fire, and poison gas. Moreover, horses contributed to human disease due to poor sanitation conditions, their manure, and their rotting carcasses. Hundreds of thousands of horses died, their corpses lining the roads to the fronts, not only from poor feeding and care, but also of exhaustion, drowning, getting stuck in mud, or falling in shell holes. They were affected by saddle sores, lameness, colic, glanders, strangles, scabies, equine influenza, equine infectious anemia, epizootic lymphangitis, anthrax, and ringworm. Better care (enough feed, more rest, time to acclimatize, and hoof care) prolonged horses' lives more than improved medical knowledge did. Women replaced stable boys to take care of horses in the remount depots in Britain, and many claimed they were superior to men in calming and training horses.

World War I stimulated the development of new types of veterinary hospitals, complete with ambulances. These field and station hospitals could handle significant numbers of ill and injured animals. As equine ambulances, horse trailers were first introduced on the western front. The German Army entered World War I without military horse hospitals. Due to the huge losses of horses and prevailing infectious diseases, the German War Ministry decided to divert resources into a system of horse hospitals in 1915. This system grew to 478 hospitals in which almost 1.4 million horses were treated. In the autumn of 1914, the veterinary school of Vienna was involved in establishing three permanent military equine hospitals near that city. Most other countries and particularly Britain, Italy, and Switzerland had organized a system of field animal hospitals much earlier. For instance, the British Army Veterinary Corps (BAVC), which was established in 1906, established mobile field veterinary hospitals, available at every cavalry and infantry division, to recover horses from injuries, diseases, and shell shock, so that they could be sent back to the front as soon as possible. In total, 18 BAVC hospitals treated more than 725,000 horses during the war, of which 530,000 were healed. A typical veterinary hospital in France could take 2,000 patients. In Egypt there were also separate hospitals for camels, which were used along with horses in desert battles.

Private organizations, especially animal welfare groups and charities, also contributed to the network of animal hospitals during this war. These advocates for humane treatment of animals linked patriotism to animal welfare: they enlisted public support to "Help the Horse to Save the Soldier" while popularizing the idea that all horses deserved better lives. At Geneva, the countries at war inaugurated the "Purple Cross Service" whose aim was caring for wounded army horses. In the United States the "American Red Star Relief," in partnership with the U.S. War Department, played the same role for military horses. In the UK, the Royal Society for the Prevention of Cruelty to Animals (RSPCA) asserted that it had saved thousands of horses, worth almost twenty million pounds. Another British organization with the long Victorian name "Our Dumb Friends League operating under the sign of the Blue Cross" became simply the "Blue Cross" in 1950. The Blue Cross symbol corresponded to the Red Cross, used for human medical relief, thus linking the well-being of soldiers to that of their animals. For fund-raising, the Blue Cross used one of the most famous images of the war, entitled "Good-bye Old Man": a soldier comforted his dying horse in battle as shells exploded around them. The Blue Cross Fund established both horse and dog hospitals near the front lines in France and Italy. This organization employed its own veterinarians, which treated more than 50,000 horses in France alone. (The name Blue Cross is still used today, although the society's services have been extended to other animal species as well.)

The need for veterinarians to care for the animals in these hospitals expanded the profession's activities dramatically. The German War Ministry initially assigned 766 veterinary officers to its first horse hospitals. However, this number grew to 5,354 army veterinarians – almost 75 percent of all veterinarians in Germany. Diverting this many veterinarians away from the home front demonstrates the importance of these horses to the German government and the war effort. This was not unique to Germany. The Italian Army Veterinary Corps began the war with 219 veterinarians in May 1915, but at the end of the war this figure had grown more than ten times to 2,819. The Veterinary Service of the French Army counted 552 veterinarians in 1914; but during the war this figure grew to about 3,000, of which 134 died. The BAVC had learned some lessons from the disastrous Boer War. Better trained and equipped, the BAVC vets tried to improve the care for war animals (and they were joined by civilian veterinarians with broader experience). In August 1914, the BAVC started the war with 164 veterinary officers. During the war, a further 1,356 were commissioned from among civilian vets, and by 1918 almost half of the veterinarians in the UK were serving in the Army. For European veterinarians, World War I was the unifying experience of that generation.

The Global Animal Economy

Like previous wars, World War I caused dramatic translocations of animals, fodder, and animal products. The worldwide supply of freshly recruited horses and animal fodder (grass, oats, hay, and straw) proved decisive for warfare, and veterinarians played important roles in this global economy. They inspected animals at ports, ran remount stations, provided medical and surgical care, and advised on daily rationing of various types and sizes of horses and mules. One important factor in the German defeat was its shortage of horses, due to the blockade by the Allied Forces that made it impossible to import enough animals. To provision the armies, the combatant governments purchased animals from remote locations thousands of kilometers from the battlefields. Moving these supplies across oceans and continents required vast expenditures on ships and rail transport, even from nations not officially involved in the war.

Huge armies required meat and other food products, and cattle and other food-producing animals traveling long distances, then confined close together in high numbers, sparked fresh epizootics. In Europe, rinderpest and contagious bovine pleuropneumonia reappeared and caused outbreaks in several places. Newly established in Poland after the Balkan Wars, rinderpest wiped out most of the cattle there in a huge outbreak after the war ended. Rinderpest surged in many other parts of the world during the war years. In Palestine, outbreaks occurred in 1913 and 1915, imported by animals from Damascus and Turkey. In Southeast Asia, the disease circulated from China through Vietnam and Hong Kong to the Philippine islands, causing epizootics between 1915 and 1920. This was an ongoing problem for the Philippines, which needed draft animals for the rice fields; the U.S. invasion had brought the disease in 1900 and cattle populations were just recovering when the wartime outbreaks began. Diseases traveled with horses, also. "Shipping fever" (pleuropneumonia) plagued animals confined for weeks on ships, spreading rapidly once the sick horses landed. Surra (equine trypanosomiasis) was endemic in Burma, Thailand, and Vietnam in equines. Once again, the Philippines suffered when the Americans brought surra-infected horses to the islands. Within a decade, surra killed up to 80 percent of the nation's horses, ponies, and mules, crippling transportation. However, by that time the Americans were preoccupied with the horse economy back home.

When the war broke out, the United States possessed 27 million horses, donkeys, and mules, while the number of vets (most caring for horses) had reached 8,163. North America, although officially neutral at this point, sold and shipped half a million horses to Europe by March 1915. By the time the United States entered the war, it had already supplied over 1 million animals (including 350,000 mules) worth about $200 million to the Allies. After entering the war in April 1917, the U.S. Army set up a remount system in France with 17 depots where about 200,000 horses and mules brought in from the United States, Britain, France, and Spain were received and maintained. The U.S. Army had one horse for every three soldiers. A huge market for U.S. and Canadian farmers had developed, but buyers from the European and U.S. armies were critical. They inspected the animals and carefully selected the most fit. Horses were rejected for war service if they had lung problems, lameness, or infectious diseases like farcy, glanders, melanosis, and mange. Veterinarians were supposed to issue the official certificates of health, but a thriving "black market" also existed for horses. U.S. sellers dumped tens of thousands of inferior horses in Canada, destined for transportation to Britain. Thousands were found unfit and died in veterinary hospitals before disembarking to Europe. These animals would have been slaughtered for meat in Europe, but Americans had a cultural prejudice against eating horse meat. Nonetheless, the demand for horses seemed unlimited, and the price for a healthy American horse almost doubled. Farm owners in the middle of North America increased horse breeding and production, hoping to make money on the wartime horse economy.

The magnitude of the global equine economy is clearly shown by the final balance sheet at the end of the war. Britain entered the war with 25,000 horses. By August 1917, the British Army counted 591,000 horses, 213,000 mules, 47,000 camels, and 11,000 oxen. It is estimated that the British, French, German, and Austrian-Hungarian armies together had about 3 million horses at the battle fields. The British Army used about 1.2 million horses (468,000 horses purchased in the UK, 136,000 in Australia, and 429,000 in North America) and mules during the war, of which 484,000 sadly died in battle. During campaigns in East Africa, the British Army lost about 31,000 horses, 33,000 mules, and 32,000 donkeys. Most of these animals died of diseases, especially African horse sickness (caused by a virus spread by insects). Due to the lessons learned during the Boer and Balkan wars, horses were better trained and acclimatized before shipment to the battlefields in France and Belgium. Veterinary care had improved so that fewer horses died from disease and starvation. Nevertheless, it is estimated that about 1.5 million horses of the combined British and French perished during World War I. Half of the French Army's horses died (over 1 million); the German Army lost about 1 million horses. More animals died due to the harsh circumstances, such as lack of fodder, than the actual number fallen in battle. Another sad result was that after the war thousands of horses did not return home but were slaughtered instead. Transporting them was too difficult and expensive, and governments feared the horses could spread diseases.

Thousands of camels were used in warfare, fulfilling the role of cavalry and carrying heavy loads in Palestine, the Jordan Valley, the Sinai Peninsula, Egypt, and northern Africa. Camels were also expensive, worth about 10 Turkish gold pounds per animal. These robust animals are better adjusted to the desert climate than horses and mules. For instance, they can close their nostrils during sandstorms, and they can survive without water for a week. However, camels have specific needs and care. They are sensitive to cold and suffer fungal infections when their hooves get wet. When they must eat fodder from the ground instead from a bucket or manger, they swallow a lot of sand, causing colic. Throughout World War I camel-mounted troops were used in the desert campaigns, such as by the Imperial Camel Corps in Egypt with a frontline strength of almost 4,000 camels. This corps was supported by a Camel Remount Depot and a Camel Veterinary Hospital. As with horses and cattle, however, diseases were a major problem for camels in the war. Surra (trypanosomiasis), with high mortality in camels, traveled with these animals in Egypt and Northern Africa. Tick-borne anemias and viral diseases also plagued camels exposed to ticks, especially in desert and steppe environments new to them. Keeping these animals alive and well depended on the expertise of camel keepers from India as well as 42 British-trained veterinarians in the Mobile Veterinary Section of the Imperial Camel Corps. The French Army also created a special *compagnie méhariste* that cared for the *Méhari* camels used in northern Africa. On the opposing side, camels were more familiar, but there were fewer trained veterinarians to provide medical and surgical care. Only about 250 formally trained veterinarians existed in the whole Ottoman empire in 1914, and the army did not possess enough medications and instruments. Injured or starving animals usually died, contributing to the high morbidity and mortality and shortage of draft animals at the end of the war.

The Dogs of War

During World War I, dogs performed a variety of tasks. The use of dogs as military weapons dates from antiquity. The Spaniards used mastiffs and greyhounds to attack Indigenous people when they conquered the Americas. Napoleon may also have used fighting dogs. The modern use of war dogs first started in Germany. The world's first military war dog school was opened at Lechernich near Berlin in 1884. Military dog schools were established in many European countries, including Germany, France, Austria, Italy, Belgium, Russia, Bulgaria, Sweden, and the Netherlands, from 1870 onward. Ghent in Belgium became the early center for training police dogs and had also established war dog schools. Draught dogs pulling milk carts were quite common in that country. By 1914 draught dogs – particularly huge Great Pyrenees dogs – were being used to haul machine guns. Britain and the United States began to recognize the value of highly trained war dogs during World War I. In war dog schools, thousands of dogs – preferably purebred German and Belgian Shepherd dogs, Airedale terriers, mastiffs, Labrador retrievers, boxers, and Scottish collies – learned to work as a messenger, sentry, scout, patrol, or ambulance (Red Cross) dog, after which they were sent to the front. They also laid down telephone wires, detected mines, forwarded carrier pigeons, and conveyed provisions and munitions. In addition, small dogs (and cats) were important to catch the huge number of rats that lived in the trenches, eating food, spreading disease, and keeping soldiers awake.

It is estimated that in total about 75,000 military dogs were employed at the battlefields of World War I (Fig. 5.4). Germany alone used 30,000 dogs, of

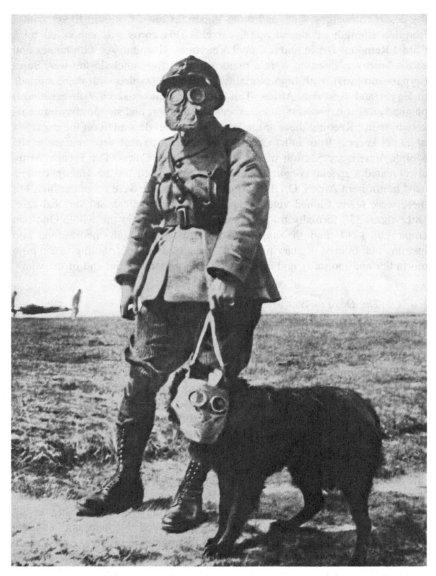

Figure 5.4 French soldier handling a war dog, both with gas masks, after the German Army started using poisonous gas in 1917.
Source: Le Miroir 7 (1917) No. 183, May 27, cover.

which 7,000 died in service. France too employed many dogs, of which about 8,000 served as sled dogs in the mountain areas. More than 4,000 wounded German soldiers and 2,000 French soldiers were saved by Red Cross dogs (*Sanitätshunden* in German and *chiens sanitaires* in French). Strict guidelines for the use, feeding, and care of war dogs were drawn up. In the kennels attached to veterinary hospitals, veterinarians performed regular inspections to avoid the spread of contagious diseases among dogs. There they also treated sick or wounded dogs that returned from the front. Veterinarians working for the Blue Cross treated over 10,000 dogs in the charity's French hospitals during World War I. Not all this care benefited the animals, however. Veterinarians also performed surgery to cut the vocal cords of dogs, mules, and horses, so that these animals could not make noise to expose the positions of their troops. Vets also cropped dogs' ears and removed part of the tail, practices that continue for some breeds today.

War circumstances strongly affected human–animal relationships. On the one hand, millions of animals were sacrificed under gruesome circumstances. On the other hand, many soldiers found comfort in the companionship of animals, and animal welfare groups linked their cause to patriotism. To commemorate the many animals that had died, various memorials were erected worldwide. Novels, poems, movies, plays, and documentaries have also featured the tragic fates of animals in World War I. A few stories were more positive: some war animals were decorated for their efforts and courage, by which many soldiers were saved. For instance, the French Army lauded message-carrying pigeons who had saved many lives by transferring crucial intelligence. The most famous World War I dog was Rin Tin Tin, a young German Shepherd with shellshock found by an American trooper. He took this "prisoner-of-war dog" to the United States, where it played the main role in twenty-six popular films. Descendants of Rin Tin Tin were used in a training school for dogs destined for the U.S. Army in World War II. Although military veterinarians mostly cared for horses, injured dogs also were patients at military veterinary hospitals. The U.S. veterinary profession benefitted at home from the good publicity.

Problems with Veterinary War Efforts

World War I amplified some of the problems facing the veterinary profession at this time. Despite the hard work of military veterinarians, the world's domestic animal population plummeted during the war years. The profession was outmatched by the overwhelming need for animal care. Along with healing wounded and infected war animals, army veterinarians had to inspect food destined for the military, train more veterinarians, conduct research, and support agriculture. Twenty percent of the veterinarians in the U.S. Army were primarily food inspectors. Veterinary food inspectors worked in special army slaughterhouses and inspected canned food supplied by factories. In their home countries, lecturers and students in veterinary schools were also involved in activities that supported the war efforts, such as the development and production of anti-pyogenic serum at the veterinary school in Turin. But in many schools, education and research were severely disrupted because so many teachers and students were enlisted into the military. Agricultural production declined due to outbreaks of livestock diseases and because so many horses served in armies. Veterinary practice also encountered problems due to shortages of (imported) drugs, instruments, and bandages. There were simply too few veterinarians to do the necessary work, and they lacked the resources they needed.

Shortages of formally trained veterinarians and veterinary supplies meant that animal health care at home depended even more on traditional and local expertise. Farmers and livestock raisers reverted to home remedies and experienced (albeit unlicensed) animal doctors. The problems they addressed included not only the usual injuries, illnesses, and difficult births, but also the issue of diseases spread by the global animal economy. This was especially true in areas around the world colonized by Europeans. Unfortunately, modern veterinary regimes had worked to destroy traditional livestock-raising practices and folk animal healing. For example, one effect of the "modernization" of animal breeding and veterinary medicine was the loss of breeds adapted to local (in some cases, harsh) conditions and the disempowerment of the people who knew how to keep them alive and well. This effect was painfully obvious in much of the vast African continent and in Southeast and South Asia. Imported European animals often did not survive well in their new environments. They imported diseases that killed native animals, causing tragic famines and mass deaths. As historian Lotte Hughes has argued, to Indigenous peoples these imported diseases (rinderpest, most notably) represented a type of "infection by colonialism" that destroyed their cultures.

Colonial regimes, which could have adopted local knowledge and encouraged training of local people to increase the veterinary workforce, usually failed to do so despite the need for more veterinary professionals. The list of "native" people in colonial areas who acquired a formal veterinary education during this period was short. One of these was Charles de Boissiere (1866–1949), a native of Trinidad and Tobago who served as the Government Veterinary Surgeon there during World War I; another was the South African Jotello Festiri Soga (Chapter 4). Veterinary schools were established in India, where members of the Goan ethnic group predominated as students, and in Burma and Java; but numbers remained small. More common was educating "para-veterinarians," or assistants recruited from the local population, which was also done in India and several other areas. In the process, the "modern" veterinary regime often failed to incorporate crucial local knowledge about animal health. For example, Dutch veterinarians working in Java had never seen water buffaloes and knew nothing about these animals' husbandry or diseases. Water buffaloes were the key draft animals in Java, yet veterinary officials and instructors ignored them. Characteristic of colonial powers' prejudices against Indigenous expertise, these were lost opportunities to gain knowledge and improve veterinary services.

Modern veterinary medicine's basis in the biomedical sciences was its great strength, but science also had a dark side: research on biological and chemical warfare agents. This type of warfare in various forms had existed since antiquity, but its use increased in World War I. The French Army fired teargas at German troops. German chemist and Nobel Prize–winner Fritz Haber performed research on chlorine gas, which was first used on a large scale by the German Army in April 1915. Also, the French, including chemist and Nobel Prize–winner Victor Grignard, studied poisonous gases intensively. Later in the war, chemical weapons like phosgene and mustard gas grenades were used by both armies. These poisonous gases caused immense human and animal suffering, although poisoning of horses was less frequent because their noses were positioned higher than soldiers in the trenches. Gas masks for soldiers, horses, and dogs were developed to protect against such attacks. As for biological weapons, German biomedical scientists, including veterinarians, became involved in developing microorganisms (plague, cholera, anthrax, glanders) that could infect enemy humans and animals. For instance, from 1915 onward German agents secretly inoculated shipments of horses and cattle in American harbors with disease-producing bacteria. These activities were part of an international network of German operatives who attempted to use anthrax spores and the causative bacteria of glanders to sabotage animal populations in France, Argentina, Mesopotamia, Romania, and Norway. These German sabotage campaigns never seriously affected the supply of military livestock and horses. However, they accelerated scientific research in several nations, which developed biological weapons that would be used later during World War.

After the War: Veterinary Internationalism

After World War I ended, the global map was redrawn in Europe, where nine new independent nations were established. Veterinary schools were established in these nations: Brno, Czechoslovakia (1918); Riga, Latvia (1919); Zagreb, Yugoslavia (1919); and Sofia, Bulgaria (1923). The modern Turkish Republic, with Mustafa Kemal Atatürk at its head, was founded in 1923 from the former Ottoman Empire. A new University at Ankara began veterinary instruction at its Higher Institute of Agriculture in 1933 (joining the older school in Istanbul). Uprisings, economic crises, and the aftermath of "war imperialism" began to undermine colonial regimes around the world. The diversion of the world's animal economy to providing war animals meant that agriculture suffered. The former Ottoman empire, for example, lost about half of its draft animals during the war, leading to severe shortages of horses, camels, and oxen for agriculture. This problem created hunger and tremendous resentment and probably contributed to the end of the empire. Wars and revolutions continued to affect livestock production significantly. For instance, in 1914, the bloodiest year of the Mexican Revolution (1910–1920), 1.5 million people died. This led to abandoned farms, destroyed infrastructure, and a loss of half the nation's cattle, bringing livestock numbers back to the level of 1880. It took 30 years to recover production at the 1914 level. The Russian Civil War (1917–1920) destroyed the rural economy and led to a huge loss of livestock and horses, mainly by spreading infectious diseases. The same happened during the Turkish War of Independence (1920–1922) and the Spanish Civil War (1936–1939). These conflicts often disrupted the veterinary infrastructure and caused outbreaks of livestock diseases.

Fears of a rinderpest pandemic led nations to cooperate on international control strategies after the war ended. Rinderpest was again spreading in Europe, as the Bolshevik armies and their infected cattle crossed the Caucasus, entering the Ukraine, Latvia, and Lithuania in 1917, and invading Poland in 1920. Due to international veterinary efforts, particularly from Denmark and France, that epidemic was finally eliminated in 1923. (Since then, Europe has been free of epidemic rinderpest, except for an outbreak in eastern Turkey in 1991 that was contained by the Turkish government.) In 1920, rinderpest had also traveled in cattle and wild animals exported from endemic areas in India and Somalia to nations such as Belgium and Brazil. These outbreaks triggered the first International Conference of Epizootic Diseases of Domestic Animals (Paris, 1921), which included representatives of 43 countries. The 1921 conference, with French veterinarian Emmanuel Leclainche (1861–1953) as chairman, called for an international organization to coordinate campaigns against infectious animal diseases. With Leclainche as its first director, the Office International des Épizooties (OIE) [World Organization for Animal Health] was established in Paris in 1924. Since then, the OIE has remained the world's leading organization responsible for collection and dissemination of knowledge on epizootic diseases and their control.

This solidarity was typical for the post–World War I era with the rise of a series of new international governmental and non-governmental agencies, with the League of Nations (LoN) at the center. As a result of the Versailles peace treaty, this organization was established in 1920 with the task of resolving international conflicts before they could lead to warfare. The 1925 Geneva Protocol banning chemical and biological weapons was a result of the

League's efforts. In 1927, the LoN appointed an expert group of veterinarians whose task was designing regulations and measures to facilitate international traffic of animals and animal products; coordinating campaigns against contagious diseases (including inspection and disease-free certification); and guaranteeing the safety and quality animal-origin foods in international trade. Their conventions, codes, and standards were adopted by 15 countries. Later, their work formed the basis for international veterinary legal regulations of the European Union, the United Nations, and the World Trade Organization.

Conditions in the 1920s and 30s reflected the dramatic changes accelerated by the war. Postwar agricultural economic depression led to cutbacks in government-sponsored veterinary expenditures in Europe and the UK. Horse prices, which had increased during the war, plummeted, and numbers of animals continued to decrease as war losses were not replaced. In the United States, equine-oriented veterinarians watched anxiously as the horse economy collapsed due to the ascent of motorized transportation. Most private, equine-oriented veterinary schools were forced to close, and numbers of vets declined by the end of the 1920s. Most veterinarians made a modest living, treating all species of animals in small private businesses. Around the world, veterinarians and animal healers directly affected by the war worked hard to restore livestock and control diseases. Several nations in the Global South successfully developed their home industries, raising animals for meat export markets. By the end of the 1920s, for example, Argentina was the world's biggest beef exporter, supplying 61 percent of the global total, while New Zealand and Australia took over as the world's top mutton exporters at 45 percent.

Despite the difficult conditions, those conducting research made some important advances. For example, Filipino veterinarians developed a successful rinderpest vaccine in 1934 that could be easily deployed in their country: it was a dried formulation that did not require refrigeration, and each animal needed only one injection to induce acceptable immunity. During World War I, German researchers had created a synthetic drug, "suramin," to be used against human trypanosomiasis or "sleeping sickness." Veterinarians in Northern Africa and India tested and adapted suramin after it became more widely available in the 1920s, to treat surra (trypanosomiasis in horses and camels). These discoveries (and many others) helped with the slow process of restoring livestock herds after the war.

Large-scale campaigns to control animal diseases, carried out by governments and non-governmental organizations, also helped to increase numbers of healthy animals. The campaign to eradicate hog cholera (classical swine fever) using veterinary vaccination and slaughter of infected animals occupied many veterinarians in the midwestern United States. Bovine tuberculosis (bTB) and brucellosis, the two milk-borne zoonoses, are also good examples. Beginning in 1917, the U.S. Bureau of Animal Industry coordinated a bTB control campaign that employed large numbers of veterinarians. Over time, this program's goals became more ambitious: from control, it became an "eradication" program aiming to wipe out bTB (deemed a success when it ended in 1940). The sugar-growing corporations of Trinidad and Tobago hired veterinarians to control bTB in the water buffaloes that were essential draft and food animals. The program included licensing milk vendors, applying tuberculin testing, and slaughtering or isolating infected cows. Between 1920 and 1950, the infection rate in water buffaloes dropped from about 40 percent down to less than 10 percent. Campaigns in several European countries, still recovering from wartime devastation, were planned and started during the 1920s and 1930s. The British government began its bTB eradication program, which continued until 1960.

For brucellosis, the Scandinavian countries' governments sponsored the first control and eradication campaigns. Norway was the first nation to eradicate the disease, followed by Sweden. Denmark began its program in 1937, with national legislation and a tax on meat and cattle exports to pay for the cost. The United States estimated that the dairy and beef cattle industries suffered $125 million loss in productivity in one year alone, 1934. However, the U.S. Department of Agriculture's campaign to control brucellosis did not start until the 1950s, after the Bureau of Animal Industry had been dissolved and its veterinarians reassigned. In the 1970s, brucellosis became the target of a global eradication campaign. However, bTB and brucellosis are still problems in many parts of the developing world today.

During the 1930s, the global economic disaster (the Great Depression) challenged hard-won gains in animal health and disease control. In the United States, many newly graduated veterinarians expecting to work with livestock could not find employment. Some began working in companion animal clinics in cities; some found work at universities or in industries; and others left veterinary medicine. Governments could not afford to hire veterinarians, conduct large-scale anti-disease campaigns, or compensate farmers for mandatory slaughter of infected animals. In the Philippines, for example, horse owners whose animals tested positive for glanders had been compensated for the animal's value. Once this compensation program ended in 1932, horse owners refused to test their animals, and glanders incidence increased. Desperate to prevent costly disease outbreaks in cattle, the Philippines stopped importing live animals. Another problem was funding veterinary education. New schools were especially vulnerable when the government withdrew funding since students could not afford high tuition fees. In Burma, for example, a veterinary school built at Insein in 1925 for Indigenous Burmese students and assistants closed between 1929 and 1933.

Despite the financial issues, several new veterinary schools were founded during the 1930s. In Tehran, Iran, the Higher School of Stockbreeding was converted to a Veterinary Faculty in 1932; and in Norway, the Norwegian School of Veterinary Sciences (Oslo) began taking students in 1934 (eventually including some from Finland, Iceland, and other countries). In Kabul, Afghanistan, veterinary sciences have been taught since 1932, while the British began veterinary instruction in Khartoum (Sudan) in 1938. In Central and South America, a trio of schools were established in the 1930s: Manabí Province and Quito, Ecuador (1931); Maracay, Venezuela (1938); and Santa Cruz, Bolivia (1940). The government of Venezuela hired experts from Chile, Uruguay, Argentina, North America, and elsewhere to design the curricula and national programs for veterinary hygiene; the school was named Escuela de Expertos Agropecuarios y Prácticos en Sanidad Animal. (Since the American veterinary leader Daniel Elmer Salmon guided the Uruguayan school's founding, North American models of education influenced the Uruguayan and Venezuelan professions.)

World War II

Despite what many people had hoped, World War I was not "the war to end all wars." At the war's end, the Allies levied severe penalties on Germany, angering the hungry and impoverished population. The Great Depression, failing diplomacy and appeasement within the League of Nations, and the rise of fascism and militarism in Germany, Italy, and Japan also contributed to the outbreak of another global war. Militarism, nationalism, and racism fed each other in East Asia following World War I. The situation was inflamed by European nations' poor treatment of their Asian allies. China, one of the winning Allies, was denied the right to its own (formerly German-occupied) territory; and the treaty ending the war excluded a "racial equality" clause requested by Japan (also an Allied nation). In 1931, nationalist Japanese forces invaded Manchuria, the northeastern provinces of China. This incident began the Pacific War (1931–1945), in which Japan gained vast agricultural lands in northern China. Japanese veterinarians and agricultural officials justified the invasion based on the idea that they were bringing "modernity" to "backward" Manchuria (a justification also used earlier in the annexation of Korea). Manchuria quickly became a testing ground for veterinary scientific colonialism: establishing breeding farms and laboratories, the Japanese developed new hybrid breeds of livestock and conducted research on diseases such as glanders and anthrax in wild and domesticated animals. These agricultural activities assisted Japanese settlement in Manchuria, and their success encouraged the Japanese government to consider expanding its control over other Asian nations.

By 1940, Japan had joined the Axis Powers – Germany (now under the National Socialist government, or Nazis) and Italy – with a tripartite agreement. Italy's invasion and annexation of Albania in 1939 had triggered a series of military conflicts, drawing several nations into battles in southern and central Europe. The conflicts in Europe, the Pacific, and elsewhere combined into the twentieth century's second global-scale war, World War II (1939–1945). Again, animals played crucial roles in this global conflagration, and veterinarians worked in both military and civilian capacities to safeguard food supplies and keep war animals healthy.

Animal Warriors in World War II

After World War I, countries reacted differently to the question about mechanization of their armies. In some countries, national horse breeding programs with government sponsorship continued their activities at a peacetime level because equines had proven to be so important. In the USSR for instance, cavalry units were not reduced. In other countries more emphasis was placed on mechanization – for instance, in Britain, where after a rapid demobilization the Army Veterinary School reduced in size and finally closed in 1938. A year later the British Army was fully motorized. The U.S. Army only had about 50,000 military horses in 1941, when that nation entered the war; this was about 1 horse for every 134 soldiers (as compared to 1 horse for every 3 soldiers during World War I). In Germany, the Nazi regime started to mechanize the *Wehrmacht* as part of war preparation in the mid-1930s. The images of the successful *Blitzkrieg* in which Poland, Belgium, the Netherlands, Luxembourg, Denmark, Norway, and France were defeated, featured motorized tanks, armored vehicles, and airplanes. Most of the defeated armies still had cavalry divisions – for instance, Poland, where 200,000 mounted troopers were powerless against German infantry divisions with tanks and modern machine guns. The last of these futile cavalry battles took place near Moscow in 1941, when 2,000 mounted troopers of a Red Army cavalry division with drawn swords rode into an artillery barrage of the German infantry. All men and horses of the Mongol cavalry were tragically killed, with no casualties to the Nazis. The era of frontal cavalry warfare had ended, but horses continued to be used for other purposes. The "modernization" propaganda of this era effectively hid the ongoing participation of animals in the war, although at much reduced levels compared with World War I.

German (Nazi) propaganda was designed to intimidate its enemies, and it featured motorized tanks, airplanes, and lethal machine guns. These technologies altered warfare forever. However, as Richard DiNardo and Austin Bay have shown, this image of mechanized warfare that did not involve any animals is incorrect. Surprisingly, the basic means of transport in the German Army was still horse drawn, with about half the German Army still relying on horses to move supplies, artillery, and troops. Next to mechanization, the *Wehrmacht* had quietly maintained remount stations and had mobilized many horses after the rapid expansion of the army began in 1935. As the war unfolded, the German Army confiscated all horses in the conquered territories (such as Czechoslovakia and Poland); by 1939, the German Army included 590,000 horses. After the campaign of May 1940, in which about 53,000 horses were used, heavier breeds of horses were also confiscated from the Netherlands, Belgium, and Normandy (France). These horses were transported to the east for hauling artillery during the invasion of the Soviet Union in June 1941. By that time, the *Wehrmacht* had sent more than 625,000 horses to the eastern front. This number of animals was about 30 percent of the horses used during World War I, and the army had to maintain veterinary forces to care for them.

After a rapid territorial gain in 1941, the German tanks and armored vehicles got stuck in the autumn mud and snow in the USSR, a country with an immense area and limited paved roads. The Soviets defended their territory using scorched earth tactics, destroying roads, bridges, and railways. Horses thus remained crucial in maintaining army supply lines over huge distances. Shortages of drinking water, fodder (and cotton feed bags), and medications, as well as the harsh winter of 1940–1941, devastated the Germans' horses. Almost 180,000 animals died or were incapacitated by outbreaks of equine pneumonia, influenza, glanders, and mange. In army veterinary hospitals designed to treat 500 horses at a time, veterinarians struggled to care for 1,000 to 3,000 patients. The German Army counted about 700 veterinary officers in 1939. By 1945, this number increased to 5,650, which was more than half of the total number of veterinarians in Germany at the time. As a rule, each army veterinarian cared for 300, later 450, animals, of which 70 to 80 percent were cured – a remarkable record. These vets also ran mobile research units for food and feed inspection, as well as for x-ray and biomedical analyses. Similar to World War I, the major cause of death was not injuries; most horses died of exhaustion, lack of water and (bad) fodder, colic, and scabies.

The German Army used a total of 2.75 million horses and mules during World War II, of which 1.2 million were requisitioned from Germany and the occupied countries. The German reliance on horses had a deep impact on European agriculture. Particularly in countries where most horses were confiscated for the army, agricultural output decreased by 20 to 40 percent. By February 1945, 1.2 million horses remained in the German Army. The devastation of animal populations in the USSR was even more severe. The horse population in the Soviet Union dropped from 21 to 7.8 million between 1940 and 1943, despite the Soviet Army's best efforts to keep them alive. A visitor to the Soviet veterinary hospitals was impressed by their modern equipment and veterinary practices. The Cossack warriors of the Soviet cavalry played a significant role in the defeat of the German invasion by attacking and harassing the Germans behind enemy lines. To support the Cossacks, veterinary equipment and drugs were sent to Russia from Britain.

The other Allied forces also depended on horses and mules as draught and pack animals while moving through terrain too rough or muddy for trucks. The Greek Army used more than 200,000 mules in its battle against the Italian invaders in 1941. The British Royal Army Veterinary Corps (RAVC), which increased in numbers from 85 to 519 veterinary officers between 1940 and 1945, had to take care of 6,500 military horses, 10,000 mules, and 1,700 camels in 1942 alone. The RAVC was also responsible for the procurement and health of war dogs. The British Army used airlifted pack horses and mules as essential means of transport, particularly in Palestine, Syria, Greece, Eritrea, Italy, and Burma. In 1943, the British began jungle warfare against the Japanese in Burma. With no good place to land airplanes, the army dropped pack animals and dogs by parachute from the airplanes. The vocal cords of these animals had previously been removed under anesthesia, so that they would not reveal their positions to the Japanese. During this campaign the British Army also used 1,600 elephants, captured from the Japanese Army, for transport and to clear trees and shrubs that prevented the army's movements. Bullocks were used as pack animals and as "meat on the hoof." Unfortunately, animals suffering from severe battle wounds could not be evacuated and, instead of receiving treatment, had to be shot. The Japanese also used horses, donkeys, and mules on a large scale.

As they had during World War I, dogs continued to play various important roles on the battlefield. They were sent first into caves and tunnels created by the enemy; carried messages; and took supplies to isolated troops. Almost ten times more dogs participated in World War II than in the World War I. Most countries had large military dog programs. The Red Army was quite successful in training dogs to find explosive mines before soldiers or vehicles could detonate them. In 1943 alone, Russian mine-detection dogs found 529,000 German mines. The dog "Zhucha" became the champion by pinpointing 2,000 mines in 18 days. As a living "anti-tank weapons," dogs in the Red Army were also trained to destroy German armored vehicles and tanks by carrying and igniting bombs under them (a suicide mission for the dog).

Unexploded mines and bombs were only one problem for the lands occupied by the armies. Numbers of livestock decreased considerably due to requisitions, strict rationing, a loss of export markets, the import blockade for animal feed and disease, and starvation. Farmers shifted from livestock to producing grains for hungry human populations. Disease outbreaks increased when armies moved through the land with huge numbers of war animals. Under war or occupation circumstances, veterinarians had difficulty maintaining effective control measures against diseases such as bovine tuberculosis.

For all countries involved, veterinary practice back at home became more and more difficult during the war due to shortages of veterinarians, supplies of fuel, equipment, disinfectants, and drugs, since the armies used up most of the veterinary resources.

Food Inspection in Wartime

Armies required huge food supplies, and given the scarcity of animals in war-torn areas, the military had to purchase, store, distribute, and transport provisions for its soldiers. Complex supply chains sustained the armies of both sides, the Allies and Axis powers. Veterinarians were at the forefront of maintaining these supplies, especially for meat, milk, eggs, and canned foods. In the U.S. Army, 90 percent of the army vets were primarily food inspectors (compared to 20 percent during World War I). They inspected enormous amounts of food in both civilian and military settings, including 142 billion pounds of meat and milk products, between 1940 and 1945. The United States ran 11 laboratories domestically and 23 abroad (from Iceland to Morocco to the Philippines) in military areas to provide bacteriological and chemical testing of food supplies. By August 1945, the U.S. Army Veterinary Service included over 2,000 officers and about 8,000 enlisted soldiers working as technicians. In the field, they worked alongside bacteriologists, physicians, and technicians and their duties included epidemiological studies (human and animal diseases); inspections of animals and microscopic inspections of food; and the development, manufacture, and standardization of sera and other biological treatments. A few veterinarians managed to conduct bacteriological, pathological, or epidemiological research along with their duties.

War circumstances showed two very different faces of human–animal relationships. On the one hand, hundreds of thousands of horses, donkeys, and mules were used and sacrificed on the battlefield. Livestock were killed to feed hungry armies and were targeted with biological weapons or animal diseases. (Horses were also killed for their meat.) Tens of thousands of dogs served and died in the combating armies, often killed by mines or explosives. On mainland Europe, starving people killed and ate dogs (and cats). On the other hand, however, during the bombing of London in 1940, Blue Cross volunteers tried to rescue horses, dogs, and cats from the ruins alongside Red Cross personnel trying to save injured people. Soldiers adopted pet animals. One nation, Germany, even prioritized animal welfare (as we will see). Amid these events, veterinarians tried to keep war horses and dogs healthy; worked to prevent livestock diseases; and attempted to maintain the safety of the food supply. Veterinarians used their scientific knowledge to increase animal health and public health. However, we must also understand the ways in which scientific knowledge could be used against humans and animals. World War

II stimulated the dramatic growth of state-sponsored programs to develop what one physician called "public health in reverse": biological weapons.

Biological Warfare: The Dark Side of the Biomedical Sciences

The civilian populations of war-torn nations suffered terribly under the "Total Warfare Doctrine" common to both sides during World War II. The goal of this doctrine was to destroy the socioeconomic infrastructure of the enemy: cities, factories, stations, railways, roads, bridges, and even farms and homes. In World War II, an estimated 20 million soldiers died. But almost twice that number of civilians, 38 million, died from bombing, disease, starvation, massacres, and genocide. World War II involved the whole population of warring nations in Asia, Europe, and Africa, and any weapon could be used against civilians. Although microbiological knowledge was a crucial tool for improving human and animal health, it had a dark side. Biological toxins or infectious agents such as bacteria, viruses, insects, and fungi could be used to deliberately incapacitate or kill humans, animals, and plants. Biological weapons (BW) offered opportunities to infect water and food as well as the human and animal population of the enemy.

After World War I, military authorities in several countries had continued or initiated programs for the development of BW on a large scale. These programs existed because nations feared that their enemies were developing BW. All these nations' governments had signed the 1925 Geneva Protocol, which forbade the use of chemical and biological weapons. But the Geneva Protocol had a major flaw: it allowed nations to defend themselves if BW was used against them. Fearing that enemies *would* deploy these weapons, several nations secretly developed their own BW to use in retaliation if necessary. Next to plague, anthrax, and glanders, the rinderpest virus was categorized as a potential weapon of mass destruction. For instance, Britain included this virus in its secret BW program during World War II. The United States and Canada, Britain's allies, worked on a rinderpest vaccine. The British also manufactured cattle feed containing anthrax spores and tested aerosolized anthrax on sheep isolated on an island. During World War II, BW programs grew much larger in Britain, Canada, France, Germany, Italy, Japan, the Soviet Union, and the United States. All of these BW programs depended on the expertise of veterinarians, microbiologists, chemists, physicians, and other scientists.

Of the nations with BW programs, only Japan used these weapons on a large scale. The people and animals of Japanese-occupied territories, especially in Manchuria, suffered as these weapons were developed and tested in secret facilities there. The Imperial Japanese Army used biological (and chemical) weapons against Chinese soldiers and civilians, killing probably tens of thousands. For example, in 1940, the Japanese Air Force released ceramic bombs full of fleas carrying bubonic plague over the city of Ningbo. The extent of Japanese biological warfare, and the widespread participation of Japanese scientists in it, has only become known since the war ended. Other isolated BW attacks occurred: the Soviet Red Army probably infected rats with tularemia (rabbit fever) and released them behind German lines during the siege of Stalingrad. At least 50,000 German soldiers became ill with fever, headache, swollen lymph nodes, and fatigue. The practical problem with BW was the potential for infection beyond the enemy, either back into the home army or the civilian population, and this fact probably deterred wider use of these terrible weapons. However, for scientists (including veterinarians), the bigger problems with BW were moral and ethical ones.

Moral and Ethical Problems for Wartime Scientists

Despite the many benefits of scientific research, biological warfare programs were a grim example of how scientists could lose their ethical beliefs under political pressure. The dark side of science included not only the BW programs, but the twisting of scientific ideas into lethal political ideologies. Many German scientists and intellectuals believed the pseudo-scientific racial ideology of the German National Socialist Party (Nazi Party). Based on an earlier British and American perversion of Darwinian ideas, the Nazi racial ideology divided people into a hierarchy of imaginary "races" similar to ideas about animals belonging to inferior or superior species. According to Nazi racial ideology, certain groups of people, including the "Aryan" leaders of Nazi Germany and their followers, were deemed the "superior men" (*Übermenschen*). Jews, the ethnic Roma and Slavic peoples, people of African or Indian descent, homosexuals, and the mentally ill were considered "inferior men" (*Üntermenschen*). This fanatic and racist doctrine dehumanized many people. The ultimate result was the Holocaust (*Shoah*), the German government's carefully planned and deliberate genocide of six million Jews, Roma, and other peoples during World War II.

This Nazi doctrine of dehumanization reframed the meaning of "animal" and "human." It also depended in part on changes in human–animal relationships. Animal welfare became an important component of Nazi propaganda, while Nazi authorities stressed the fact that veterinarians should prioritize animal protection (Fig. 5.5). Under the Nazis, animals were often treated much better than the stigmatized so-called inferior humans. The Jewish procedures of ritual slaughter and vivisection of animals for scientific research were forbidden. Instead, people belonging to the so-called inferior groups were used as laboratory animals in horrible medical experiments conducted in German-run concentration camps. These crimes against humanity did not only occur in German-occupied territories. Racist ideologies also flourished within the

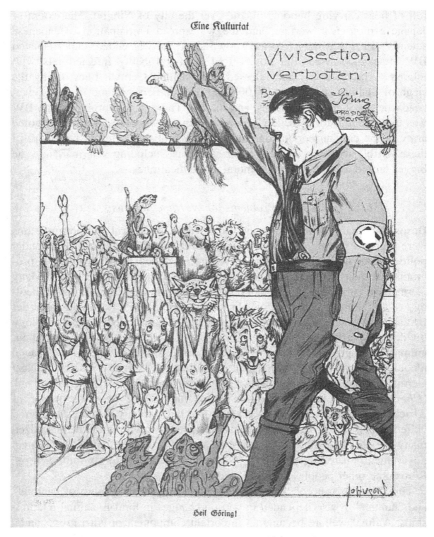

Figure 5.5 The animal world salutes Hermann Göring. Cartoon in
Kladeradatsch, September 3, 1933.

Japanese Imperial government and its army. While occupying parts of China,
Korea, and Southeast Asian countries, the Japanese Army targeted and killed
millions. Cruel experiments on humans were also conducted by Japanese
Army scientists, using people considered to be members of "inferior races."

Some of this research was even published after the war. (The authors claimed the experimental subjects were monkeys, but the evidence is clear that humans were subjected to experiments.) In the infamous Unit 731 in Manchuria, horrific biological weapons tests were conducted on prisoners of war and captured local people as well as on animals. It is important to recognize that these activities were not the work of a few depraved individual scientists. On the contrary, a tour of duty in Manchuria was part of the training and work of large numbers of Japanese scientists (including physicians and veterinarians) between the late 1930s and 1945.

History shows that biomedical researchers, including veterinarians, have played an important role in the development of biological (and chemical) weapons. It is difficult to understand how veterinarians, physicians, and scientists could have participated in such horrible activities. They had lost their moral compass due to nationalism, patriotism, or certain political or ideological agendas. In addition, some found their justification and motives in scientific prestige, employment, increased resources, and safety during wartime. The military leader of Unit 731 urged Japanese scientists to partici-pate in experiments with biological weapons (on humans as well as animals) for the scientific thrill and unique opportunities to conduct research that was usually prohibited. Not only voluntarily, but often under terror and pressure, scientists were forced to engage in this kind of research. Often, they or their families were threatened with imprisonment or death. For example, some scientists who tried to refuse a tour of duty in Unit 731 were threatened with execution. For any or all these reasons, some scientists who were educated to honor and protect the lives of humans justified the use of their knowledge for the explicit goal of injuring or killing civilians *en masse*. Others collaborated with brutal regimes and occupying armies. Faced with the moral dilemma of using or abusing their professional knowledge, they made choices that we view with horror today. How could this have happened? To understand their choices, we must consider the words, actions, and contexts of historical people.

Professional Accountability: Facing Our Past, Working for a Just Society

Like other scientists, veterinarians always work within a societal context, differing from time and place. Particularly during wartime, terror, or under totalitarian, racist, and intolerant regimes such as that of the Nazis, working conditions could be extremely difficult and dangerous. As we have seen above, these circumstances existed during both world wars. Similar to the majority of the population, most veterinarians followed a strategy of survival and quietly continued their local work. However, veterinarians in public service and leadership positions found themselves faced with the moral dilemma of whether to resist or to collaborate with a brutal regime such as the Nazis. This meant that many cooperated to some extent to prevent worse things from happening. Others were forced, or chose voluntarily, to engage with acts of war varying from supporting war activities, actively joining the military, or even developing weapons of mass destruction. As one U.S. veterinarian who helped develop BW later remembered, Americans expected to be attacked at any time and many felt desperate to help. Patriotism (saving the nation) and fear were powerful forces during times of war.

Sociological and psychological research has shown that after a war, most people want to forget the tragedies and losses they suffered and instead focus on recovery and return to normal life as soon as possible. Only later – often decades later – will most people reflect on their behavior during wartime. This also happened within veterinary medicine, where the behavior of the profession as a whole (and certain individual veterinarians in particular) was only examined in Germany 50 years after the war ended. In the 1980s, members of the History Section of the German Veterinary Medical Association had the courage to reflect on the behavior of their profession under Nazi rule in the period 1933–1945. They acknowledged the fact that more than 57 percent of German veterinarians were members of the Nazi party – the highest percentage of all academic professions. The inquiry included the activities of veterinarians in the nations occupied by the German Army as well as vets at home. By openly discussing how veterinarians contributed to the terrible events of World War II in multiple places, it was possible to make meaningful comparisons from different points of view and account for veterinarians' offenses. In Austria, this self-examination has recently begun. Like Germany, most veterinarians collaborated with wartime aggression; for example, 65 percent of the professors at the Vienna veterinary school belonged to the nationalist political party working with the Nazis. In other Axis countries this topic is still taboo and not discussed openly.

On the other side, countries belonging to the Allied coalition saw themselves as on the morally correct side of the war. Therefore, the veterinary profession in these countries mostly discussed the merits of veterinary heroes. Only much later did their veterinary histories critically evaluate the activities of veterinarians. There were questions about which veterinarians in the army, administration, education, and practice had collaborated with the enemy, and which were resistant. Historians wrote about the tragic fates of Jewish veterinarians in Germany and in the Nazi-occupied countries. Finally, despite taking a professional oath to guard animal health, some Allied veterinarians had participated in developing biological weapons deadly to both humans and animals. No matter which side veterinarians found themselves on during World War II, they had to make many difficult decisions – decisions that might haunt them later.

As a veterinary student or veterinarian, you might wonder why you should know about these histories of the profession under totalitarian regimes. Isn't that something of the past and not relevant in modern society? Unfortunately, this is not the case. Similar regimes still exist today. Many people still suffer from inequality, discrimination, racism, and suppression based on political, socioeconomic, or religious doctrines. Therefore, it is important to become aware of the fact that circumstances similar to both world wars still exist or might recur. Moreover, even in peacetime, as medical professionals, veterinarians must make difficult ethical decisions, such as whether to euthanize a patient. These daily ethical decisions may seem to have nothing to do with war, but we are shaped by our behavior. It is easy to state that one would never have cooperated with suppressive Nazi, communist, or apartheid regimes. But it is difficult to imagine daily life and work under such circumstances. Each of us must think hard about this question: "What would I have done in this difficult situation?" For instance, how would you have reacted if the authorities banned Jewish or Black students and professors from universities, or from the veterinary profession? Unfortunately, some of us may have to face difficult questions like this someday.

Each of us plays a role in ensuring a just and ethical society, as well as working for the improvement of animal health. As educated and trained professionals, veterinarians have leadership responsibilities during peaceful times and during crises such as pandemics, economic recessions, food shortages, or conflicts. Studying the events of the two world wars bring this fact into sharp focus, and they help to guide us as we face similar challenges today. Professional accountability to society played and still plays an essential role within the veterinary profession. Therefore, we believe that veterinary education must include how the ethical, cultural, and political context shapes veterinarians' activities. This is one of the major lessons to be learned from history – and from this book.

Veterinarians in the New World Order, 1945–1960

After the defeat of the Axis powers (Nazi Germany, Italy, and Japan), a new political order developed that divided the world into communist (led by the USSR) and capitalist (led by the United States) blocs. Tensions between the two blocs led not only to the so-called Cold War but also to armed conflicts in nations such as Korea and Vietnam. The postwar period also witnessed decolonization conflicts and the subsequent independence of numerous new nations, including the former battlefields of Eritrea and parts of Libya in eastern and northern Africa. Major concerns of governments worldwide included postwar recovery and feeding the human and animal populations. Veterinarians had to find their way against this changing background. Those who had served abroad with the military had new insights into the global animal economy, animal diseases, and laboratory procedures.

This was true in terms of veterinary education and knowledge exchange, also. In Germany, world veterinary literature had almost ceased due to Nazi policies and the difficulties of wartime circulation. When the Allied armies arrived, they found German veterinarians to be very interested in foreign research developments; the school at Hannover, although damaged, began functioning again. For the first couple of years, students were required to help with the labor of rebuilding the German veterinary schools. Textbooks and journals imported from the Allied nations helped to restock veterinary libraries. On the Soviet side, veterinary education in Czechoslovakia, Poland, Hungary, the Baltic countries, Romania, and other occupied countries was reorganized according to the Soviet educational model. New schools were rapidly established as well. For example, "Veterinary Sciences" was one of three faculties comprising the first university in Mongolia, established at Ulaanbaatar in 1942. By the mid-1950s, about 50 veterinarians graduated from this school each year. With Soviet support and oversight, the Mongolian government established 24 large and 480 smaller veterinary clinics/hospitals around the country by 1947, with national laboratories and scientific research institutes soon after that. Controlled by Soviet-style Five-Year Plans, animal breeding and disease prevention were crucial to making Mongolia a productive, "modern" nation because animal products were a major source of wealth.

Recognizing the declining role of horsepower, veterinarians continued to shift away from equine medicine, and many explored new niches. The role of horses and mules in the armies quickly decreased due to further mechanization. The same happened in agriculture. In the United States, the change from horsepower to tractors was stimulated during the war. Farmers got higher prices for their products, while tractor manufacturers were encouraged to increase their production as part of the war-related rapid industrialization. Generally, tractor power overtook horsepower on American farms around 1945. Elsewhere around the world, this transition took place later as part of the postwar recovery process. Instead of equine medicine, veterinarians found more employment in increasing animal production, veterinary public health, and the food supply to support an economy that initially was characterized by scarcity. They worked in eradication schemes to control livestock diseases and those that also infected humans, such as bovine tuberculosis and brucellosis. In their clinics, veterinarians began using new therapies, drugs, tools, and animal husbandry technologies (herd health and preventive medicine), while more and more pet animals became new patients, particularly when prosperity started to grow again in the 1950s.

Postwar Recovery: International Organizations

Besides the human tragedy and casualties of the war, a considerable part of the agricultural and industrial infrastructure had been destroyed in several African, Asian, and European nations. In Europe, postwar governments concentrated on denazification (removing all Nazi collaborators) and reconstruction. Denazification included purging collaborators from all veterinary institutes (both professors and students) and veterinarians in private and public services. This process divided the veterinary profession, and it took decades before relations between colleagues were restored again. The USSR faced vast challenges in recovering its livestock and agricultural economy, especially in the former battlefields of Ukraine, the Baltics, and the trans-Caucasus region. In Eastern Europe and Asia, the Soviet Army had liberated nations from German, Italian, and Japanese occupation but then set up Soviet-allied governments after the war. Veterinarians in these satellite states were confronted with the growing political and socioeconomic influence of the USSR. The authoritarian Soviet-controlled regimes regulated veterinary education and veterinary practice along socialist lines. The U.S. Army occupied Japan and other areas in Asia, and it took over the registration and regulation of veterinarians. Reconstruction in war-torn nations, from China to Europe to Eritrea, included emergency efforts to rebuild livestock production. Standards of living were low, and the food supply was insecure and scarce; in Europe, food rationing lasted through the 1940s. Many countries could no longer afford to pay for the necessary imports of such things as raw materials, foods, capital goods, and machines from their gold reserve and export income. Imports and rationing of animal feed hindered animal production, and veterinarians struggled to survive. A total economic collapse was feared.

In response to these problems, some vets from the less-affected nations (such as the United States) joined the international organizations working to rebuild war-torn nations' economies and infrastructure. The United Nations Relief and Rehabilitation Administration (UNRRA) coordinated the shipments of cattle and other livestock from the United States to suffering nations, and it hired veterinarians to accompany these animals and keep them healthy on ocean voyages. These animals were to help reestablish livestock breeding and increase the local food supply. American veterinarian Martin Kaplan (1915–2004) joined UNRRA and was assigned to the problems of livestock production in Greece. Kaplan transported donated American cattle and purchased Arabian stallions for horse breeding; helped restart laboratories to manufacture vaccines; and worked with Greek veterinarians to rebuild their practices. Kaplan next joined the international Food and Agriculture Organization (FAO), doing similar work in several European countries, particularly in Poland. These veterinarians brought new techniques and pharmaceuticals, including sulfonamides to treat infections. Sulfas and other recently discovered antimicrobials promised to revolutionize the treatment of animal infections, but they were scarce and too expensive to use in many places around the world.

In 1947, the American secretary of state George Marshall (1880–1959) announced a plan for extended economic aid to all European countries. This "Marshall Plan" was launched to restore the economy by removing essential shortages and promoting international economic cooperation. Another motive behind the plan was the hope that economic reconstruction of Europe would prevent the spread of communism due to hunger and distress. In the period 1948–1952, the Organization for European Economic Cooperation divided $14.6 billion of Marshall aid among 17 countries. Apart from infrastructure recovery, rebuilding industry, and research programs, modernization of agriculture and livestock production was financed. Much emphasis was placed on restoring and increasing animal production under increasing pressure from rapid postwar population growth. This brought about some fundamental changes in veterinary medicine. Due to imports of animal feed, crop seeds, fertilizers, tractors, milking machines, and other machinery, Marshall Plan aid enabled the growth of livestock numbers and animal production. Rationing measures on most consumption and production goods as well as animal feed were removed by 1950 in Europe. International cooperation stimulated economic recovery by trade liberalization within the European Economic Community framework from 1957 onward.

The other crucial international agencies coordinating the recovery of animal economies were the FAO and the World Health Organization (WHO). As historian Michael Bresalier has argued, the FAO and the WHO began cooperating after the war to use agricultural development to increase global food production. In 1946, the FAO conducted their first *World Food Survey*. The *Survey* counted food-producing animals in nations such as India and assessed livestock levels of health and fertility. The *Survey* found that parasitism, disease, poor nutrition, and other problems plagued the world's cattle, sheep, goats, and other milk and meat producers. FAO/WHO officials decided to encourage consumers to ingest more milk products and eat more meat, which would also increase farmers' income. Experts, including veterinarians, worked around the world to impose modern (largely U.S. and European) breeding, feeding, and disease prevention practices designed to make livestock more productive. While overall food production did increase after World War II, these "development" strategies unfortunately required local farmers to abandon their own knowledge and practices. This change meant the loss of local expertise, the conversion of the world's populations to eating higher on the food chain, and, in some places, damage to environments. Farmers' relationships to their animals often changed, also, due to the greater degree of state intervention in agriculture. Without doubt, farmers had their own ideas about how much of the new development regime they would accept; but the postwar economic reality pushed them to participate.

Veterinarians, who had already moved away from horse medicine to focus on cattle and other livestock, enthusiastically embraced the FAO/WHO livestock programs. Martin Kaplan became a leader in these efforts, joining the WHO in 1949 and establishing a special Veterinary Section within the Division of Communicable Diseases. In the United States, veterinarian James H. Steele (1913–2013) had proposed a Veterinary Public Health Division of the U.S. Public Health Service in 1945, which he led from the Centers for Disease Control and Prevention for many years. In this way, veterinary disease problems were attacked alongside diseases of human populations, and veterinarians were employed to do this work. In many countries, governments supported animal production by establishing and financing several institutes, programs, and knowledge transfer. Research was carried out on animal feeds, new intensive livestock production systems particularly for poultry and pigs, breeding, artificial insemination, blood-typing, and vaccination. By labor-saving mechanization and an increase in scale, animal husbandry was rationalized. Veterinarians played important roles in scientific research of modern livestock production systems. The increase in scale and the concentration of large groups of production animals that went hand in hand with industrialized intensive livestock farming (factory farming) involved a higher risk of outbreaks of animal diseases. Consequently, the postwar rise of herd-health management brought about a shift from a curative to a preventive approach for veterinary practitioners.

Herd Health, Maximizing Production, and Encouraging Consumption

As historians have demonstrated, plans implemented in the aftermath of the war were the basis for regimes of agricultural development deployed around the world during the next half century. The "right" way to feed the world was the modern, technocratic way, based on government-controlled regimes of imported experts. International organizations and Soviet- and U.S.-controlled occupation governments decided that the global food crisis could only be solved by increasing the amounts of calories and (especially) protein per person. One direct way to accomplish this goal was to urge people to eat more animal products. Veterinarians would play a key role in this shift by breeding highly productive animals, overseeing animal husbandry, controlling animal diseases, and overseeing production of foods like milk, butter, cheese, ghee, meats, and eggs. Many of these roles fell under the rubrics of "herd health" and "preventive medicine," which emphasized working with large numbers of animals and making decisions based strictly on economic value. This orientation replaced the clinical care of individual animals, and it also linked veterinary medicine to human medicine and public health.

The goals of herd health are to raise large numbers of animals cheaply, in less space, and quickly. The herd became a "production unit," managed by veterinary advisors. Veterinarians in the United States and other areas saw the intensification of animal agriculture as an opportunity, beginning with the poultry industry. Raised indoors in very high densities, rather than outdoors in small flocks, in the United States poultry went from an expensive rarity to a cheap source of protein in the 1940s and 1950s. Around the world, veterinarians helped restructure animal economies for intense production, even in places where people had not previously consumed large amounts of meat. The U.S. occupation governments in Japan (1945–1951) and Korea (1945–1948) are good examples. Official reports at the end of the war noted that the Japanese did not eat much meat, had a very small livestock industry, and lacked the pastureland necessary to develop large herds. Horses and bovines were draft animals, not primarily sources of meat; meat animals were ducks and other poultry and swine. Before the war's devastation, Japan had a well-functioning veterinary disease control regime. U.S. veterinary forces worked alongside Japanese veterinarians to restore disease control, import fodder and grains, use more intensive breeding operations, prevent animal diseases from being imported, and, most importantly, to dramatically increase production of meat, milk, and eggs. They standardized food inspection, pasteurization, and refrigeration according to U.S. models.

In South Korea, the removal of Japanese personnel at the end of the war left few graduate veterinarians to administer national-level food production and inspection. U.S. Army officers took control of veterinary education at Seoul National University, where they trained Korean veterinary students according to the U.S. model. The Korean population had traditionally used poultry, dogs, and other smaller animals for meat; but the 35-year Japanese occupation had completely wiped out the dog population and the two major poultry farms. Vaccinating large numbers of cattle against rinderpest and battling outbreaks of diseases such as anthrax and rabies were the first animal disease problems confronted by the U.S. veterinarians. Next, the Americans replaced older regulations and laws. Since about 15 percent of the cattle tested positive for bovine tuberculosis, they began a tuberculosis control program modeled on that of the United States. Stimulating dairy production was another major goal, despite the fact that the Korean people traditionally did not consume much dairy.

Around the world, experts from the FAO, WHO, and other organizations targeted protein-calorie malnutrition by focusing on the production of foods that were highly digestible and contained larger amounts of high-quality proteins needed by human bodies. Most U.S. and European physicians, nutritionists, and veterinarians agreed that foods of animal origin supplied the highest-quality protein per unit of weight, and that incorporating animal protein into a person's diet increased the conversion of plant foods into nutrients for growth. By supplying the animals, the livestock industry was essential to this program. Postwar veterinarians contributed to the drive for increasing meat and milk consumption by increasing livestock production and by battling animal and zoonotic diseases.

Increasingly, these activities changed the bodies of the animals themselves through breeding programs, new feeding regimens, and specialized housing. Chickens, turkeys, and ducks for meat were bred to have huge breast muscles. Cows that produced the most milk were the foundation for dairy herds. Scientific diets stimulated maximum growth in the shortest time, or more eggs or milk produced per animal. Confining animals inside buildings enabled the diet, light, and temperature to be controlled for maximal production. Crowding animals together, however, encouraged the spread of diseases. Veterinarians, using a herd health approach, battled disease problems both before they occurred (preventive medicine) and during active outbreaks and epizootics. The newly developed pharmaceuticals, vaccines, and antimicrobials promised a new era of veterinary control.

New Tools and the "Therapeutic Revolution"

One major accomplishment of researchers in various places around the world was the development of new drugs and vaccines, some of which were quickly adopted internationally (see Table 5.1). For example, salvarsan (originally developed to treat human syphilis) worked well against African trypanosomiasis. In 1911, German Army veterinarian W. Rips proved that it was also successful in the treatment of contagious equine pleuropneumonia (caused by bacteria). Traditionally, veterinary education also included training in pharmaceutical preparation. Veterinary practices maintained their own pharmacies. However, more and more (international) pharmaceutical and chemical companies started to provide veterinarians with their products in a direct way, or through agents. In addition, national serum and vaccine institutes developed and distributed vaccines that were used by vets in their practice.

As more microorganisms were discovered, the search for chemical preparations to treat infections by microbes intensified. German pathologist and bacteriologist Gerhard Domagk (1895–1964) and his colleagues investigated several potential chemotherapies against bacterial infections. In 1935, they demonstrated in mice and rabbit experiments that sulfonamides (Prontosil) were effective in treating blood poisoning caused by high mortal doses of bacteria (*Staphylococcus aureus* and hemolytic streptococci). This discovery was the basis for producing sulfa drugs, the first type of antibiotic with strong antibacterial effects against several common bacteria. Veterinarians and physicians quickly began using sulfa drugs in their practices. For veterinarians, figuring out the correct dosage for different species of animals and different infections was the first concern. For example, sulfonamides attacked streptococcal bacteria responsible for mastitis in dairy cattle. The right dose of sulfas, sometimes orally and sometimes infused into the affected teats, cleared up the infection right away. To many veterinarians, sulfas seemed like miracle drugs; but more of these "magic bullets" were to come.

The development of antimicrobials was a collaborative international effort, and penicillin is an excellent example. English physician Alexander Fleming (1891–1955) had published an article in 1928 in which he described his (coincidental) observation that a species of fungi, *Penicillium*, had a bactericidal effect. Initially, neither Fleming nor the medical community recognized the potential of this discovery. However, Ernst Boris Chain (1906–1979), a Jewish German biochemist who had moved to England in 1933, and Australian pathologist Howard Florey (1898–1968) noticed Fleming's discovery and obtained financing from the Rockefeller Foundation to develop a pharmaceutical from Fleming's fungus. Chain and Florey worked at the University of Oxford (UK) and there they elucidated the chemical structure and therapeutic efficacy of a compound they called "penicillin." Initially, however, penicillin could only be produced in small amounts at great expense. Recognizing its potential, scientists at British and American universities and pharmaceutical companies cooperated to produce penicillin on a large scale by the end of World War II, saving the lives of many soldiers on the battlefields. Physicians quickly tested penicillin on any infection they thought might respond to it: pneumonia, urinary tract infections, sepsis, and many others.

The increasing availability of antimicrobials changed veterinary practice, although these changes often happened slowly. In the United States immediately after the war ended, large commercial laboratories such as Lederle Laboratories, Park-Davis, and Merck began manufacturing forms of penicillin that would be useful to veterinarians. Industrial production of penicillin by pharmaceutical companies increased from a few milligrams in 1940 to almost 200 tons in 1953. Penicillin-G, the dried crystalline form, had the advantage of not needing refrigeration. It could be made up in doses for any size of animal (although dosing horses, cattle, and other large animals was very expensive at first). Penicillin-G was also shipped around the world. The companies advertised their new products, and veterinary journals published articles instructing veterinarians how to use these medications in their practices. These articles advised veterinarians that simply treating an animal, based on one's experience, was not sufficient. Different antimicrobials attacked different species or groups (Gram positive or Gram negative) of bacteria, and veterinary practitioners were instructed to always microscopically examine and stain samples from sick animals before treating them. Common problems such as mastitis or infected wounds would then yield to the proper antimicrobial treatment. This "therapeutic revolution" not only changed veterinarians' usual procedures; it also raised their expectations for their ability to treat sick animals successfully. Animal owners' expectations for their veterinarian increased, also; the late 1940s and 1950s were a new era for veterinary medicine.

The increase in animal production and lowering production costs during a period of global reconstruction and food scarcity were the main reasons for the widespread adoption of antibiotics in veterinary medicine in the 1950s–1960s. Biochemists accidentally discovered that these antimicrobials also increased the growth rate of young livestock when added as supplement to animal feed, particularly for pigs and poultry. Antibiotics were also used as a food preservative. In 1962, 14,000 tons of penicillin was produced in the United States, and about 46 percent of this amount was used in agriculture. Besides penicillin, 350 other antimicrobials had been isolated by 1957, including bacitracin (1945); chloramphenicol and streptomycin (1947); chlortetracycline (1948); and oxytetracycline (1949) . Many of these antimicrobials were used as feed supplements and as preventive medicines against infectious diseases and parasites that plagued animals crowded together. Production statistics rose dramatically: cows produced more milk, hens produced more eggs, and meat animals grew faster (so they could be slaughtered at younger ages). These were tremendous economic benefits to the animal feed industry (and, by extension, to their consulting veterinarians).

However, the use of antibiotics in animal production, particularly as growth promoters, was not undisputed. By 1950, scientists already warned that microbes evolved resistance to antimicrobials. New antimicrobials had to be developed, but scientists feared that microbial evolution would happen faster. The use of these antimicrobials as growth promoters was especially dangerous, since low levels of these chemicals in animals' bodies and environments encouraged the development of resistant strains of pathogenic microbes. Physicians used the same drugs to treat infections in their patients, and they worried that the widespread use of these drugs could leave residues in food of animal origin. Then drug-resistant strains of microbes would affect human patients. Within about forty years, they were proven correct as antibiotic resistance has increased steadily in human populations. Veterinarians noted that part of the problem was a lack of regulation: in some places, farmers could obtain and administer these drugs without a veterinary prescription.

Despite these problems, the new antimicrobials, anthelmintics (parasite killers), and vaccines available after the war revolutionized veterinary practice. Veterinarians could now effectively treat individual patients with pneumonia or other serious infections with simple injections or oral medications. Chemoprophylaxis as a routine whole-herd treatment made even more impact. Internal parasite infections, from the amoebas to the roundworms, could severely affect or even kill young animals. External parasites, including mites and fleas, were also serious problems. The development of new chemicals for prevention of parasite infections promised to improve animal health dramatically: hexachloroethane against liver flukes, and the benzimidazoles against trichinosis, tapeworms, whipworms, roundworms, and protozoans *Giardia*, *Coccidia*, and *Cryptosporidium*. Chemical companies developed liquid dips and dry powders to apply externally, to repel or kill insects including mites, ticks, fleas, and flies. Formerly life-threatening infections could now be routinely controlled. Finally, new vaccines were being developed that enabled disease *control* campaigns to become disease *eradication* campaigns.

From Control to Eradication: Battling Animal Diseases

In various countries, organized campaigns against contagious livestock diseases had started already before the war, often on a local level. But by the 1950s these campaigns were carried out by well-organized, nationwide programs whose goals were increasing from *control* (allowing low levels of the disease) to complete *eradication* (no disease). Along with vaccines and pharmaceuticals, diagnostic tests for animal diseases were developed and improved. Farmers were compensated for losses they suffered by being forced to slaughter their animals that tested positively. Millions of animals were tested, and thousands were slaughtered. Apart from bovine tuberculosis, organized eradication campaigns against brucellosis, foot and mouth disease, warble fly, swine fever, *Salmonella pullorum*, and Newcastle disease were quite successful in many areas. Sometimes, cull-and-slaughter strategies were applied; in other cases, newly developed vaccines were used, for instance in the case of foot and mouth disease. Two important facts are illustrated by these early eradication campaigns: (1) moving from "control" to "eradication" required a combination of techniques, including an effective, safe, and widely available vaccine; (2) however, if the vaccine was a modified live formulation, the problem was that diagnostic tests could not distinguish between infected animals and vaccinated animals. Having a vaccine did not guarantee eradication.

Nonetheless, vaccines were crucial tools, and they were developed by scientists working around the world. Researchers working in African and Asian institutes contributed to the evolution of a colonial scientific culture, thereby extending the growing international veterinary scientific community. For example, French veterinarians working in Algeria created an early successful sheep pox vaccine in 1911. Historian Karen Brown has shown that during this period the nature of research at the Onderstepoort Veterinary

Institute, near Pretoria, South Africa, exceeded just progress in biomedical procedures, because diseases were studied in the context of the local ecological factors (weather, soil, and nutrition). This was also the case with research in the Veterinary Institute in Buitenzorg in Java, Indonesia. In South Africa, the etiologies of diseases such as lamsiekte (botulism), geeldikkop, and African horse sickness were revealed; in Indonesia this was the case with surra, dourine, and Newcastle disease. Based on this scientific and veterinary knowledge, governments imposed regulations and designed control and eradication programs. The successful eradication and control of various diseases increased the prestige, institutionalization, and legitimacy of the veterinary sciences.

The development of intensive livestock production and the organized campaigns against animal diseases also changed daily work for practitioners and the function of veterinarians active in research and management in the 1950s. The campaigns brought along a lot of diagnostic and preventive work for practitioners, as well as the introduction of antibiotics and new types of veterinary drugs like sulfonamides. In addition, veterinarians played an active role in information campaigns for farmers, assisting veterinary services with the development of all kinds of publications, films, and propaganda. These activities resulted in more employment of veterinarians in private practices, the pharmaceutical industry, as well as in government services and animal health services, sometimes for decades. Avian influenza (or true fowl plague), spread from northern Italy around the world, represented a big challenge for veterinary medicine. This highly contagious and acute viral disease is virulent for all bird species and has led to huge losses of poultry worldwide. Effective vaccines were developed, but stamping-out and carcass destruction have remained the most important control strategies. Large numbers of veterinarians worked on campaigns against these diseases.

Another good example is rinderpest, the world's cattle killer. After the huge outbreak of rinderpest in Europe in the 1860s, this disease was kept under control there by stamping-out and trade policy measures. However, this policy failed during the Balkan War and World War I and its aftermath. After 1924 the Office International des Épizooties (OIE) guidelines were followed in many countries, and by 1930 eastern Turkey was the only region in Europe where rinderpest was still endemic; but the disease reappeared periodically around the world. In 1950, the Inter-African Bureau of Epizootic Diseases was founded with a directorial plan to eliminate rinderpest from Africa. Working in the Muguga Laboratory of the East African Veterinary Research Organization (Kenya), veterinarian Walter Plowright (1923–2010) and R.D. Ferris developed a new rinderpest vaccine from bovine kidney cells in 1957. This tissue-culture rinderpest vaccine was stable, safe, and cheap to produce. Along with restrictions on moving cattle and slaughtering infected animals, the vaccine greatly accelerated rinderpest control in African endemic areas.

The other cattle disease that became the subject of targeted eradication was foot and mouth disease (FMD). Despite the low mortality (2 to 5 percent), FMD represented the most severe animal plague after the rinderpest. For instance, more than 7 million animals were infected in Germany between 1889 and 1894, leading to economic losses due to loss of weight and meat and milk production. A major epizootic spread at the end of the war in South America, especially in Brazil; and war disruptions caused outbreaks in many other places also. The DDR (East Germany) was the first country in the world to introduce an annual vaccination against FMD in 1950. In the same period, Dutch veterinarian Herman Salomon Frenkel (1891–1968), director of the State Veterinary Research Institute, had developed an effective vaccine, produced on a large-scale *in vitro* virus cultivation. This vaccine was not only used in European countries but also by the USDA during anti-FMD campaigns in Mexico, 1946–1954, to stop the spread of the South American epizootic. However, as we will discuss in Chapter 6, this live-virus vaccine created a problem for control and eradication programs. The problem is that diagnostic tests cannot differentiate a vaccinated animal from an infected one, due to the action of the live virus vaccine on the animal's immune system. Fearing the spread of infection, officials might order the slaughter of a vaccinated animal that tested positive. This problem could lead to bans on moving or exporting animals, and huge economic losses for the livestock industry.

Classical swine fever (also known as "hog cholera"), another major epizootic disease, also illustrates this problem with eradication strategies that include both testing and live virus vaccines. Both acute and chronic forms of this notifiable viral disease occur. The virulence may vary from severe, with a high mortality, to mild or even subclinical. Sources of infection are living pigs and raw pig products. Effective preventives became available with work conducted in the United States by chemist and physician Marion Dorset (1872–1935) and other researchers. Between 1903 and 1906, Dorset and colleagues determined that swine fever was caused by a filterable virus and developed a "hyperimmunization" technique that protected non-immune pigs. However, between 1914 and 1924, outbreaks of swine fever still cost American farmers $415 million. In 1934, Dorset developed a vaccine with 90 percent effectiveness; but this was a modified live virus vaccine. Along with this vaccine, cull-and-slaughter remained an important eradication strategy throughout the twentieth century. By 1970, the U.S. government prohibited the vaccine due to fears of infection and positive testing, and finally the disease was eradicated by destroying every animal that tested positive and strictly regulating imports. Because of its potential economic damage, swine fever was (and still is) a feared disease in countries with a high pig production. For example, during an outbreak in 1961 in the Netherlands more than 320,000 animals were killed to prevent the disease from spreading. By 1990, the combination of culling and prophylactic mass vaccination had *almost* eradicated the disease in Europe, but the European Union banned the use of the vaccine unless in an emergency. The reasoning was that animals that tested positive could not be moved or exported to other countries – and vaccinated animals tested positive. Ironically, the very scientific development that enabled disease control also potentially threatened the livestock economy.

Finally, some diseases still resist scientists' efforts to develop effective vaccines against them. African swine fever is an infectious viral disease in domestic and wild swine, which primarily originated in sub-Saharan Africa. It was first described in Kenya in 1910. The clinical symptoms are very similar to those of classical swine fever, while infection occurs directly or indirectly by contaminated feed or certain ticks. During the twentieth century, African swine fever spread to Latin America and Eastern Europe. African swine fever control relies on slaughtering infected and exposed animals alone. There is no effective vaccine against this disease, despite efforts over decades to develop one. It continues to plague swine production today: it appeared in China in the summer of 2018 and spread through Southeast Asia, where it has caused meat shortages.

During the mid-twentieth century, many contagious animal diseases were eradicated or controlled by government-sponsored campaigns using culling plus prophylactic measures. These successes owed a great deal to scientific research and discoveries in laboratories of veterinary schools and of public or private pharmaceutical, biomedical, and veterinary institutes worldwide. This interdisciplinary research would increase animal health and thereby the production of livestock and food of animal origin. But some disease eradication campaigns have failed. In some parts of the world, bovine tuberculosis stubbornly persists. Both sheep and goat poxes were successfully controlled in most European countries by attenuated vaccines, but remained endemic in many African, Middle Eastern, and Asian countries. Why could the same disease be controlled in one place, but continue to kill animals in others? Obviously, control and eradication strategies and success have differed from one place to another. But another important reason that eradication campaigns failed was that many diseases of domestic animals (and humans) were closely related or identical to those in wild animals. If a disease is established in wild animal populations, it is very difficult to prevent its introduction into local domesticated animals (and even human populations). This fact became clear with ecological studies of various diseases during the twentieth century.

Disease Ecology

Ecological approaches to disease, which developed in the early to mid-1900s, recognized that some diseases regularly circulated between humans and wild and domesticated animals. The source of the circulating infection was the *reservoir* – the animal species in which the disease was constantly present or "enzootic." If a disease had a wild animal reservoir, it was very difficult or impossible to eradicate that disease without killing *every* susceptible wild animal (and vector). If the reservoir species was a wild rodent, or bat, for example, it was simply impossible to eliminate all these animals. Other wild animals were too valuable to exterminate, such as those species important for tourism and hunting. Contact between wild and domestic animals, such as rats or other rodents living in barns or stables, reintroduced the disease periodically. To control these diseases, three strategies were adopted: (1) eliminating vectors, (2) developing vaccines, and (3) creating "buffer zones" between wild animals and humans and their domesticated animals.

The first strategy, eliminating vectors, was crucial for many diseases of the Global South and warmer areas in temperate zones. Ticks, fleas, mosquitos, midges, and biting flies were known to spread animal diseases since the 1890s. The blood-borne parasites that caused anaplasmosis, babesiosis, and anemias killed untold numbers of animals. Mosquitos and midges spread Rift Valley fever, bluetongue, and African horse sickness. Ticks carried Texas cattle fever, African swine fever, encephalitis, and hemorrhagic fevers. Some arbovirus diseases, such as equine encephalitis and sleeping sickness, were also important zoonoses. By the mid-1900s, scientists had begun to use the new insecticides (such as DDT) to kill disease vectors over large territories. Developed during World War II and used for delousing armies and refugees, at first these insecticides seemed to be miraculously effective. They have been crucial tools in campaigns against vector-borne diseases. However, insects developed resistance to them over time and the chemicals often damaged the environment, sometimes even driving species (some birds) extinct in treated areas. Like the search for antimicrobials, the search for new insecticides continued throughout the 1900s.

A good example of the second and third strategies is rabies. Besides dogs and cats, this disease can also be spread by wild animals like bats, raccoons, skunks, and foxes; almost all mammals are susceptible to the rabies virus. People have battled rabies for centuries by reducing the numbers of stray dogs and isolating and killing infected animals. Until dog and cat licensing and vaccination campaigns were introduced during the twentieth century, killing large numbers of dogs was the only effective tactic to protect humans. But Louis Pasteur and Emile Roux developed the first prophylactic for humans, from adult mammalian brain tissue, in the 1880s. They first tested it on animals, so the idea of vaccinating domesticated dogs slowly took hold. The phenol-inactivated vaccines developed by Fermi (1908) and Semple (1911) began to be used in domestic dogs in the 1920s. By the late 1930s, chloroform-killed vaccines were being advertised and sold by pharmaceutical companies such as Parke, Davis & Company and Sharpe & Dome in the United States. Safe, stable, and effective vaccines were affordable enough that ordinary veterinarians could use them.

These vaccines were a key to rabies control programs. After both world wars, rabies epizootics in Hungary were controlled with mass vaccination campaigns. Japan also conducted large-scale, successful anti-rabies campaigns in the 1920s. In the district of Osaka, for example, a 1926 campaign using military personnel included registration and rabies vaccination for dogs at police stations. The cost of a vaccine was 50 copper coins (*sen*) for a large dog and 25 *sen* for a small dog (Fig. 5.6). Although safe and effective vaccines have not been easy to develop for animals, by the 1960s modern modified-live and inactivated parenteral vaccine preparations were widely available. Epidemiologists realized that regular vaccination of pet animals decreased the number of human infections by providing an "immune buffer" separating susceptible human populations from wild reservoir species like bats. Advised by veterinarians such as Karl Friedrich Meyer (1884–1974) and Martin

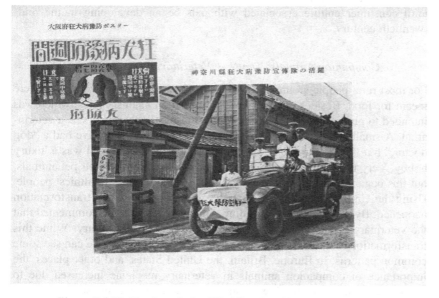

Figure 5.6 "Rabies Inoculation Week" and "Military Group Activity for Rabies Prevention Propaganda," Osaka District, Japan, 1926.
Source: 日本帝国家畜伝染病予防史. 大正・昭和 第1篇 [History of Prevention of Livestock Infectious Diseases of the Japanese Empire. *Taisho / Showa Vol. 1]* (www.dl .ndl.go.jp/api/iiif/1903868/manifest.json) Image p. 506. Courtesy: Prof. Myung-Sun Chun, College of Veterinary Medicine, Seoul National University, South Korea.

Kaplan, the WHO began global efforts to control rabies with buffer vaccination of domesticated animals. Eliminating all the wild reservoir species harboring rabies was impossible, they acknowledged, and vaccinating all humans was not feasible either. By putting dog licensing and rabies vaccination laws in place, public health officials and veterinarians created a barrier of immunity in the domestic dog population and human cases dropped quickly in the protected regions. Since the late 1970s, various oral anti-rabies vaccines have also been tested and deployed for wildlife using baits. However, no methods have been developed that can successfully vaccinate all wildlife. Prophylactic vaccination in rabies-endemic areas, along with licensing of dogs and eliminating street dogs during epizootics, remain the major anti-rabies strategies today.

Rabies and other vaccinations became a mainstay of veterinary practice focused on dogs and cats. As wealth grew in many areas during the 1960s and 1970s, companion animal veterinary care also grew rapidly. Veterinarians had always treated some pet and working dogs, and in places such as the United States specialty urban animal hospitals for dogs and cats had existed since the late 1800s. But these hospitals and clinics were rare in most places until consumer culture associated with pets began developing in the mid-twentieth century.

Companion Animals: The New Veterinary Frontier

For most rural people around the world, dogs were valued as workers or were meant for food. Besides the occasional vaccination against rabies, which was intended to protect people as well as dogs, these animals rarely saw a veterinarian. A small number of pets belonging to urban elites may have had a "dog doctor," but this was unusual. Spending money on a pet animal was a luxury hobby. Very few people purchased food or medical care for their pet animals, but this began to change in the early 1900s for the world's wealthiest people. Using the United States as a case study, we can see how this transformation happened. By the late 1930s, a leading American veterinarian commented that the veterinary profession was "going to the dogs" in his country. While this transformation did not develop in the same way everywhere, we can see some common patterns. In Europe, Britain, the United States, and other places, the importance of companion animals in veterinary medicine increased due to several factors: (1) increasing urbanization, wealth, and consumer culture; (2) changing human–animal relationships; and (3) veterinarians' need to find new patient populations as working horses disappeared.

During the early to mid-1900s, affection for companion animals combined with increasing wealth to create a new consumer culture devoted to pets. The animal heroes of World War I, such as the dog Rin Tin Tin, starred in popular stories, books, and films in the United States and Britain that were exported around the world. Managers in meat production companies realized that they could make money from products made especially for dogs. This also solved the problem of what to do with offal and the bodies of horses being slaughtered as they were replaced by mechanization: use the meat that people did not eat in special food for pets. The dog food industry targeted owners' sense of love and responsibility for their "faithful friends," and advertisements urged people to think about their pets as "family members." Pet food companies helped owners believe that spending money on pets exhibited their own wealth and high moral values. This was so important to the rising middle and upper classes that, even during the devastating economic depression of the 1930s, pet food sales in the United States continued to increase. Pet animals were no longer just a luxury but were becoming almost a necessity for the modern family living in the cities and suburbs.

Changing human–animal relationships, and the increasing sentimental value of pets also drove this developing consumer culture. Popular animal welfare societies, which had worked to protect horses and dogs in cities since the late 1800s, laid the foundation for the moral and sentimental importance of pet animals. As horses began disappearing from city streets, organizations such as the Society for Prevention of Cruelty to Animals focused on dogs (and other pets). They argued that cruelty to these animals led to cruelty against people, and that it was especially important to educate children to be kind to animals. By keeping a pet dog or cat and caring properly for it, children learned proper behavior. This was not a new idea, but it became important to people seeking upward mobility into the middle and upper classes. These people could demonstrate humanitarianism toward animals (and other humans) with good treatment of their family's pets. Instead of being valued only for economic reasons, companion or pet animals were valuable because their owners loved them.

Pet owners increasingly sought high-quality medical care for their animals. Any veterinarian could treat parasites or injuries, but owners looked for a "pet doctor" who cared about the welfare of their animals and used the latest scientific knowledge to provide specialized medical and surgical care. Veterinarians needed to be "sympathetic scientists," and they also needed to learn how to interact with pet owners. Treating livestock and other large animals required brute strength and disregarding the animal's comfort; but treating pets was just the opposite. The veterinary profession had traditionally served the commercial interests of livestock owners and the public health, not humored useless and pampered pets. Most veterinarians viewed pets as feminized and frivolous, and beneath the dignity of a professional man. This changed as veterinary leaders and individual practitioners realized the economic benefits of pet practice. For those vets in urban areas, or who were not interested in livestock, pets replaced horses as their main patient population.

Owners would spend more money on pets, also, which allowed veterinarians to use more of the new technologies and medications in their practices. The early companion animal veterinarians modeled their practices on those of physicians, and their specialized animal hospitals were designed to operate like smaller human hospitals.

However, even in the 1940s, veterinarians learned very little about dogs, cats, and other companion animals during their education. Veterinary schools' curricula still focused mainly on food-producing animals, although some schools offered courses in canine medicine and surgery as early as the 1920s. The demand for pet animal treatment, the willingness of pet owners to spend money on their animals, and the availability of new vaccines and antimicrobials drove changes in veterinarians' training. Anatomy courses increasingly used dogs as the "standard" animal for training veterinary students. Anesthetic regimens and specialized techniques were developed for smaller animals. Energetic leaders in small animal veterinary medicine and surgery gave presentations and demonstrations of techniques for blood analysis, nutrition, and castration and abdominal surgeries, and many practicing veterinarians learned in this way. By 1950, schools located in urban areas around the world not only began to change their curriculum but also provided treatment for large numbers of dogs and cats. These developments were responses to the changing veterinary marketplace.

The growing influence of pharmaceutical companies in veterinary medicine also encouraged this slow shift toward dogs, cats, and other small animals. Scientific innovations, such as vaccines and antimicrobials, were tested on dogs and other animals in laboratories. Early vaccine research targeted not only the canine disease rabies but also other filterable virus diseases such as distemper that could be models for human diseases. For example, the British National Institute for Medical Research established a program to produce a vaccine against canine distemper after World War I. After a great deal of work, Patrick Laidlaw and G.W. Dunkin developed a killed-virus vaccine and follow-up immune modulator that they field-tested in Britain. In the United States, Pitman-Moore and Lederle Laboratories began producing this vaccine and advertising to pet owners that their dogs needed it. Pharmaceutical companies partnered with the veterinary profession, ensuring that only veterinarians could administer the vaccine. Creating proper standards of care for pet animals included the annual visit to the veterinarian, where a physical examination, deworming, and distemper and rabies vaccinations were increasingly expected by owners. This preventive medicine approach was endorsed by public health authorities (worried about rabies), veterinarians (who gained economic benefit), and pet owners (who wanted to care properly for their pets). In the 1960s, veterinarians responded to cat owners' desire for state-of-the-art treatment for felines also.

The development of small animal veterinary practice drove increasing specialization in veterinary medicine. For example, vets could specialize in feline medicine and surgery; and they founded professional associations and journals devoted to cats. Not only species but also particular sciences developed as veterinary specializations: cardiology, dermatology, and others within internal medicine; veterinary pharmacology to support the rapidly growing demand for pharmaceuticals; and radiology and anesthesiology to support surgery. All these specialties (and others) established their own post-graduate education standards, examinations, and specialty status such as holding a diploma from the American College of Veterinary Internal Medicine (just one example). Many nations began developing their own set of specialties within veterinary medicine and surgery during the 1960s, and these specialists became the teachers and professors in the veterinary schools. As the rise of companion animal medicine accelerated worldwide in the second half of the twentieth century, veterinary training and the veterinary workforce transformed as the profession adapted to new social conditions and responded to new challenges in animal health.

Conclusions

From this survey of the period 1900–1960, we can conclude that:

1. Until the 1920s, horses represented the most important clientele for veterinarians in society and agriculture as well as for the military. Most veterinary schools' curriculum was built around the horse as a model animal. With high densities of horses in urban areas, city veterinarians often specialized in horses.
2. Numbers of horses in urban areas began to decrease dramatically in the early 1900s as they were replaced by motorized vehicles, trains, and other modes of transporting goods and people. Although horses and donkeys were still common in many parts of the world, there were fewer animals overall. The reduction of urban horse numbers economically threatened the urban veterinary profession. Private veterinary schools focusing on horses began to close during the 1920s.
3. Numbers of horses in rural areas decreased more slowly, because the new machines were expensive. Small farms used horses for a longer time, and even larger farms kept a horse for particular tasks. Oxen and water buffaloes remained important for agriculture in Asia; mules, oxen, and cattle were still important in most African societies. Urban veterinarians searching for employment turned to treating livestock and worked in the food production industry; working for the government; or supporting global trade in animals and animal products.

4. Military use of horses, mules, and oxen continued to be important through the end of World War I (1914–1918). National armies employed many veterinarians to manage, care for, and heal army animals used for hauling supplies, cavalry, and hauling artillery. Modern technological warfare during World War I required more horses and mules than any preceding war. Moving fodder, cattle, and other food animals around the world caused disease epizootics. Rinderpest, glanders, shipping fever, and other diseases spread rapidly. In all nations affected by the war, veterinary education, training, and employment shifted to support the war.

5. Major developments in the biomedical sciences, especially in immunology and virology, increased the tools veterinarians could use to understand and control animal diseases. Brucellosis and bovine tuberculosis were two diseases targeted for veterinary control by many nations.

6. World War I accelerated the development of biomedical technologies, including biological and chemical weapons. After the German use of these weapons during the war, many nations began working on weaponizing the causative agents of glanders, anthrax, and other diseases for use against animals and humans.

7. International cooperation among veterinarians, which had begun already during the 1800s, intensified after World War I as organizations such as the Office International des Épizooties (OIE) [World Organization for Animal Health] were established. Still, economic conditions were very difficult for veterinarians and most tried to work in small-scale food animal or livestock practices.

8. World War II (1939–1945) still used a surprisingly large number of horses, oxen, dogs, and other animals for military purposes, mainly as draught and pack animals. Dogs carried messages, took supplies to isolated troops, and located explosives. In some armies, half of the nation's veterinarians served in the military forces during and after the war.

9. Veterinary involvement in war and the development of biological weapons raise important questions about the moral, ethical, and professional consequences of these activities. To prepare veterinarians to meet these challenges and make decisions, veterinary education must include how the ethical, cultural, and political contexts shape veterinarians' activities.

10. After World War II ended, veterinary schools and veterinary institutions in many parts of the world were destroyed. Food supplies were low and agricultural production was not functioning. International veterinary cooperation not only helped to restore the global food supply but also emphasized highly industrialized production that did not always fit the needs of local people. Some animals (poultry, pigs) were forced to adapt to crowded indoor conditions due to intensive "factory farming." Veterinarians helped to make this type of animal production possible by

advising farmers on animal breeding and husbandry and controlling diseases.

11. New tools, such as antimicrobials and new vaccines, made it possible to control and even try to eradicate animal diseases. Ironically, some of these tools actually caused problems, such as the fact that animals vaccinated against foot and mouth and other diseases then tested positive (as if they were infectious). Therefore, traditional methods of testing and slaughter-and-culling remained important in disease control programs. The ecological understanding of animal diseases was also crucial. A disease with a wild animal reservoir could not be eradicated; but by vaccinating domestic animals (such as dogs against rabies), human populations could be protected against zoonoses.

12. During these years, more veterinarians treated companion (pet) animals, especially in urban areas. Companion animal practice grew with the development of consumer culture in the middle and upper classes. Pet owners expected scientifically trained veterinarians to provide the same services for pets that their owner could expect from physicians. This included the use of the latest technologies, vaccines, and antimicrobials.

Question/Activity: What major scientific discoveries or developments occurred in your country or region of the world? Can you connect these scientific developments to epizootics or outbreaks of animal diseases? How were these scientific ideas different from the beliefs of animal owners? When did veterinary practice for companion animals or pets develop in your nation?

6   Food, Animals, and Veterinary Care in a Changing World, 1960–2000

Introduction

Throughout the past sixty years, veterinarians have been quite successful in maintaining and expanding their position and role. The profession has shaped, and been influenced by, some major transformations due to economic, political, cultural, and technological developments. These have included new regimes of food production and the changing global economy; decolonization and the dissolution of nation-states; changing roles for women and feminization; and the digital technologies that have spread around the world. Animal production, food inspection and controlling infectious livestock diseases, all shaped by increasing international cooperation, remained important veterinary concerns in the late 1900s and early 2000s. Reemerging diseases and new (zoonotic) diseases such as bovine spongiform encephalopathy (BSE, or "mad cow disease") in the 1980s, caused by prions, and the coronavirus diseases SARS and COVID-19 have represented new challenges. Moreover, veterinarians in some areas were confronted with increasing criticism from consumers and the general public and a great deal of media attention after massive outbreaks of swine fever, avian influenza, and foot and mouth disease (FMD) around the millennium year 2000.

In this chapter, we analyze the late twentieth century by focusing on selected themes about veterinary medicine: ongoing changes in food-animal production and consumption; animal disease outbreaks; and women in the veterinary profession. We begin with the ongoing development of intensive animal agriculture, or "factory farming," characterized by dense populations of confined livestock and poultry. How did the veterinary profession respond to the needs of these animals? And how has the profession responded to public criticism aimed at the practices of factory farming and food production? We also recognize that, in many areas of the world, veterinary practice is largely in the hands of animal owners and local healers. We sketch how these local experts provided necessary care, knowledge, and continuity, and how the continuing problems of small-scale animal production interfaced with the expectations of the global economy. We also consider how veterinarians have had to respond to the environmental problems created by food production: infectious diseases in animals and humans, pollution, the impacts on wild populations of animals, and the production of greenhouse gases contributing to climate change.

Repeatedly occurring food scandals, including the illegal administration of antibiotics and growth hormones, contributed to the poor image of factory farming and the meat industry as well as of the veterinarians involved. The latter were seen as having been active in increasing livestock production while ignoring the negative effects of intensive farming, and residues of antibiotics in food, animals, humans, and the environment resulted in problems with antibiotics resistance in humans. In the twenty-first century, veterinary authorities would be forced to reduce the amount of antibiotics used in livestock production and companion animals (pets) significantly. By that time, critics argued that the limits of mass production in the livestock industry had been reached. Both the livestock industries and veterinary profession were faced by challenges of concerned consumers, animal rights activists, and environmental lobbyists, especially in Europe.

The development of veterinary public health continued to play an important role in the professionalization process of veterinary medicine. This discipline also changed significantly during the past half century along with technological innovations in the globalizing animal production chain, which became longer and more invisible to consumers. In countries with large-scale factory farming, traditional meat inspection was gradually replaced by new surveillance strategies with (electronic) identification and traceability systems, "from farm to fork." Farmers and veterinarians in developing countries with fast-growing populations remained focused on providing food of animal origin for local markets, one reason being that international trade rules made it difficult for them to export animals and food to consumer countries.

In 1960, the parts of the world most affected by World War II were recovering in varying degrees. We begin with the ongoing problem of feeding the human populations of the world, to which one solution was the development of intensive animal agriculture, or "factory farming," characterized by dense populations of confined livestock and poultry

Feeding the Fast-Growing World Population with Food from Healthy Animals in the 1960s and Beyond

Between 1960 and 2020, the world's human population more than doubled. In some areas, this coincided with an increased standard of living. Those people with higher incomes spent more money on luxuries, including more food of animal origin in the diet. There is a strong relationship between per capita meat consumption and average gross domestic product (GDP). The richer people are, the more meat they consume. Although poverty has certainly continued to affect many people around the world, in many regions, food security has increased due to cheaper and more widely available meat, milk, yoghurt, cheese, eggs, and other animal products. The growing demand for substantially more food of animal origin on the global market stimulated small-scale as well as intensive livestock production. Of course, increasing livestock production had traditionally been an important challenge for the veterinary profession. However, meeting this huge demand required major technological and logistics changes in large-scale production systems for milk, dairy, eggs, meat, and farmed fish as well as scientific innovations in controlling diseases that continued to plague animal production.

This increased food production came with a price, however. Confining large numbers of animals indoors makes them vulnerable to diseases and undesired stress behaviors because of crowded conditions, while also causing large-scale waste disposal problems and contributing to the production of greenhouse gases (climate change). During the twentieth century, factory farming has made animal products cheaper and more widely available around the world, and veterinarians have contributed greatly to these developments. But this major transformation in food-animal production has encountered criticism from environmentalists and animal protectionists. They have argued that it is unethical to see animals as industrial "production units" instead of living, sensitive creatures. The call for returning to small-scale extensive (organic) farming, which had continued elsewhere in the world, became louder. How did veterinarians respond to these challenges and subsequent problems?

Spectacular Growth of Animal Production

During the past 60 years world population grew from 3.0 to 7.8 billion. Feeding this vast number of people became a priority for governments worldwide. Thanks to scientific and technological innovations, sufficient food is produced – in principle – to feed the whole world population. Unfortunately, due to inequality, political conflict, wars, and poverty, still not all people are able to benefit. Let's have a look at the amazing growth of animal production during the past six decades. Statistics from the United Nations Food and Agriculture Organization (FAO) reveal that meat production on a global scale has more than quadrupled in the period 1961–2018 (Fig. 6.1). Meat production increased in all regions. In Europe and North America, the output more than doubled. However, the biggest change took place in Asia, where meat production increased 15-fold. Asia is now the most important meat-production region in the world. Asian nations supply 42% of the world's meat, up from only about 12% in 1960. This huge growth was due to several factors, most importantly for our purposes the increasing use of factory farming methods and state support of smaller-scale livestock production farms.

Global meat production, 1961–2018

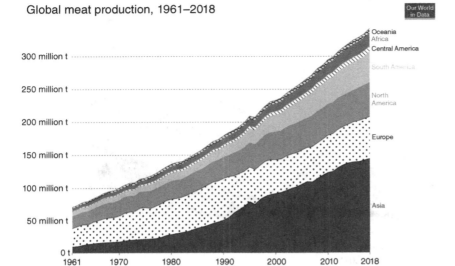

Figure 6.1 Global meat production (in million tons) in the period 1961–2018. *Source:* FAO.

The annual production of more than 300 million tons of meat requires the slaughter of billions of individual animals every year. For instance, in each of the past few years an estimated 50 billion chickens were slaughtered to feed the world. This figure even excludes male chickens and unproductive hens killed in the egg production sector. As for pigs, almost 1.5 billion were slaughtered to meet the growing demand for pork and processed foods like bacon, ham, and sausages. This figure has *tripled* in the past half century. The number of slaughtered cattle and buffaloes also increased, although at a lower level than chicken and pigs. Half a billion sheep are killed annually for mutton production, while during the 1990s the number of goats slaughtered overtook the number of consumed cattle. The contribution of meat from geese and guinea fowl, camels, horses, ducks, and wild game was much lower; however, still considerable (Fig. 6.2). As for seafood, it is virtually impossible to estimate the number of individual fish and shellfish that were caught. In 2016, not less than 150 million tons of seafood were produced for human consumption. About half of this amount came from fisheries, while the other half was produced on land by aquaculture. Particularly in Scandinavia and China, large salmon, trout, and shrimp farms have been developed that send fish products around the world.

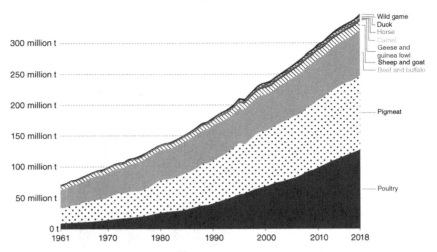

Figure 6.2 Global meat production by livestock type in the period
1961–2018.
Source: FAO.

The enormous growth in the production of food of animal origin was only
made possible by an extension of livestock worldwide. The distribution of the
different kinds of livestock over the various regions of the world in the year
1961 is listed in Table 6.1. Europe and the Americas then counted many
horses, bovines, swine, and poultry, while Africa had relatively more camels
and goats. Typically, Australia and New Zealand had high numbers of sheep.
The stock numbers for bovines, buffaloes, donkeys, mules, sheep, and goats
were highest in Asia. There, the number of pigs was relatively low, but Asia –
and particularly China – rapidly became the world's leader in the number of
pigs, chickens, and sheep in the following decades. Today, Brazil and India
possess the highest number of cattle. New Zealand counts 8 sheep per inhabitant, Uruguay 3.7 cows per inhabitant, and Brunei 40 chickens for every
person. Between 1970 and 2000, particularly, pigs, ducks, and poultry in
confinement industrial production accelerated. This was based on ever-
growing global livestock numbers (Table 6.2). The global average stock of
chickens living at any one time is about 20 billion, which means about
3 animals per person on the earth. This huge number is followed by 1.5 billion
cows, and sheep and pigs both around 1 billion. The total number of production animals living at any one time outnumbers the number of humans 3 to 1.
According to a recent census of the world's animals, 96% of mammals living
on the earth are either humans or domesticated animals (only 4% are wild); and
70% of all birds living on the earth are domesticated poultry. Although humans

Table 6.1. *Number of livestock (in millions) in Europe, Africa, Americas, Asia, and Australia & New Zealand in 1961. Based on Reinhard Froehner, Kulturgeschichte der Tierheilkunde. Ein Handbuch für Tierärzte und Studierende. Vol 3, Geschichte des Veterinärwesens im Ausland (Konstanz: Terra Verlag, 1968) pp. 423, 459–460, 532, 643, 656.*

	Europe	Africa	Americas	Asia	Australia & New Zealand	Total
Horses	23	2.4	24	14	0.7	64.1
Donkeys + mules	5	11	15	19		50
Bovines	187	116	296	329	23	951
Buffaloes	0.5	1.8		93		95.3
Camels	0.3	7		3		10.3
Swine	156	0.3	139	22	2	319.3
Sheep	261	123	162	213	202	961
Goat	24	76	40	173		313
Poultry	1 348	193	860	886	21	3 308

Table 6.2. *Global livestock populations in 1961, 1970, 2000, and 2010. (Sources: Froehner 1968; FAOSTAT, February 23, 2012.)*

	1961	1970	2000	2010
	(million)			
Bovines	951	1 081	1 315	1 428
Buffaloes	95	107	164	194
Camels	10	16	22	24
Sheep	961	1 063	1 059	1 078
Goats	313	377	747	921
Pigs	319	547	899	965
Turkeys		178	449	448
Ducks		256	948	1 187
	(billion)			
Chickens	3.3	5.2	14.5	19.4
Total	6	8.8	20.1	25.7

Sources: Reinhard Froehner, Kulturgeschichte der Tierheilkunde. Ein Handbuch für Tierärzte und Studierende. Vol 3, Geschichte des Veterinärwesens im Ausland (Konstanz: Terra Verlag, 1968) pp. 423, 459–460, 532, 643, 656. https://aboutzoos.info/images/stories/images/ Livestockpopulationsize_trend_Table.jpg; UN Food and Agricultural Organization, production data. www.faostat.org

are only 0.1% of life on earth, we are causing the biggest changes in the composition of the earth's animals due to our vast production of livestock. This fact has generated numerous problems and challenges, some of which we will return to at the end of this chapter.

Veterinary Contributions to the Increased Food Production

The staggering increase in food production described above could not have been possible without the contribution of agricultural and veterinary sciences. In 1961 there were more than 161,000 veterinarians active worldwide; in 2018 there were more than half a million. Since it was a traditional area of their professional activities, veterinarians worked hard to facilitate the enormous growth of food production described above. Much emphasis was put on developing intensive livestock production systems. Governments supported research on animal husbandry, genetics, meat, and dairy quality and optimizing feed conversion. Research institutes were established in which multidisciplinary research programs were carried out to improve production and quality. As a result, new types of large stables were built with more attention to hygiene, ventilation, and climate control. Further mechanization and automation of feeding, milking, and drainage of manure enabled higher production with fewer personnel. A new generation of drugs was developed, particularly antibiotics and vaccines, to control the diseases that spread in high-density animal populations. New reproduction practices such as artificial insemination and caesarean sections became widespread. All these factors contributed to a higher level of herd health.

Intensive livestock raising began with smaller animals, such as mink and poultry; but the principles of running a successful "factory farm" were soon being applied to pigs and even large animals such as dairy cattle. The key to profit on these farms was treating animals almost as machines to produce eggs, furs, meat, and milk. Overall, individual animals were far less important, but the conditions of housing, nutrition, and sanitation were crucial. In poultry houses, infections such as pullorum disease (an intestinal infection spread from hens to chicks through the egg) could wipe out an entire flock of young birds at one time. Close confinement spread coccidiosis and other infections, which also could kill most or all the birds rapidly. Disease was the major problem faced by intensive animal farms.

Factory farming was not possible for many species of domestic animals until new pharmaceuticals became cheap and widely available after World War II. Veterinary pharmaceutical companies produced sulfathiazole, sulfaguanidine, and other effective antimicrobials. After research demonstrated that feeding low levels of these antimicrobials prevented outbreaks of coccidiosis, they were sold as feed additives for poultry confinement houses. By the 1950s, these chemicals made large-scale poultry production possible both by preventing disease and the (related) antibiotic growth effect. Young animals fed low levels of antibiotics gained weight faster, matured faster, and produced more eggs. Along with vitamins, hormones, and others, these feed additives increased the efficiency of the "animal machine" and made more money for the farmer/producer.

Veterinarians, who had previously ignored chickens because individual animals were not worth the price of medical care, realized they could provide preventive care for whole flocks. Vets were unhappy that farmers could purchase the sulfa feed additives directly (not through the veterinarian). However, there were other services that only vets could provide. Veterinarians still controlled most vaccinations – and vaccines were the other essential disease-prevention tools for large poultry houses. Newcastle disease and other viral infections plagued poultry operations, and veterinary researchers worked hard to find effective and cheap vaccines that could be used for large flocks. Veterinarians also provided the diagnostic laboratory tests needed to identify the cause of infections. The other role for veterinarians was to inspect flocks of poultry and poultry products (eggs and meat). As poultry production dramatically increased, so did the need for veterinary inspectors.

By the 1950s, new technologies and pharmaceuticals were also allowing big changes in dairy production. Milking machines and modern milking houses led to bigger herds and, eventually, to partial confinement of dairy animals. Improved nutrition, antimicrobials, hormones, and vitamins in the feed all contributed to faster growth and much higher milk production. By the 1960s, many larger cities around the world regulated the quality of milk and the conditions under which it was produced. Veterinarians were needed to create disease prevention and control plans, to provide reproductive consultation and services, and to inspect animals, milk, and meat. Cows in large herds were susceptible to mastitis, uterine infections, displaced abomasum, and diseases such as brucellosis, tuberculosis, and leptospirosis. Veterinarians vaccinated animals against these diseases, performed surgeries, carried out pregnancy checks, evaluated semen for artificial insemination, and treated mastitis. The largest farms scheduled their veterinarian for regular monthly visits to carry out most of these procedures on a schedule and provide information for detailed records on the herd and individual animals.

Production in both cattle and pigs was further increased by feeding hormones as growth promoters. Antibiotics were also added to animal feed as disease preventatives and growth promoters for meat- and dairy-producing animals. Between 1962 and 2002, selective breeding and genetic modification techniques were used to make pigs more economically productive: the proportion of muscle for the most popular cuts of meat was dramatically increased (Fig. 6.3), and breeders selected sows who gave birth to the largest numbers of

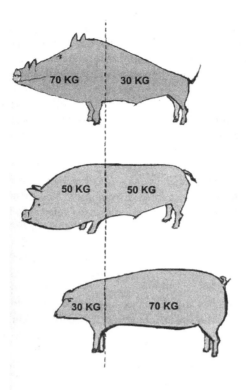

Figure 6.3 Drawing showing the changes in the body proportions of pigs over time due to selection, crossbreeding, and genetic modification.
Source: Modified from Hjalmar Clausen, "Svineracer og svineproduktion i et udvidet europaeisk faellesmarked," *Nyhedstjeneste BP Olie-Kompagniet A/S* 23 (1972) 71: 1–19. Image p. 6.

piglets. By 2002, the average sow produced 50% more piglets, which on average ate 33% less feed, produced 50% less manure, and produced 33% more pork than did the pig of the 1960s. Genetic, hormonal, feeding, and other modifications materially changed the bodies and production capacity of pigs, an example of human-managed evolution. These techniques were so successful in poultry and swine that they were quickly applied to other livestock species as well. The modern system of large-scale livestock production has been built on these modifications to animals' bodies, physiology, and environments.

Veterinarians as Herd Health Experts

To expand their role for large-scale livestock production, veterinarians had created a new type of practice: "herd health." They educated themselves about the most important management problems for chickens, pigs, and dairy cattle. They learned to read and use new types of records and to make clinical judgments based on what was best for the whole herd and not just an individual animal. They made themselves the experts on a wide range of subclinical diseases that could reduce animals' productivity and owners' profits. They learned about the latest vaccines and procedures in newly established professional journals and professional education workshops. Eventually, veterinary schools began including instruction on caring for large-scale herds and animals in confinement, and this type of work had become a new specialization for some veterinarians. However, some worried that this type of work made vets into specialist technicians rather than independent analytical experts. Anyone could be trained to do ordinary technical work such as injections, putting vets out of a job. The producer's desire for profit also conflicted with the veterinarian's responsibilities for animal welfare and food safety – a conflict that veterinary journals rarely discussed until the 1980s or even later. The veterinary profession continues to debate aspects of the veterinarian's role in herd health today, but high-intensity livestock production dominates the global markets and veterinarians provide crucial services to maintain it.

However, in most parts of the world, livestock were (and still are) raised in small numbers and with hand labor. While large-scale farms increasingly supplied global markets, small-scale livestock production remained very important locally and regionally. Small-scale dairy farming practices are not the same everywhere, obviously. But usually, these farmers kept ten or fewer animals (usually goats or cattle), which they milked by hand and cared for themselves. Beginning with local breeds that could survive local diseases, farmers took advantage of dairy development programs to crossbreed with imported animals to increase milk yields. The major health problems for these farmers continued to be parasitism, vector-borne diseases (such as East Coast fever in eastern African regions), and bacterial infections, with high juvenile mortality. Veterinary care, often provided by government veterinarians, began with vaccination programs against the local diseases that most threatened people (such as brucellosis) and the animal economy (such as rinderpest). Vets also provided advice and education, anthelmintics and antimicrobials, and the coordinated response to epizootics. Sometimes they performed surgeries or treated individual animals. Finally, vets provided the inspections and certifications necessary for small-scale owners to sell their animals' milk, meat, and other products to the markets. These veterinarians, especially the government-employed ones, addressed herd health for smaller herds.

The herd health approach was designed to increase the supply of foods of animal origin, for both local areas and the global market. With international efforts after World War II and large-scale development projects in decolonizing nations in the 1950s and 1960s, the veterinary profession concentrated on solving local problems to help the global food supply. Veterinarians were also involved in developing national and international legislation aimed at increasing production, quality, and safety of livestock. They drew up inspection procedures, quality standards, and safeguard clauses to facilitate national and international trade in live animals and food of animal origin. The European Economic Community (EEC) consulted veterinarians for its directives on the trade of live animals (pigs and cattle), for example. International trade within the EEC was strongly stimulated by the regulated trade of fresh meat and the higher quality of food products. Similar standardization and regulations were also established within the Office International des Épizooties (OIE), Food and Agriculture Organization of the United Nations (FAO), and the Veterinary Public Health Division of the World Health Organization (established in 1949). These measures facilitated trade in animals and their products on a global scale, and they standardized expectations for production.

Becoming herd health and preventive medicine managers meant also changing veterinary education. Animal husbandry with the subdisciplines of breeding, genetics, statistics, animal handling, and farm management obtained a more prominent position in the veterinary curricula over time. New fields such as food science, technology, and legislation were incorporated to provide the students with adequate knowledge of the food chain, quality control, and (inter)national trade. Veterinary schools and associations were in the process of specialization at this time. Those students and practitioners who were especially interested in livestock practice and herd health formed groups such as the World Association for Buiatrics (cattle practice), which in 1960 joined together the existing Danish, Austrian, German, and Norwegian associations. By the 1970s, cattle-practice specialty associations had formed in Australia, North America, Britain, France, Uruguay, the Netherlands, Italy, Argentina, and Mexico. The Federation of Asian Veterinary Associations (FAVA), founded in 1978, also had a specialty group for bovine and herd health veterinarians.

Another route to specialization was to attain a species-specific certification in clinical practice, reflecting advanced training and successfully passing examinations. These specialists had expertise in dairy animals, beef cattle, and other types of clinical practice beyond the knowledge of most practicing veterinarians. They were certified by the national government and national societies (such as the American Board of Veterinary Practitioners, under the American Veterinary Medical Association). Modeled after the specialty Colleges in academic subjects (pathology, microbiology, etc.), expert clinicians (including herd health veterinarians) could now attain a higher status. Since the late 1970s, clinical specialty certification (of various types) has grown to include more nations and regions and more categories (such as swine health management and exotic companion animals).

Veterinarians working with cattle, poultry, swine, and other farm animals became even busier during the 1970s and 1980s, with the resurgence of epizootics. Foot and mouth disease, swine fever, Newcastle disease, and encephalitis, as well as many other diseases, appeared more frequently to challenge governments, livestock owners, and veterinarians. These outbreaks could almost always be traced to the increasing global trade and travel in animals and animal products. In the next section, we will describe how these events led to new programs of veterinary preventive medicine and veterinary public health.

Diseases Are Social Events: Global Disease Challenges and the Veterinary Response

The huge increase in global animal economies, including higher concentrations of livestock populations and international traffic in live animals, animal feed, and food of animal origin, led to outbreaks of familiar and new animal diseases and zoonotic infections among humans. These diseases spread and circulated quickly due to modern international transport technology and large-scale systems, as well as changes in the food chain. Veterinarians worldwide responded to these challenges with further developments in preventive veterinary medicine. In the 1970s–1990s, preventive veterinary medicine sought to serve high-density livestock production and veterinary public health by controlling diseases. However, the veterinary profession also needed to respond to social attitudes and cultural beliefs on the part of consumers of meat, milk, and other animal products, as well as people concerned with ethics and animal welfare. These groups placed limitations on the power of the livestock industry to control food production. Veterinarians sometimes felt that they were caught in the middle of debates about livestock production and, especially, how to respond to disease problems.

Strategies for Controlling Animal Diseases in the Global Economy

Annual statistics on livestock production, as well as on the health status of livestock, and outbreaks of animal diseases can be found in archives of ministries of agriculture and national veterinary services in most countries around the world. This also goes for international (veterinary) organizations, notably the OIE. Since the 1920s, the OIE has provided information about the state of the art of preventing and controlling animal diseases and zoonotic diseases. Guidelines drawn up by international veterinary experts are used as standards by national veterinary authorities. Well known are the former OIE A- and B-lists with classifications of animal diseases. A-list diseases had three characteristics: (1) the potential for very serious and rapid spread across national borders, (2) serious social or public health consequences, and (3) major economic importance in the international trade of animals and animal products. These diseases required an international control strategy. B-list diseases had socioeconomic and/or public health importance within countries, regions, or even only on the one-farm level.

In 2005, OIE established a single list of notifiable terrestrial and aquatic animal diseases that replaced the former lists A and B. In cooperation with the World Trade Organization, OIE created and manages the World Animal Health Information System (WAHIS). In 2020, it provided actual information on 117 animal diseases, infections, and infestations such as rabies, BSE, anthrax, Q-fever, FMD, classical swine fever (CSF) and African swine fever, Newcastle disease, glanders, bovine babesiosis, equine influenza, salmonellosis, and many others. The OIE and its partners coordinated the international campaign against rinderpest, the first animal disease eradicated from the globe in 2011 (discussed later in this chapter). The rinderpest eradication campaign has served as a model for campaigns currently undertaken by the OIE against other important animal diseases, such as CSF and FMD. The combination of test and slaughter of infected animals and vaccination (if a good vaccine exists) are central strategies of anti-disease campaigns. Additionally, highly contagious diseases such as CSF and FMD also require preventive culling: "ring-culling" of all animals on infected farms, quarantine of the area, and prohibitions against moving animals. Because humans can spread the disease on shoes, boots, clothing, and vehicles, both animal and human movements are often restricted in the quarantined areas. Although necessary to control the disease, these strategies are economically and psychologically devastating to farmers and livestock producers.

Despite experience with eradication and vaccination strategies in the 1940s and 1950s, CSF and FMD outbreaks continued to occur in Europe in the second half of the twentieth century. Outbreaks of bovine tuberculosis and brucellosis remained limited. In case of outbreaks of CSF (classical swine fever), infected farms were isolated, while pig markets, moving animals, and imports were prohibited. An eradication cull-and-slaughter policy with (some) compensation to the farmers was carried out. In some heavily infected areas, healthy pigs were immunized by a live, attenuated vaccine (developed in rabbits) combined with injection of immune serum. CSF remained a problem in Central and South America, Europe, and Asia and parts of Africa. North America, Australia, and New Zealand remained free of the disease. Large outbreaks of CSF occurred in Germany (1993–2000), Belgium (1990, 1993,

1994), Italy (1995, 1996, 1997), and the Netherlands (1997–1998). The outbreak of a severe epidemic of CSF in February 1997 in the Netherlands and the mandatory cull-and-slaughter policy led to the destruction of 11 million pigs using ring-culling (infected farms and preventive killing) at a cost of US $2.3 billion to the livestock sector. Due to quarantine lockdown measures in infected areas, even more money was lost in the economic sectors of tourism, the hospitality industry, and recreation. Many farmers and local businesses never recovered. This tragic event represented the biggest CSF outbreak ever in the European Union (EU) as a whole.

As with CSF, outbreaks of FMD continued to occur in the second half of the twentieth century. Depending on the scale and region, eradication and/or vaccination strategies were followed. More effective vaccines against the different strains of FMD were developed and applied in various countries. Annual vaccination schemes against FMD were conducted by government veterinarians or private practitioners, often assisted by veterinary students. However, only domesticated bovines were vaccinated, since regular vaccinations of huge amounts of wild animals or slaughter pigs with a short life cycle was practically impossible and too expensive. FMD remained a continuous problem in parts of eastern and southern Africa, especially due to imported animals (although wild animal populations were often blamed as the source of "endemic" FMD). In Europe, between November 1961 and August 1962 more than 320,000 pigs were killed to stop FMD in the Netherlands. In 1967 another FMD epidemic caused huge economic losses in Western Europe. Fortunately, the annual vaccination approach was quite successful in many countries, with very few bovine cases. Despite this success, the European countries changed strategies in 1991: they decided to stop vaccinating cattle against FMD. Instead, the eradication/ring-culling and quarantine strategies alone would be used against FMD. This decision illustrates the high stakes of animal disease control policies. Why was a vaccination strategy that seemed successful abandoned in Europe in 1991?

The Mathematics of Devastation: Foot and Mouth Disease (FMD)

To answer this question, it is important to remember the situation in the late 1900s. International relationships depended in part on positive trade relationships, including the trade of animals and animal products. A disease outbreak could threaten good diplomatic relationships as well as cause economic devastation. CSF was a good example: major importing countries like Japan and the United States had no CSF, and these countries tested samples of European pork for CSF. A positive result condemned the whole shipment and sometimes led to a complete ban on animal products from European countries with endemic CSF or other diseases. Bans on "infected imported meat" caused economic hardship and anger in the country of origin. Another example was the international incident between Argentina and the UK in the late 1960s, when British importation of some infected Argentinian meat almost led to a diplomatic crisis. Veterinary historian Abigail Woods has called these FMD-related international crises "manufactured plagues" (see Further Reading) because an agricultural problem that could have been contained was magnified into an international incident. Veterinary concerns quickly got overruled by the economic and diplomatic implications. International political changes, such as the formation of the EU, meant new rules for the global market in animal products. Scientific considerations were also important, especially the qualities of the tests and the vaccines. For example, animals that had been vaccinated against FMD become seropositive, the same as infected animals; testing could not tell the difference between them. In addition, the existing modified live vaccines against FMD could cause outbreaks if the vaccines were not carefully produced.

Given these problems, agricultural and veterinary economists were employed by the EU to determine whether it was more cost-effective (for the government) to vaccinate all animals or to stop vaccinating and rely on early warning and quick cull and slaughter in the case of new outbreaks. These economists developed mathematical models that simulated outbreaks. Based on the results of their models, they recommended that it was cheaper for governments to stop vaccinating against FMD. This decision left all European animals susceptible to FMD. If an outbreak began, a rapid and overwhelming response would stop it. Of course, this would necessarily destroy a lot of animals and cause economic (and social) damage to farmers and livestock producers. Despite the availability of effective vaccines against CSF and FMD, the EU non-vaccination policy was issued in 1991. This policy dictated EU member states to apply a cull-and-slaughter policy in case of outbreaks, and it also influenced other countries exporting animals and meat to the EU. Any imported animals or products that were seropositive for FMD were rejected. Since vaccinated animals were seropositive, countries that used vaccination could not export animal products to the European market.

The non-vaccination policy led to tensions and concerns within the veterinary profession, particularly between practitioners who worked with farmers and the official (government) veterinarians responsible for the cull-and-slaughter policy. Veterinarians complained that they had to kill thousands of animals, even after new vaccines were available to solve the problem. With these so-called DIVA [Differentiating Infected from Vaccinated Animals] or "marker" vaccines, it was possible to differentiate between field-virus infected and vaccinated animals. This scientific development could have solved the problem. However, national and international trade rules overruled veterinary science. The number of outbreaks increased within Europe, culminating in a major catastrophe in 2001, when an epizootic began in Britain. Ironically, this devastating FMD epizootic started in Britain by feeding swill containing infected meat to pigs, exposing the importance of regulating not just animals but also imported animal *feeds*. Next to Ireland and Denmark, Britain was one of the EU nations most in favor of non-vaccination legislation. Britain would pay a huge price for this legislation.

From February 2001, FMD quickly spread to farms all over Britain, where 2,000 cases were reported in the initial wave of the outbreak. The British government, despite farmers' lawsuits, still viewed the cull-and-slaughter strategy as the right response. As Abigail Woods has shown, this strategy reflected the EU's policy, and it was also viewed by the British government as a morally upright policy that would force farmers to act for the overall common benefit to the market, but at their own expense. Angry farmers and upset rural people watched as the government condemned and slaughtered their herds. The epizootic was stopped only after the killing of more than 6 million cows and sheep. Economic losses for agriculture and the food chain were estimated at about £3.1 billion. By transportation of infected animals from the UK, the disease spread to Ireland and from there to farms in France and the Netherlands. Besides Britain, the Netherlands became the worst affected country with more than 265,000 animals killed by the strict preventive cull-and-slaughter policy applied. The economic damage amounted to some 2.8 billion Dutch guilders. As terrible as the FMD outbreak had been, this disease was not new; and it did not cause dangerous infections in humans. The world would not be so lucky with the next major disease outbreak, which again occurred in Britain and again reflected the importance of animal feeds and fodder.

Making the Cows Go Mad: Bovine Spongiform Encephalopathy (BSE) and the Prion Diseases

The history of BSE is an excellent example of how the veterinary perspective has enabled primary scientific discoveries in biomedicine. BSE was also a major social and political problem in Europe, specifically Britain, in the 1980s and 1990s. BSE is a fatal neurodegenerative disease of cattle, and it is categorized as a transmissible spongiform encephalopathy (TSE). Animals slowly develop progressive central nervous system signs, including aggression, nervousness, pacing, rubbing, licking, ataxia, trembling or fits, anorexia, coma, and death (thus the common name of "mad cow disease"). The first infections of this disease in British ruminants probably occurred in the 1970s or even earlier, but no unusual cases or deaths were reported at the time. Only in 1986, when veterinary pathologist G. Wells at the Weybridge Central Veterinary Laboratory in England noticed the unusual lesions in the brains of animals that died with these symptoms did veterinary authorities become alarmed. The brains of affected animals were full of holes, and they looked like sponges, leading to the name of the disease (*spongiform*). Definitive diagnosis was made at postmortem, and with Wells' publication of two cases in 1986, veterinarians and pathologists began to look for these brain lesions in animals that died with central nervous system signs and symptoms. Pathologists and bacteriologists also sought the cause of the disease, looking especially for viruses that caused encephalitis. They were puzzled when they could not definitely find a causative organism. Based on the brain lesions, pathologists had a theory that this "new" disease was in fact closely related to some well-known diseases in other species that looked similar, such as scrapie in sheep. The unique veterinary perspective that these diseases were probably related and caused by similar infectious agents proved crucial to the medical under-standing of the TSEs (and the discoveries that would lead to two Nobel Prizes).

In the 1980s, veterinary pathologists did not at first realize how important their research would become; but relating "mad cow disease" to scrapie in sheep was the first step in a major scientific discovery. Scrapie, or "trembles," in sheep had been categorized as a puzzling disease thought to be caused by an unidentified "slow virus" – a transmissible virus or agent that developed in an infected animal over long periods of time, eventually causing neurological symptoms and death. Because scrapie often appeared in inbred herds, some thought it was partly a heritable disease. Sheep herders, veterinarians, and scientists had been aware of scrapie since at least the 1700s, and by the mid-1800s they understood it as a disease that could be transmitted through the placenta of infected ewes to their lambs. In 1898 at the Toulouse (France) veterinary school, Charles Besnoit (1867–1929), M.Ch. Morel, and colleagues described the characteristic holes or vacuoles in the brain tissues of animals that died of scrapie. They noted that infected materials from lamb births could also expose other animals to the disease.

By the 1930s, Toulouse veterinary researchers Jean M. Cuillé (1872–1950) and Paul-Louis Chelle (1902–1943) concluded that scrapie was caused by a "nonconventional agent" that was not a virus. They successfully inoculated healthy animals (intraocularly) with scrapie-infected brain tissue and patiently waited almost two years for the disease to appear in the inoculated animals. When the animals became sick with classic symptoms, Cuillé and Chelle had proved that scrapie was a transmissible disease. However, they still could not identify a causative agent. Veterinarian D.R. Wilson at the Moredun Institute in Edinburgh, Scotland, had demonstrated some puzzling attributes of scrapie: it could not be prevented by trying to kill the mysterious infectious agent with ionizing radiation or heat; and scrapie also seemed to have a genetic compon-ent, with the infectious agent infecting much higher percentages of some breeds and families of sheep (W.S. Gordon's research). Finally, veterinarian

I.H. Pattison discovered that goats were 100 percent susceptible to scrapie, thus establishing its ability to jump between species.

The next important development that would eventually link scrapie to BSE and other similar diseases occurred halfway around the world, with humans as the affected population. In Australia, the physician and virologist Frank MacFarland Burnet (1899–1985) had established an important center of research devoted to infectious and zoonotic diseases and the immunological response of hosts. One of Burnet's colleagues, physician Carlton Gadjusek (1923–2008), began investigating *kuru*, a central nervous system disease of humans in Papua New Guinea. Able to demonstrate characteristic brain lesions, Gadjusek and colleague V. Zigas could not isolate an infectious agent but published reports about the disease in 1957. An American veterinary pathologist, William J. Hadlow (1921–2015), quickly noted the similarities to scrapie in sheep, publishing a paper that theorized *kuru* and scrapie to be manifestations of the same disease process in different species. Hadlow's observation stimulated Gadjusek's lab to try inoculating chimpanzees with *kuru*-infected brain tissue and, crucially, to wait patiently for two years for the disease to manifest in the experimental animals. This was the first transmission of the disease between humans and non-human primates, and Gadjusek won the 1976 Nobel Prize in Physiology or Medicine for this work.

Pathologists were also already linking *kuru* to Creutzfeldt-Jakob disease (CJD), named for the two German neurologists who had characterized it in the 1920s. By the late 1960s, veterinarians had demonstrated that scrapie, a similar disease in mink (Aleutian disease), *kuru*, and CJD belonged in the same category of diseases: the transmissible spongiform encephalopathies (TSEs). CJD had also been reported in people receiving transplants of central nervous system tissues and growth hormones from cadavers. The evidence was building up: these diseases could freely pass between humans and between humans and animals, not only chimpanzees but also laboratory mice and other species.

CJD was transmitted by injecting, implanting, or feeding infected materials, and this is exactly what happened with BSE in cattle in the 1980s. Cattle feed was commercially produced using poorly rendered offal from sheep and cattle slaughtered for meat. The practice of recycling meat-and-bone meal, derived from slaughterhouse waste and dead animals in rendering plants, goes back to the early twentieth century. This was considered very profitable for a cleaner environment and the production of cheap, protein-rich animal feed. By the 1970s, infected carcasses were certainly being used to produce cattle feed, bone meal, gelatin, and tallow and in pharmaceuticals for both humans and animals. By the mid-1980s (the incubation period of the transmissible spongiform encephalopathies is very long), a major outbreak of BSE appeared in cattle in Britain. Veterinary investigation revealed that the animals had been infected by commercial feeds produced from infected animal carcasses, probably after changing the rendering process to a lower temperature and pressure around 1980.

The BSE outbreak heightened investigations into both the zoonotic aspects of these diseases and the race to find the causative agent – and this discovery would be the biggest breakthrough in disease biology in a century. American neurologist and biochemist Stanley Prusiner (b. 1942) and colleagues had shown that the cause of BSE was something entirely new: rather than a living microorganism, the causative agent was misfolded proteins known as prions. (Prusiner won the Nobel Prize in Physiology or Medicine in 1997 for this research.) Finding the process by which normal proteins became "infected" and misfolded created a new branch of disease pathology. These prions were not alive; and that explained why they survived ionizing radiation. They had to be injected or eaten and had to pass through the blood-brain barrier. They took a long time to convert proteins in the central nervous system tissue to the pathological forms that, once they built up, caused the characteristic symptoms. Finally, they could easily travel between species because they were not living organisms that had to adapt to new hosts. This explained the close connections between transmissible encephalopathies in multiple animals and humans.

The development of the prion theory coincided with the British BSE outbreak, which became a crisis for the British government at the end of the 1980s that lasted for twenty years. Concerned that humans could become infected with a form of BSE, the British government removed the most dangerous meat from the food supply in 1989 and outlawed the use of cooked animal parts in cattle feed. Government officials then reassured the public that the meat supply was safe. However, panic broke out in 1996 when some people in Britain began to show signs of CJD, and their infections were traced to earlier ingestion of contaminated animal products. They showed the classic signs and symptoms of CJD, but some of these victims were young people. This is very unusual for classical CJD, which is almost always diagnosed in elderly people. This variant was thus named "new variant CJD" (vCJD) and it was definitively linked to BSE in British cattle using molecular genomics in the late 1990s. (We now know that the same agent caused both BSE in cattle and vCJD in humans, and humans became infected through the food supply.) In the 1990s, there was great fear that everyone who had eaten meat in Britain could die of this new disease, which spread to other countries where infected British bone meal had been added to animal feed. Trying to eradicate the infection, the British government ordered that every animal older than 30 months in the national herd be immediately slaughtered. About 4.7 million cattle were killed and their bodies burned on huge pyres during the weeks-long culling. The photos of the pyres and upset farmers appeared in media around the world. The EU banned exports of British beef from 1996 to 2006, and nations around the world banned imported animal products from Britain. Along with the FMD outbreaks, BSE destroyed the livelihoods of farmers who had raised cattle for the beef market. Trade controversies, called the "beef wars" in the popular media, fed British anger and bitterness against both the UK government and the EU.

Around the world, importation restrictions against British beef have continued until recently, due to the long incubation period of vCJD and fears that more people could begin to show signs of the disease. In humans, as with other animals, prion diseases are fatal. The signs in humans include personality changes, memory loss, problems walking, and coma. In 2020, fewer than 250 people have been diagnosed with vCJD since its appearance in the 1990s and the vast majority have been British citizens. Since 2000, new vCJD cases have been declining in Britain. However, new cases could still be diagnosed for some time to come, due to the long incubation period. Research has shown that the genetic makeup of the infected people determines which types of prion proteins are developed, and some types take longer than others. This explains why early scientists thought that CJD could be partially inherited. Fortunately, vCJD is extremely rare and will probably remain so. But the TSEs, nicknamed the "zombie diseases," remain greatly feared by the public.

To protect the human food supply, the European Union and other countries adjusted feeding and rendering regulations and banned feeding meat and bone meal to cattle. In U.S. and EU slaughterhouses, the brain, spinal cord, intestines, eyes, and tonsils from cattle were classified as "Specified Risk Materials" that must be disposed of at high temperatures (incinerated or digested at high pressure and temperature). These measures resulted in an interruption of the transmission cycle and a strong reduction of BSE cases. Infectious prion particles were never found in whole muscle tissues, such as beef roasts and steaks. New, strict regulations on the production of mixed-tissue products, such as sausages, have been developed in many nations. Importation of food and products derived from cattle and sheep are highly regulated around the world. These measures have slowed the spread of BSE and probably greatly reduced cases of TSEs in animal species that are part of the global economy.

However, it was much more difficult to restore faith in the various government officials who were involved in the BSE crisis, and the veterinary profession also experienced some criticism. BSE and vCJD redefined what was "natural" by turning the public spotlight on large-scale animal production and forcing it to change. BSE exposed the practice of feeding dead animal products to cattle, which are naturally herbivores that do not eat meat. Journalists and the media closely scrutinized the animal industries, and consumers were shocked and disgusted to learn the details of where and how their meat was produced. The BSE crisis changed public opinion. Politicians and the public alike were opposed to the idea of making herbivores eat the remains of their sisters, which was unnatural and "cannibalism. The "cannibalism" idea was encouraged by salacious media accounts about *kuru*, the disease Carlton Gadjusek had studied in Papua New Guinea. Gadjusek had found that *kuru* was spread by funerary practices of New Guineans, who respectfully ingested parts of the deceased person (including the brain). *Kuru* disappeared after these practices were outlawed. To British citizens in the 1990s, modern prejudices fed the horror of equating vCJD with *kuru* in "uncivilized" people who engaged in "cannibalism." Critics charged that the government (and farmers and veterinarians) should have known that such practices were wrong and would spread diseases.

These criticisms also influenced the pet food industry. Pet owners were shocked to learn that their beloved companions had been fed recycled parts of various species of dead animals in canned pet food ever since rendering plants became active during the 1900s. The fact that pets were fed with offal from slaughterhouses and meat factories did not fit into the ideology of a highly civilized society. This practice was also widely denounced as "unnatural." However, these pet owners were not aware of the history: for centuries, pigs and dogs had been fed animal carcass remainders obtained from knackers' yards and slaughterhouses. This fact did not eliminate the public's criticism of pet food production practices, however. During the 1990s and early 2000s, concerns about the use of offal in pet foods contributed to the increasing production of commercial "natural" and vegetarian foods for dogs and other pets. These products allowed owners to feel that they were not supporting what they considered to be pet food companies' immoral, dangerous, and disease-spreading production practices.

The number of TSEs will undoubtedly continue to grow in the future, with new variants being discovered in domesticated and wild animals, and even humans. The spread of these diseases in the modern era has been driven by the practices of the global commercial livestock economy, particularly including materials from animal carcasses in animal feed and in a wide range of products used and consumed by humans. These practices not only have increased profits for companies selling these products, but have also increased the development of, and our attention to, these diseases. Another example is the recent recognition of "chronic wasting disease" in North America, in herds of wild and captive elk and deer. This disease is also a TSE that is similar to scrapie. CWD is a potential zoonosis since these animals are hunted and their meat is consumed by humans. First described by Colorado State University veterinarians Beth S. Williams (1951–2004) and Stewart Young in 1978, chronic wasting disease has been increasingly detected in parts of the midwestern United States and Canada, where it is spreading. Cases of CWD have recently been discovered in Swedish and Norwegian reindeer and caribou, and it is now likely to spread across Eurasia in wild cervids. Scientists have probably uncovered only a few of the diseases caused by transmissible prions in susceptible wild animal populations.

Changing Societal Context: Challenges to Animal Production Methods

In Europe, the crises around BSE, CSF, and FMD made clear that these outbreaks were strongly influenced by a changing societal background. Until the 1970s, outbreaks of epizootic diseases were mainly considered to be a problem in the agricultural sector, and they drew little media or popular attention. Most consumers were only interested in keeping meat and milk prices low. They were not very concerned with controlling animal diseases or ensuring animal welfare. However, the systematic killing of millions of healthy animals during the BSE, CSF, and FMD outbreaks, with images of burning piles of livestock, generated great opposition throughout society, particularly in high-income countries. The modern media, which had become less distant and more critical during the late 1900s, were responsible for putting these diseases in the spotlight in newspapers and on radio, television, and the Internet, thereby enhancing the negative image of factory farming held by the wider public. Faced with popular protests, politicians were forced to reevaluate their policy toward environmental sustainability in livestock production, disease control, and animal welfare. The public response also showed the large gap that had developed during recent decades between the urban consumers and the producers living in the countryside. Modern factory farming had moved far from urban life, to be invisible behind the walls of huge barns and slaughterhouses. This was also the working environment of veterinarians who specialized in preventive medicine and food safety. Therefore, public criticism also extended to them. Veterinarians were accused of facilitating and making money out of animal production, without paying enough attention to animal welfare and ethical production practices. Since these outbreaks, and under negative public pressure, the veterinary profession in Western countries has begun reappraising its role in factory farming.

The way in which farmers, the meat trade, the meat and dairy industries, veterinarians, the media, and the wider public responded to outbreaks of epizootics showed that long-standing legislation could still be changed. Measures dealing with livestock health, which are firmly dictated by national and international trade interests, eventually turned out to be negotiable when critically discussed by the various actors in society. For instance, since 2003 a European Union Directive on FMD has changed its position on eradication methods based on large-scale culling (which was very controversial). The EU now allows a combination of culling on infected farms and protective ring vaccination of healthy animals surrounding the infected area (instead of killing them). Many national governments have begun to regulate the livestock industry in terms of animal welfare and environmental pollution. For example, the Dutch government has issued several recent regulations on milk quotas and reducing numbers of animals (and manure and nitrogen output) per meadow and stable area, resulting in a decrease of livestock numbers. While this does not completely reverse the high-density methods of livestock production, it certainly influences those methods and changes them to some degree.

Another example is legislation concerning antibiotics used in veterinary practice. This legislation is a response to pressure from medical authorities who blamed the widespread use of antibiotics in veterinary practice as a major cause of resistance to antibiotics used in human medicine. The governments of Sweden, Denmark, the Netherlands, and (recently) the United States have banned the addition of antibiotics to animal feed. Antibiotics are still commonly used in animal feeds, with varying regulations, in the Americas, parts of Asia, and many African countries. In most African countries, antibiotics can be purchased without a veterinary prescription. The penicillins, tetracyclines, aminoglycosides, and fluoroquinolones are the most widely used. A recent study in Rwanda showed that over 90% of farmers use antibiotics routinely, mainly as a feed additive to prevent diseases, in intensively raised poultry and other animals. According to the OIE, antibiotic use is mostly unregulated in African countries such as Rwanda. Livestock production is crucial for feeding the population and, in most areas, is a significant part of each country's gross domestic product. These conditions are common around the world. By 2030, antibiotic usage in animal production is estimated to increase worldwide by 50% to 67%, with countries such as China, Brazil, India, South Africa, and Russia expected to be the major contributors to this trend. Antibiotic-resistant infections in human populations are likely to increase, also.

In livestock production, the problems with antibiotic resistance can be traced to several factors: the use of low levels of these drugs in animal feeds; the fact that animals are often not given a full course of treatment (to save money); and the lack of veterinary supervision that can lead to improper usage of antibiotics. Usage of low levels in animal feeds, including medications that are sporadically used to prevent coccidiosis in poultry, causes selection pressure in communities of microorganisms. After the drug has killed off the susceptible microorganisms, only the resistant ones are left to reproduce. These resistant strains take over, becoming the majority microbial flora in animal populations and their environments. Once this happens, the farmer must switch to a new antibiotic. If a sick animal receives some, but not all, of the antibiotic it needs, again the microbes will adapt and only those resistant to the antibiotic will multiply.

Finally, veterinarians have been trained to administer the correct antibiotic for the infection (this is best done using a culture of the microbes and antibiotic sensitivity testing). If farmers use antibiotics without veterinary supervision, they are much more likely to administer the wrong medication for the infection by relying on the cheapest or most familiar antibiotic. This, too, leads to the development of antimicrobial resistance. Many of the original antibiotics developed in the 1940s and 1950s are useless today due to widespread microbial resistance. Unfortunately, microbes develop resistance faster than scientists can develop new antibiotics. Human infections of antibiotic-resistant microorganisms include extensively drug-resistant tuberculosis (XDR TB) and methicillin-resistant *Staphylococcus aureus* (MRSA). These infections have skyrocketed recently, especially in certain areas of the world and among certain populations; and they can easily spread around the world. The problem of antimicrobial resistance will only become more difficult in the future, and social concerns about these infections are likely to drive further changes in livestock production practices.

Antibiotics are not the only chemicals used in livestock production that have become controversial. In the United States, bovine somatotropin (BST) was introduced in the 1990s. Administering BST, a growth hormone, to dairy cows resulted in a 10% to 25% higher milk production. Within 10 years, BST was being used in about 33% of the dairy cows in the United States. Veterinarians quickly realized that BST made cows sick, with an 80% increase in mastitis infections and udder inflammation and decreased fertility and suppressed immune systems. Moreover, if growth hormone metabolites were present in the milk, they could cause hormonal and allergic effects in people consuming the milk, especially infants and children. BST injection of dairy cows is not allowed in the EU, Canada, Australia, New Zealand, Japan, Israel, and Argentina, and it is currently being challenged in the United States, where it began. Similarly, the use of estrogens and other anabolic steroids was regulated after human health problems, including cancers, occurred in the 1980s and 1990s. Significant numbers of consumers have refused to purchase milk or products that they suspected had been produced using hormones, arguing that it was cruel to cows and unethical, and that there was not enough information to ensure the milk was safe for people to drink.

However, companies producing and distributing these synthetic hormones made a lot of money, and they pushed hard to prevent regulation of their products. Farmers also knew that these illegal substances would help them make higher profits in the short term. In European countries, farmers quietly purchased the outlawed hormones from criminal organizations (the "hormone mafia") that illegally imported the drugs from the United States. This generated huge profits for the hormone mafia, until governments appointed veterinary inspectors to investigate and stop the illegal sale and use of these chemicals. This led to a tragedy: Belgian veterinarian and government inspector Karel van Noppen, well known for his struggle against the illegal use of hormones in livestock production, was shot and killed by criminal hitmen in front of his house in 1995. This horrific event caused public outrage and protests. In response, the Belgian government enacted Europe's strictest legislation controlling the use of antibiotics and hormones in veterinary practice. Other European nations soon adopted similar laws. By 2000, it became very clear that global livestock production methods could not be determined by economic factors alone. Societal attitudes, cultural beliefs, animal health and welfare, and consumer and environmental protection all had to be considered as well (Fig. 6.4).

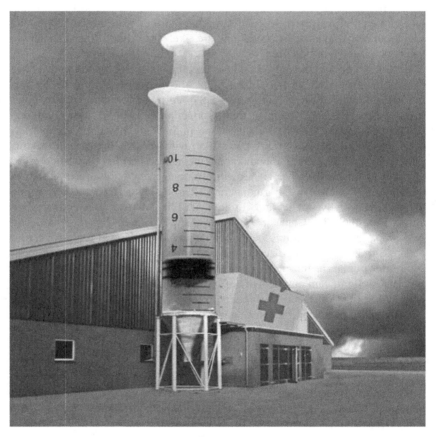

Figure 6.4 Image symbolizing the widespread use of antibiotics in livestock production. The Netherlands 2011.
Source: A. Sikkema, "Stoppen met spuiten," *Wageningen Resource* 6 (2011) September 3: 12–15.

Veterinary Responses to Disease and Public Health Challenges

Research and Control of Parasitic Diseases

With some notable exceptions, veterinary historians have focused on panzootic diseases (such as rinderpest) and have neglected the persistent parasitic and vector-borne diseases (especially those diseases endemic in the Global South). However, these diseases cause tremendous morbidity and mortality and are very persistent. For example, in sub-Saharan Africa, as well as in areas of the Middle East and South Asia, several animal diseases caused by trypanosomes cause huge losses in livestock productivity every year. Trypanosomes, protozoan blood parasites transmitted by biting flies, easily infect camels, horses, cattle, and many species of wild hoofed animals. In the 1960s and 1970s, African postcolonial nations such as Kenya and Somalia maintained veterinary research and vaccine production laboratories that were among the world's most experienced centers of research on veterinary trypanosomiasis, methods of fly control, and disease ecology. This applies to viral diseases, also. The control of various types of vector-borne encephalitis emphasizes that these diseases are constantly moving, often spreading to new geographic areas with the importation of animals and insects. They appear to be "new" diseases, and sometimes they *are* new if they manage to jump to a new host or become endemic in a new area. Usually caused by arboviruses, diseases such as eastern, western, and Venezuelan equine encephalitis and West Nile virus have been increasing in incidence worldwide.

Parasitic diseases have threatened the domesticated animal economies of most of the world's nations. It is a mistake to think that parasitic diseases are only problems of low-income societies in the Global South; they affect large commercial livestock operations everywhere. Parasitic diseases have increased due to human activities, especially increased buying, selling, and moving animals as part of the global economy. Two excellent case studies in veterinary history show how widespread these problems are and how the veterinary profession has responded to them: the eradication (1960s–1990s) of screwworm infection in the Americas, and the global campaign against *Echinococcus* infection in dogs, sheep, and humans (1960s through today). These case studies highlight several themes in the veterinary response to diseases in these decades: the mobilization of new technologies; the importance of international relationships and economic partnerships; and the necessity of cooperation and education between veterinarians, farmers, and ranchers who raise livestock.

Screwworms are parasitic flies that lay their eggs in wounds and under the skin of warm-blooded animals: cattle, horses, pigs, sheep and goats, dogs, cats, wildlife, and (rarely) humans. Once the eggs hatch, the larvae burrow into and consume the flesh of the host, causing tissue damage, itching, and pain; up to 3,000 larvae have been discovered in a single wound pocket. The infected animal suffers terribly: it stops eating, yields less milk, stops moving, and can die in a week or two. Once the larvae mature, they drop off the animal and pupate in the soil. Within 14 days, fresh flies hatch and seek more animal hosts. Screwworms, an ancient problem, had traditionally been attacked by livestock owners using both topical and environmental methods. Animals' wounds were smeared with oil mixed with tobacco to ward off the flies and suffocate any hatching larvae. Livestock owners also burned smoky fires to protect their animals from the flies. However, it is very difficult, if not impossible, to remove all larvae from wounds of an infected animal, and insecticides must be reapplied every few days. These strategies are not practical with large numbers of animals. As cattle ranches became large "production units," especially during World War II, unprotected cattle were crowded together in open feedlots, and screwworms caused great suffering, morbidity, and mortality in the Americas.

In the 1930s, veterinarians and entomologists decided that prevention of screwworm infection would only be possible with eradication of the insects. Screwworms were injuring and killing so many animals in the southern United States, especially along the border with Mexico, that the U.S. and Mexican federal governments partnered with the FAO to sponsor an eradication program. In the 1950s, entomologists tested an innovative but untried technique: irradiating screwworms to make them sterile, then releasing them into the wild. The sterilized flies would mate with the wild population, but the eggs would not be fertilized, and no fresh flies would hatch. In theory, the wild screwworm population would die out. Borrowing the idea from genetics research, the entomologists used U.S. Army war-surplus medical X-ray machines to irradiate flies. They determined the dose that would sterilize but not kill the insects, preserving their ability to mate. They raised large populations of sterilized male insects, then conducted tests on screwworm-infested islands: they released the sterile males on Sanibel Island (Florida, USA) and, cooperating with the Dutch government, on Curaçao (Netherlands Antilles). By the end of three weeks, the screwworm population was disappearing rapidly, and the remaining individuals were sterile – thus eradicating the population of flies on both islands. (However, without continuously releasing fresh sterile flies, screwworms returned to Curaçao, and eradication began again in the 1975.)

The sterile-insect approach was a major innovation in entomology and in veterinary control of insect-borne diseases. Using this technique, screwworms were eradicated from a vast territory in the southern United States by 1966. Since 1991, Mexico, Belize, Guatemala, El Salvador, Honduras, and Nicaragua have also eradicated screwworms, as have areas in northern Africa. Anti-screwworm campaigns are active in Central and South America today. The technique is considered friendly to the environment, since no chemicals are used. The successful North American eradication campaign depended not only on the new technology, but also on cooperative international agreements between Mexico and the United States and between adjoining Central American nations. The screwworm-free zones are maintained today with buffers of sterile insects covering a vast territory, over 2,000 kilometers of the Mexican–U.S. border. Fresh sterile insects are produced at a factory in Chiapas, Mexico, owned by a joint Mexican–U.S. commission, from which they are transported and released in the buffer zone every few weeks. Governments have declared that they continue to participate in this international program for several reasons: saving more animals on the plains and pampas encourages livestock producers to avoid cutting down forests to create new pastures; the program helps to ensure enough food both for the nation and for export; and it saves farmers and governments a lot of money. There are difficulties: inaccessible mountainous or jungle areas can still contain flies; different local cultures and languages make communication difficult; and governments must agree to share the cost. But overall, local farmers across vast regions have supported the effort to get rid of the flies. International cooperation in the Americas has continued for more than fifty years. Without this constant maintenance of the cooperative program, screwworms would return with imported animals and insects, as they did on Curaçao.

Cooperation has also played an important role in another parasitic problem: *Echinococcus granulosus* and *E. multilocularis*, which produce hydatid cysts in mammals (including humans) and cause "hydatid disease." *Echinococcus* is a dog tapeworm whose life cycle must include an intermediate host, often livestock. The immature stages of the parasite can infect many species as intermediate hosts, including sheep, goats, cattle, pigs, horses, and wild ungulates and rodents. Humans and other mammals are accidental dead-end ("aberrant") hosts – the immature stages cannot become adults. Unable to leave the host body, the immature worms eventually cause tissue damage and clinical signs. *Echinococcus* is also known as the "bladder worm," because the cysts containing the immature worms are bladders filled with clear fluid. In aberrant hosts, such as humans, the cysts can form anywhere in the body, including the brain, becoming quite large over time, causing illness and eventually death. Infected humans suffer grotesque swellings of the abdomen, eye area, or anywhere else the cysts have grown. Hydatid disease is a particularly serious problem in children. The complex life cycle of *Echinococcus* is perfectly completed by the common practice of humans raising sheep, using dogs to herd the animals, and feeding the dogs with viscera from dead or slaughtered sheep. *Echinococcus* occurs worldwide, from the Arctic south to New Zealand, wherever dogs and livestock are kept in proximity.

By the 1850s, veterinarians and parasitologists had worked out the basic life cycle of *Echinococcus*. They advocated controlling hydatid disease by interrupting the life cycle of *Echinococcus*. In the 1860s, the Danish government started the earliest veterinary–agricultural control program in Iceland, where about 20 percent the human population was infected. This program focused on dogs as the most important definitive host. It included mandatory dog licensing, killing infected and stray dogs, destruction of infected viscera in slaughterhouses, and annual treatments of all dogs with areca nuts or arecoline. Arecoline caused intestinal contractions and defecation of the worms; however, it sometimes did not work. A much more important tool was educating Iceland's citizens to stop feeding sheep viscera to dogs. Pamphlets developed by Copenhagen veterinary professor Harald Krabbe (1831–1917), translated into Icelandic, were freely distributed around the country between the 1860s and 1890s. Farm families read them so often that children memorized passages from these pamphlets. At school, children also received special lessons about the parasite's life cycle and how to interrupt it. As a result, generations of Icelandic farmers voluntarily stopped feeding viscera to their dogs and cooperated with the government program. Iceland has successfully controlled *E. granulosis*, with the last human case reported in 1960.

At this same time, the WHO's Veterinary Public Health division, led by veterinarian Martin Kaplan, entered a cooperative agreement with the Pan American Health Organization (PAHO) and the FAO to start an *Echinococcus* eradication program. In the early 1960s, six *Echinococcus* research groups existed in New Zealand, Lebanon, Japan, Chile, and the United States (in Alaska and Atlanta, Georgia). Most of these groups were headed by veterinarians, including veterinary epidemiologist Calvin W. Schwabe (1927–2006), working in Lebanon, and veterinary pathologist Michael A. Gemmell (1926–2003) in Dunedin, New Zealand. Both worked to develop preventive hydatid disease programs. International cooperation provided money, enabled veterinarians to share research, regulated imports and exports of infected animal products, and standardized the methods used to control the disease. International cooperation also led to national government regulations requiring the destruction of infected offal and viscera (not feeding it to the dogs) and the careful inspection of all animal products for the cysts (veterinary inspection).

As with Krabbe's program in Iceland, Schwabe and Gemmell found that the most successful anti-*Echinococcus* campaigns included education, local farmers' cooperation, surveillance, and treatment and traceback of any infected dogs. In New Zealand, Gemmell incorporated mathematical modeling and surveillance. This program also focused on education, aimed at women who wanted to protect their children's health. But most farmers only began to cooperate when their profits were threatened, after exports of infected sheep livers were outlawed. Farmers then formed their own local hydatid disease control committees. These committees registered every dog, treated them and examined the stool, and treated them again if needed. Arecoline was replaced by praziquantel in the 1970s, and mobile treatment units tested neighborhood animals together. When one dog tested positive, everyone knew about it. Dogs with repeated infections, which revealed that their owner illegally fed them viscera, could be seized from their owners. This "peer pressure" approach has been quite successful in breaking the *Echinococcus* transmission cycle in the New Zealand sheep industry.

Today, over 1 million people around the world are infected with, and suffer from, hydatid disease. *Echinococcus* infections cost the livestock industry over US \$2 billion per year. The infection is currently enzootic in several parts of the world, including central Asia, China, northern Africa, and parts of South America – wherever livestock and dogs are closely associated. Control programs in China, Kyrgyzstan, Argentina, and Chile have been successful in reducing infections in enzootic and endemic areas. A vaccine, EG95, can now be used to immunize livestock. However, like screwworm, control of *Echinococcus* can only be maintained with ongoing surveillance, expense, and control activities. Social, cultural, and political cooperation are the essential components of successful control of these complex infections.

Veterinary Public Health Scenarios and the Veterinarian's Role

History tells us that from the 1960s onward, veterinarians were faced with new challenges in livestock production and controlling food quality. The profession responded with the further development of veterinary public health. Key roles were played by the American veterinarians James Steele (1913–2013), often referred to as the father of veterinary public health, and who worked for the PAHO; Calvin Schwabe, the hydatid disease researcher who also worked for the WHO; and Swiss-born American Karl F. Meyer (1884–1974). Other pioneers in this field were Italian veterinarian Adriano Mantovani (1926–2012), who worked at FAO in Rome, and Austrian-born Dutch veterinarian Dan Kampelmacher (1920–2011), who worked for the World Association of Veterinary Food Hygienists. The role of veterinarians as gatekeepers of public health was commissioned by them. Veterinarians had to comply with consumers' needs with shifting priorities from food security to food safety and finally to food acceptance.

Veterinary public health (VPH) is that part of public health activities using veterinary skills, knowledge, and resources to protect and improve human health. This term was introduced in the 1970s, when veterinary authorities recognized the importance of the veterinary contribution to preventing human diseases. As we have seen, this insight was not new, but from the 1960s onward, fundamental transformations in livestock production, food technology, the supply chain, consumption of food of animal origin, human–animal relations, and society have precipitated changes in the science, ideology, and practice of VPH – especially with surveillance strategies and state intervention. The globalizing livestock production provided many challenges for veterinarians, not only in rich countries with large-scale, capital-intensive factory farming but also in areas where transhumance and peasant farming remained dominant. Vets also had to adjust to shifting attitudes toward food of animal origin in urban consumer societies. In the development of livestock production, consumption, and VPH, three different scenarios with different roles of veterinarians can be distinguished.

In the first scenario, the food chain is short, and veterinarians play a limited role. Today, this scenario is most common in rural areas around the world, especially those of lower income. In higher-income areas, this scenario lasted for centuries, until the twentieth century. Peasant and transhumant herding, farming and home slaughter, and barter and local markets provide consumers with food. However, farmers get little profit and there is often no margin for problems in the system, which could be disrupted badly by crop failures and livestock diseases. This system is also labor intensive, requiring many people to focus on raising food. Animal healers and veterinarians provide care only when a valuable animal is seriously injured or ill. Veterinarians employed by the government or non-governmental organizations (NGOs) also provide mass vaccination and disease control. In more urban areas, as dairies and slaughterhouses are established, veterinary inspection often becomes required by the municipality. In this scenario, the main goal of veterinarians is to try to secure a steady food supply.

In the second scenario, the food chain is longer and based on more intensive farming to ensure a reliable supply of food for large urban populations. Once an adequate food supply is available, the next goal is to be sure that food originates from healthy animals (food safety). Veterinarians in this scenario carry out several activities: treat sick animals; monitor animal health at the farm level; inspect centralized slaughtering facilities; conduct traditional meat inspection; and inspect milk and dairy products (see Chapter 4). As in the first scenario, governments often employ veterinarians to maintain disease control and response, including mass vaccination.

In the first scenario, farmers and veterinarians in developing countries with fast-growing populations focus on increasing the production of healthy livestock for the provision of food of animal origin for local markets. International trade rules and quality requirements and guarantees often make it difficult to export animals and food from low-income to high-income countries, but veterinarians inspect both exports and imports. Within the interior, government-sponsored veterinary services are often robust, especially in providing large-scale vaccination campaigns and herd health. In more urban areas, traditional food inspection under veterinary control is organized. The second scenario is more common in high-income countries, where the food chain has become longer, with food production largely hidden from consumers. In this scenario, veterinarians provide assurances to consumers that the food chain provides healthy food. More and more urban consumers have demanded that their food should be healthy and originate from healthy (and happy) animals that were raised sustainably on appropriate feed, in a clean environment, and with attention to the animals' welfare. These demands have represented a big challenge for veterinarians in modern society.

Notably, these different scenarios are not chronological or place independent, and one scenario does not inevitably lead to the next. For instance, highly developed and hygienic poultry production and slaughter under veterinary surveillance take place in countries like Thailand and Brazil, next to uninspected home slaughter and unhygienic local markets that lack refrigeration. In the United States, home slaughter of both wild and domesticated animals is legal and often carried out in rural areas, alongside the vast, veterinary-inspected food production industries.

Modernizing Veterinary Food Control

While food inspection and safety are very different in different areas, the European Union provides a good model of how veterinary participation in livestock production and slaughtering may change in the future. Until the 1960s, the traditional methods of meat inspection proved to be quite successful. In general, veterinary authorities were satisfied with the way in which meat inspection had developed since regulating acts had come into being around 1900. Inspection had become much more effective because of centralized and more hygienic slaughtering under veterinary supervision. Since then, the health status of animals had improved considerably, resulting in a much lower number of condemned animals. The incidence of food poisonings had also dropped significantly due to better hygiene, and preservation and cooling technology. Indeed, by 1960 professionals in human and veterinary medicine alike had the rather triumphalist idea that thanks to progress in diagnostics, pharmacy, microbiology, and immunology (chemotherapy, vaccines, antibiotics), most infectious diseases could be kept under control. However, that optimistic vision was challenged by recurrent outbreaks of salmonella, often with human deaths. Research showed that salmonella was present not only in livestock but also in (imported) animal feed, seagulls, pigeons, animal feces, and water – in short, in the whole environment. This stimulated the study of large food cycles, as well as ways to create effective intervention measures (prevention, sterilization, decontamination, preservatives, etc.) to accomplish food safety.

With slaughtering, ever larger production units became operative from the 1970s onward, while speed of slaughtering lines increased, leaving less time for adequate inspection. As a result, much emphasis was laid on the introduction of strict hygiene codes to increase the standard of hygiene in the meat production and processing chain. However, despite these measures, infections transmitted by foods of animal origin continued to occur. One of veterinary inspectors' main problems was the presence of microorganisms such as *Salmonella* and *Campylobacter*, which do not necessarily produce clinical illness or pathological lesions. For such diseases, a more flexible system of control is required. The effectiveness of the traditional ante- and postmortem meat inspection based on incision, palpation, and organoleptic and visual inspection was questioned from the 1980s onward. Authorities and food experts recognized that end-product testing had become an outdated and inefficient form of food safety control.

Innovative frameworks were scaling up, based on risk assessment, more uniformity in inspection methods, lower inspection costs, and a rational employment of inspection personnel. After the example of the automobile industry, it became clear that the demands for safe and high-quality food could only be met via a longitudinally integrated quality control system, in which the primary responsibility for safety and quality lay with the producer. Large-scale factory farms have responded by gradually replacing traditional meat inspection with new concepts of process control and certification, such as Good Manufacturing Practices (GMP), Good Veterinary Practices (GVP), Hazard Analysis Critical Control Point (HACCP), and surveillance strategies with (electronic) identification and traceability systems "from farm to fork." The producer was responsible for implementing risk assessment of HACCP and Integrated Quality Control (IQC) in the whole production chain of food of animal origin. The framework of risk analysis was incorporated in operating procedures of the international standards organizations. Requirements have been put in place for process control in the meat and dairy industry, based on the principles of HACCP. The role of government veterinarians is to inspect the producers' system. Modern inspection requires transfer of data on the health status of groups of animals from veterinary practitioners responsible for their care to their colleagues in abattoirs and dairy and meat plants.

Related changes in slaughtering processes greatly affected the veterinary profession, particularly in terms of requiring specialized training in GVP and HACCP and in reducing the number of ordinary veterinary inspection jobs. Due to increased competition, higher inspection charges, and national and international regulations, slaughterhouses and abattoirs consolidated: smaller ones were absorbed into larger ones. This trend increased with changes in EU legislation, in which strict hygiene measures were set from 1991 onward. Many small slaughterhouses and public abattoirs could not comply with the new regulations, and they lost their "EU-Approved" status and their license to export meat. Small enterprises were closed when they could no longer compete with large-scale (international) corporate slaughterhouses. Larger units proved more cost-efficient and were quicker to incorporate new technology. As a result of replacement of public abattoirs by huge corporate slaughterhouses in Europe, the veterinary profession has lost many positions as directors and inspectors formerly available in smaller abattoirs.

The changing food habits of modern consumers also represented a challenge for veterinarians. On the one hand a huge market for "fast food" developed with globally operating companies. This food is generally safe; however, the composition and certainly the quantity of popular meat and cheese snacks consumed have resulted in an obesity epidemic and poor health among consumers in high-income regions. On the other hand, some consumers turned away from fast food and returned to so-called slow food. Next to regular supermarkets, a separate market for "organic" or naturally prepared food developed. Such food is also sold in open-air farmers' markets (often without supervision by inspection authorities) and may be labeled "biological" or "organic." Because consumers would pay higher prices for milk, meat, and eggs produced organically, some farmers turned away from factory farming to become small-scale, specialized producers of organic foods. These farmers must comply with imposed regulations, including a ban on fertilizers for animal feed production, restricted use of antibiotics, and more living space for animals. Also, some of these farmers have turned away from evidence-based Western medicine and asked for alternative or irregular veterinary treatment and medicines (homeopathy, orthomanual therapy, acupuncture, magnetism, herbal medicine, etc.). Again, this represented a challenge for veterinarians who had not been trained in these techniques. Also, veterinarians feared that diseases that had been controlled for a long time (such as trichinosis, bovine tuberculosis, and brucellosis) could reemerge in nonvaccinated and uninspected flocks and herds, because conditions for old pathogen cycles became favorable again.

In high-income countries, the public image of producers and veterinarians involved in inspection of food of animal origin has remained somewhat negative due to the adverse effects of factory farming on the environment, controversies about the ethics of meat production, and the many fraud and food poisoning scandals that have occurred. Debates about food safety culminating in international trade conflicts continue to affect public opinion today. The perceived conflict between the needs of humans, animals, and the environment has become a cause of widespread concern. In these circumstances, government authorities have been forced to take public action. However, the general public's knowledge about food safety and health risks is often limited. This topic doesn't always get enough (objective) attention in education and information via the media. When consensus among scientists and objective information from scientific research is lacking, policy making proves to be difficult. Consequently, public concern regarding food safety is fed by biased reporting from the media, mainly highlighting sensational scandals. Public distrust toward industrially prepared food and "chemophobia" concerning food additives has increased, while agriculturists and many food scientists claim that our food has never been as safe as it is today.

With increasing income, more people around the world will become consumers of animal products on a larger scale. Consumer cultures will develop in their own ways, and the region's veterinarians will need to adapt to changes in economics, consumer preferences, livestock production practices, and food safety regulations. As a society's income rises, another major change for the veterinary profession has been the increase of a relatively new patient population: companion animals, or pets, kept for sentimental rather than economic reasons. Finally, social changes have led to changes in the veterinary professional workforce itself, including the increasing gender diversity in the profession. Traditionally a profession that was largely restricted to men, veterinary medicine in many countries has only recently made educational and employment opportunities available for women. This has been one of the many changes in the veterinary workforce and veterinary practice.

How Veterinarians Work: New Paradigms in Veterinary Practice

The 1980s witnessed fundamental changes in veterinary practice. First, the demand for veterinary services in the various fields of the profession increased dramatically from the 1960s onward. Until then, most veterinary graduates found employment as an individual practitioner. However, it became increasingly difficult for an individual to practice all aspects of the profession. From the 1970s onward, the number of group practices, as well as the number of veterinarians per group practice, grew. This was mainly the case with farm animals of mixed practices; many companion animal practitioners continued to work in solo practices. In the late 1980s and 1990s, large companies began opening veterinary practices for pets, where they employed salaried veterinarians.

The importance of pets for veterinary practitioners increased significantly; toward the end of the twentieth century, most veterinarians found employment in that growing segment of the profession. This shift in veterinary practice strongly stimulated specialization within the profession. Within the larger practice units, further division of labor and species or discipline specialization was facilitated. In some countries, veterinary associations had a keen eye for market regulation as well as for self-regulation within the profession. Special postgraduate programs of education and research for several veterinary specialists on a national and international level came into being. Veterinary associations, as well as the World Veterinary Association and the European Association of Establishments for Veterinary Education (EAEVE, established in 1988) supported and aligned these programs and facilitated national and international examination, accreditation, and registration. Furthermore, some national associations also introduced a system of certification of veterinary practices. A recent development is the buying up of veterinary practices by large international investment companies – an extension of the corporate trend that began in the late 1980s.

Another change in veterinary practice was the way in which the whole chain of production, registration, distribution, administration, prescription, and application of veterinary drugs was adapted. For centuries, veterinarians had mixed their own medications with which they filled their practice pharmacy. By the last decades of the twentieth century, pharmaceutical companies supplied veterinary practices with almost all their drugs. This shift allowed authorities to better control the quantities of used veterinary drugs, as well as their residues in food of animal origin and in the environment (especially antibiotics).

As we have seen in previous chapters, next to educated veterinarians, all sorts of other animal healers were active in the field. This continued in many countries, but veterinary associations were keen on protecting veterinarians' core activities and responsibilities. They did so by lobbying for legislation (liability and disciplinary law) in which competencies and responsibilities between educated vets were protected from "unqualified" animal healing by farmers, animal owners, and auxiliary personnel such as castrators, obstetricians, animal physiotherapists, inseminators, technical veterinary assistants, embryo transporters, and animal dentists. Education, accreditation, and registration for these professionals were established and enforced. Competition also came from people offering alternative and complementary treatments such as homeopathy, acupuncture bio resonance, shiatsu, Reiki, and magnetizers, as well as manual, holistic, cranial-sacral, and aromatic therapies. The demand often came from customers who had turned themselves to such treatments. In many countries, veterinary associations disqualified all these workers as "quacks" and praised the standard of evidence-based veterinary medicine.

However, it also led to tensions within the profession when educated vets began offering alternative and complementary therapies. This very broad category encompassed traditional Chinese and Ayurvedic treatments; ethno-veterinary medicine based on botanical knowledge of Indigenous people around the world; competing Western medical systems such as homeopathy and osteopathy; and everything else that was not taught in a traditional

Western veterinary curriculum. Veterinarians who were critics of these "alternative" medical systems accused their colleagues of using them to please clients and make money, not because they believed these treatments actually worked. Certainly evidence-based Western medicine and science were the foundation of veterinarians' claim to professional autonomy; by bringing these other therapies into veterinary practice, vets might be jeopardizing their own professional position. Moreover, research done by veterinary skeptics had not shown these techniques to be successful. Although these critiques continue, and it is still not clear what role "alternative" therapies will play in veterinary medicine, the fact that consumers are asking for these services means that some vets will provide them.

Today, some veterinary schools offer courses in "Integrative Veterinary Medicine," (IVM), which combines conventional medicine with complementary and alternative veterinary medicine (CAVM). A 2011 survey of veterinary schools in Europe, Australia, New Zealand, Canada, and the United States found that almost half offered a course in CAVM subjects such as nutritional therapy, acupuncture, and rehabilitation or physical manipulation therapy. Almost a quarter of schools surveyed were conducting research in CAVM, stressing that only evidence-based therapies would be included in the curriculum. The integration of these therapies into conventional veterinary medicine has not shown any signs of disappearing over the ten-year period 2010–2020. As long as animal owners want to consider using these unconventional therapies, CAVM will probably be included in veterinary curricula and continuing education despite the controversy.

Of all these changes at the end of the 1900s, the biggest and most difficult for many veterinarians was the feminization of the veterinary profession. Although a few women had managed to become veterinarians, the profession was traditionally a male bastion that opposed educating and admitting women as qualified veterinarians.

Women in Veterinary Medicine: A Slow Start and a Fast Acceleration

Europe, the United Kingdom, and North America

In the late 1800s and early 1900s, some brave and determined women accepted the challenge of becoming a formally educated veterinarian. Scholars around the world have identified these pioneer women veterinarians and have written their biographies. They describe how these women faced a misogynistic environment at veterinary schools, followed after graduation by an unfriendly male working environment as well as reluctant clients. Women sometimes traveled far from home for veterinary education. Some historians have stated

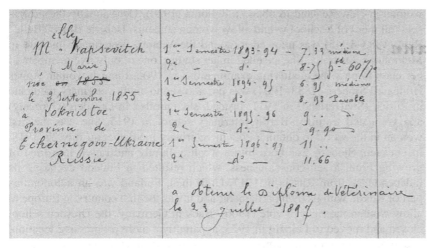

Figure 6.5 Record from the archive of the veterinary school of Alfort showing that Marie Kapsevitch (Marija Kapčevič) from Russia (Ukraine) graduated on July 23, 1897.
Courtesy: Prof. Christophe Degueurce, Director École Nationale Vétérinaire d'Alfort and Curator Musée Fragonard, Paris.

that V. Dobrovoljskaja, a Ukranian woman, graduated from the Zürich (Switzerland) Veterinary School in 1889. However, Swiss veterinary historian Marianne Sackmann-Rink (1985) searched the Zurich school's archives and could not find any record of Dobrovoljskaja or other Ukranians in the 1880s. Therefore, Marija Kapčevič, born in 1855 in Loknika, Russia (today's Ukraine), was probably the first European woman to obtain a veterinary degree, in 1897 (Fig. 6.5). She was allowed to attend the French Alfort school (1893–1897) only under a special license. Often reluctantly, veterinary schools had to open their doors for women after changes in legislation. This was the case in Germany (1913), Britain (1919), and the Netherlands (1925). But the schools established special rules and quotas that still severely limited the numbers of women allowed to study. In these ways, most European and U.S. schools affiliated with universities excluded women, although legally they were allowed to attend.

Women developed strategies to gain access to education: they used family connections and money; worked to be the top students at school; traveled far from home; or attended private schools, which were less strict as long as the student could pay the fees. For example, six of the first seven U.S. female veterinarians graduated from private veterinary schools. One of these private schools ran a correspondence course taken by Pearl Howard Dawson, the first woman in New Zealand to obtain a diploma (1920). Occasionally the professors (all men) of a school would allow women students. Isabelle Bruce "Belle" Reid (1883–1945) was allowed to attend the Victoria Veterinary Institute in Melbourne, Australia. She excelled in her studies, one of only five members of her class to pass the qualifying examinations in 1906. Finnish woman Agnes Hildegard Sjöberg (1888–1964) was not allowed to study veterinary medicine in Zürich (Switzerland) in 1911. Instead, she enrolled in Dresden (Germany) and graduated from the Berlin veterinary school in 1915. She was the first woman in the world to obtain a PhD in veterinary medicine, on July 27, 1918, in Dresden. Sjöberg was born into a wealthy family and raised in a time of growing Finnish self-consciousness, which resulted in Finland declaring its independence from Russia in 1917. Until then, Finland was an autonomous part of Russia with its own parliament; and it was the first country in Europe to allow women the right to vote (1906). Back in Germany, the Dresden school closed and moved to Leipzig in 1923, apparently a more progressive location, and three more women gained their veterinary degrees there in the 1920s: Germans Ruth Eber and Inkeri Bernhard and Finnish Airi Borustedt.

The early 1900s witnessed turmoil and many social changes associated with World War I, and women used this to help them get their veterinary education and qualifications. Another pioneer female veterinarian was Anglo-Irish Aleen Cust (1868–1937), who obtained her degree in Edinburgh in 1897. (Due to her family's opposition, she enrolled under a different name.) However, the Royal College of Veterinary Surgeons in London refused to allow her to take the qualifying examination. It was not until 1922 that she was officially registered as veterinarian, after Britain passed a law making it illegal to exclude women from working in the professions. British women demanded this law (and the right to vote), pointing to their service for their country during World War I. Aleen Cust served in a diagnostic laboratory on the battlefield during the war. Another determined woman, Polish Helena Bujwid-Jurgielewicz (1897–1980), also served during the war and graduated from Lvov veterinary school in 1923. Romanian Zoe Draganescu (?–1980), attending the Bucharest veterinary school during the war, served in the army, and graduated in 1919. Women could also begin to enroll in veterinary schools in the newly established countries such as Estonia, Latvia, Yugoslavia, and Czechoslovakia after World War I. Although these women seized their opportunity during wartime, veterinary medicine still remained one of the most strictly male professions, even as others (such as human medicine and law) admitted more and more women.

Beyond the conditions of World War I, the social and political situation greatly affected the availability of veterinary education to women, and the history of women veterinarians in Turkey is an excellent example. As Tamay Başağaç Gül and colleagues have shown in their 2008 paper, "Historical

Profile of Gender in Turkish Veterinary Education," the establishment of the Republic of Turkey (1923) included loosening the restrictions on women in the Faculties of Law and Medicine in Istanbul University, and later the Faculty of Veterinary Medicine in Ankara. Merver Ansel, who transferred to the veterinary school after two years of medical school, became the first woman graduate in 1935. Although eighteen other women followed her path before 1940, the hardships of the economic depression and World War II contributed to an employment crisis. Fewer women continued to higher education in the 1940s, and by the 1950s less than 2% of the Ankara school's graduates were women (an average of 1.4 women per year during this decade). Gül et al. also point to the rise in the 1950s of the Democratic Party, which held conservative views about higher education for women. This party lost power in 1960, and a new constitution in 1961 granted more autonomy to the universities in Turkey. These events probably contributed to the modest increase in the number of women enrolling in veterinary school during the 1960s. Still, the enrollment of women in the veterinary schools of Istanbul, Ankara, and Bursa only rose above 10% in the 1980s; and the percentage of women students overall remains under 50% today, so this process is ongoing in Turkey.[1]

After graduation, women worked in various aspects of veterinary medicine depending on their local and national circumstances. Several women were able to work in private clinical practice, treating horses, livestock, and companion animals (pets); but this was often difficult because clients were reluctant to consult a woman veterinarian. Instead, some women vets (such as Belle Reid in New Zealand) established their own animal breeding farms, raising and caring for large numbers of animals themselves. An important niche for women vets has been working in positions such as diagnostic or bacteriological laboratories, university labs or teaching, and in government employment. Several early graduates found employment this way: O.T. Markus (Tiiu Koplus), graduate of the Veterinary Faculty at Tartu, Estonia, in 1925; Jeannette Donker-Voet (1907–1979, graduated from Utrecht, the Netherlands, 1930); Jelka Bojkić (graduated from Zagreb, Croatia, 1932); Maria Luz Zalduegni Gabilondo (1914–2003, graduated from the University of Madrid, Spain, 1935); and Abide Koray (graduated from the Veterinary School in Ankara, Turkey, 1938). Industry, including pharmaceutical companies, has been another source of jobs for women, including Erzsébet Schvartz (1915–1993, graduated from the Budapest Faculty of Veterinary Medicine, 1937). These positions were not dependent on the whims and prejudices of often-conservative farmers, and women could also pursue higher degrees and

[1] Gül, R.T.B., Özkul, T., Akçay, A., and Özen, A. (2008). 'Historical Profile of Gender in Turkish Veterinary Education', *Journal of Veterinary Medical Education* vol. 35, no. 2, pp. 305–309.

specialization (such as the Doctor of Philosophy or Doctor of Science) while working.

The feminization of veterinary medicine had begun slowly in most countries. Until the 1970s or later, female veterinarians accounted for less than 5% of the profession in the Western world. Of course, there are important exceptions – countries and regions in which more women have worked as veterinarians. Today's Russian Federation, formerly the USSR, is an excellent example. During the tsarist period, some women from the Russian empire fought successfully to attend medical school and become physicians. The Bolshevik Revolution opened the doors of medical schools to women in 1918, and the percentage of women physicians and feldshers (a type of physician's assistant) increased. By 1965, about 70% of physicians in the USSR were women. Even during the Soviet period, however, numbers of women in veterinary medicine lagged behind those in human medicine, reflecting women's lack of access to education. Veterinary education was not equally available to women, and far fewer veterinarians were women in 1967: only about 30% of all qualified veterinarians were women. (Only one other profession had fewer women at that time: engineering.) However, the tiered educational system in the USSR meant that more women could achieve the lower qualification of "vet-feldsher" (veterinary assistant, requiring fewer years of education). The Soviet veterinary journal *Veterinariia* included stories about women vets, calling them "A Wonderful Collective" and "Good Workers," according to the Communist Party line. Women worked as vet-feldshers at state farms and also as specialists in laboratory sciences, meat inspection, and epidemiology. They may not have been as numerous as women physicians, but women veterinarians in the USSR were far more common than in the rest of Europe. Today, women are 79% of the veterinary workforce in the Russian Federation.

From the 1970s onward, however, the enrollment of female veterinary students in other European countries started to increase steadily from around 10% to about 70% to 90% in the first decade of the twenty-first century. Since then, this percentage has stabilized, and veterinary medicine is now the most feminized of the comparable health professions in the Western world. After the Soviet Union, it was the Nordic countries where feminization accelerated before the rest of Europe: first in Finland, then followed by Scandinavian countries Sweden and Norway. In Helsinki and Stockholm, women comprised 60% of all students in the 1975 classes. From the 1990s onward, more than 90% of Finnish veterinary students were female, and in Oslo (Norway) this average was more than 80%. As in many countries, enrolled female students in Madrid (Spain), Utrecht (the Netherlands) and the colleges in the United States began to outnumber the male students in the 1990s. In 2005, the EAEVE published data on the enrollments of female students in 26 countries. Lower percentages were in Turkey (12%), Bosnia-Herzegovina (34%), and Ukraine (47%). In France, 70% of veterinary students were women; Belgium had 71% and Britain had 72%. Most veterinary students were women in Finland (88%), Austria (91%), and Switzerland (92%) by 2005. These changes are reflected in the demographics of the profession today (2020): in Finland, 89% of veterinarians are women; in Sweden, 82%; and in Turkey, 19% of the veterinary workforce are women.

Figures for the United States and Canada show an increase of female enrollment during this time period to about 80%. Until the 1970s, few women were allowed to enroll in U.S. veterinary schools, especially after the private schools closed in the 1920s and 1930s. University-based schools kept the numbers of women at 2% or less, arguing that admitting women would deprive men of educational (and employment) opportunities and that women could not do the physical work of handling large animals. Deans and professors at American veterinary schools openly derided women, telling them to "go back to the kitchen" and to stop behaving in an "unfeminine" manner by seeking higher education. The few women veterinarians banded together in 1947 to start the Women's Veterinary Medical Association; they received hundreds of letters every year from young women asking how they could gain entrance to a veterinary school. The socially conservative atmosphere of the 1950s allowed veterinary schools to continue to reject women. Employment for women was difficult to attain and lower paid, despite federal legislation in the 1960s that supposedly barred gender discrimination. The situation only changed in 1974, when the federal government forced veterinary schools to accept equal numbers of women or lose federal funding. The next year, the numbers of women enrolled in veterinary schools doubled and have continued to rise since then.

Overall, women have become the majority of the student population in European and North American veterinary colleges (Fig. 6.6). By 2018, women accounted for almost 60% of practicing vets registered in the Western world. This trend is continuing in Europe, where the proportion of female veterinarians has risen from 53% in 2015 to 58% in 2020. There and elsewhere, this figure is likely to further increase because around 80% of students enrolling veterinary colleges are now female. While female students became dominant in veterinary colleges, in many countries, women earn less money than equally employed men. In North America, few women have been appointed as deans of veterinary schools or other leadership positions until recently. The American Veterinary Medical Association did not elect its first woman president until 1996. However, as older men retire from the profession, the profession's leadership is likely to include more women, with corresponding changes in compensation and availability of opportunities.

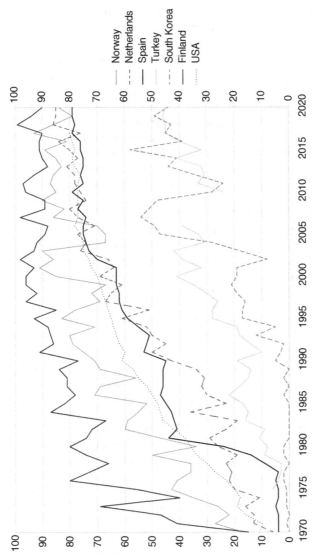

Figure 6.6 Enrollment of first-year female students (%) in the veterinary college of Helsinki (Finland), Oslo (Norway), and an average of 28 colleges in the United States. Female graduates (%) of the veterinary colleges of Madrid (Spain), Seoul (South Korea), Utrecht (the Netherlands), and Turkey (average of veterinary colleges in Ankara, Bursa, and Istanbul) in the period 1970–2007 and of Ankara (2010–2020). Courtesy: Prof. Tamay Başağaç Gül, Faculty of Veterinary Medicine, Ankara University; Prof. Myung-Sun Chun, College of Veterinary Medicine, Seoul National University; Ann Kristin Egeli, Study Advisor, Faculty of Veterinary Medicine, Norwegian University of Life Sciences, Oslo; Prof. Joaquín Sánchez de Lollano, Faculty of Veterinary Medicine, Complutense University, Madrid, and Prof. Antti Sukura, Faculty of Veterinary Medicine, Helsinki University. Data from the U.S. Internal Report Assoc. of American Veterinary Medical Colleges 1970–2017. Courtesy: Monique Tersteeg B.Sc. Department of Population Health Sciences, Faculty of Veterinary Medicine, Utrecht University.

Ethnic and Racial Diversity in Veterinary Medicine:
The United States

Other groups remain underrepresented in veterinary medicine, however – especially people of color and Indigenous peoples. Similar to the situation for women, they struggled to gain access to education. The United States, with its multi-ethnic population, presents an interesting case. The first Black (African American) graduate of a U.S. veterinary school was Henry Stockton Lewis, Sr. (1858–1922), who graduated from the Harvard University Veterinary School in 1889 (this school closed in 1902). Eight years later, two more Black men earned veterinary degrees. The first, Robert F. Harper, graduated in 1897 from a private veterinary school, the short-lived Indiana Veterinary College (1892–1924). His colleague, Augustus Nathaniel Lushington (1869–1939), completed a degree in agriculture at Cornell University and graduated from the University of Pennsylvania Veterinary School in 1897. Lushington, born into a poor family on the island of Trinidad, worked his way to the United States. After attaining his veterinary degree, he worked in private practice in Philadelphia, taught Veterinary Sanitation and Hygiene at a college, then practiced for the rest of his life in Virginia, where he experienced severe racial discrimination. His alma mater, the University of Pennsylvania, graduated four more Black men in the early 1900s. Another early leader in veterinary education for Black men was The Ohio State University. The initiative of these students, and the willingness of veterinary administrators to enroll them in these two schools, defied the racism that characterized U.S. society at the time. Although the first Black meat inspector, Cornelius Vanderbilt Lowe (University of Pennsylvania, graduated in 1909) was hired in 1910 by the U.S. government's Bureau of Animal Industry, the more conservative American Veterinary Medical Association did not elect its first two Black members until 1920.

Cornelius Lowe, while working for the U.S. government c. 1910–1945, traveled around the southern and midwestern United States, giving speeches about the opportunities in veterinary medicine. Black students later remembered that they were astonished to see a Black veterinarian, and they began to see veterinary medicine as a possible career. Very few could afford the cost of moving far from home, however. In 1945, the historically Black university Tuskegee Institute (now University), in Alabama, established its own veterinary school to provide opportunities for people of color to get a veterinary education. The first Black woman to graduate from a U.S. school of veterinary medicine was Alfreda Johnson Webb, who graduated from Tuskegee and qualified in 1949. After earning a master's degree in anatomy, Webb worked as an instructor at two universities during her career and was active in politics. She immediately joined the Women's Veterinary Medical Association. Today, the Tuskegee University College of Veterinary Medicine has graduated nearly 3,000 veterinary students, many of them Black or people of color. Despite the success of the Tuskegee school, in 1973 only 2.2% of American veterinary students belonged to minority groups and even today (circa 2020) this number is only around 30%, with only 4% identifying themselves as African American or Black.

The history of Native American (American Indian) people working as veterinarians in North America is a topic that needs further research. Indigenous peoples' expertise, particularly with botanical treatments, is well documented from the early days of European contact and this has been the basis of most veterinary care. The U.S. Census listed three Native American veterinarians in 1910 and only five in 1930, three of whom worked on reservations. (These were probably non-graduate practitioners.) Few White veterinarians ventured onto reservations, and owners and local healers provided veterinary care for the millions of animals owned by Native Americans. For potential veterinary students growing up on the reservations, the road to veterinary school was long and hard. They had to overcome poverty, limits to early education, and the shock of living far from home in a discriminatory culture. Ethel Connelly, who grew up on the Blackfeet Reservation in the state of Montana, graduated from the Colorado State University Veterinary School in 1989, the first Native American woman to do so. She remembered how difficult it was to complete her education, eventually returning to the reservation where she has cared for all species (except snakes). Today the Native American Veterinary Association supports Native American students and veterinarians.

In 2020 and beyond, leaders of the veterinary profession in the United States and the American Veterinary Medical Association are pledging to continue working to increase diversity in the veterinary profession. Some improvements have been made, but there is much work to do. Research by the Association of American Veterinary Medical Colleges (AAVMC) on students enrolled in U.S. veterinary colleges in 2009 found that 4% of students identified as Asian, almost 4% as Hispanic, 2.4% as African American, while only 1% identified as Native American. In 2020, about 12% identified as Hispanic, 8% as Asian, 5% as multi-racial, about 4% as African American, and about 1.5% American Indian/Native Alaskan. This situation is not unusual, and veterinary medicine remains one of the Western world's most ethnically homogenous professions.

Women and Indigenous Africans in Veterinary Education, on the African Continent

Dutch veterinarian Katinka de Balogh, who is affiliated with FAO and who has worked as a lecturer for many years in Africa, has pointed out the main differences between activities of Western and African female vets. While most students in Western countries find employment in clinical practices, in Africa most veterinarians work in the government structure and are generally occupied with disease prevention and control, as well as administrative activities. Fieldwork is not popular and has a lower status than administrative tasks, which is preferred by male vets. Female veterinarians in Africa are mostly working in government service in urban areas, in diagnostic and research laboratories, or as staff in veterinary and agricultural colleges. Generally, the salaries at these institutes are quite low, another reason why their male colleagues have gradually shifted to veterinary work in the private sector.

Next to the old African veterinary schools in Cairo (1827), Pretoria (1920), and Khartoum (1938), Africa counted 25 veterinary schools in 2000; most of these were established after 1960 when many former colonies became independent states. Veterinary faculties were established in Angola, Congo, Ethiopia, Kenia, Mozambique, Nigeria, Tanzania, Uganda, Zambia, and Zimbabwe. Nigeria has five veterinary colleges, and many of their graduates work in other African countries. Some African students, such as Jotello Festiri Soga (Chapter 4), graduated from veterinary schools in Europe (often the former colonial nation). After 1960, African schools admitted more African students, but many were also trained elsewhere: France, the UK, Japan, and the United States; or the USSR, Romania, Hungary, DDR (East Germany), and Cuba. The long stay abroad made it more difficult for female students, particularly for those with children. In South Africa, the Medical University of South Africa (MEDUNSA), including a veterinary faculty, was opened near Pretoria in 1976. This university accepted only Black South Africans; their compatriots of Indian origin were excluded both from Onderstepoort and MEDUNSA. After apartheid was abolished, the MEDUNSA veterinary faculty was absorbed into Onderstepoort in 1996.

Feminization of veterinary medicine also occurred in African nations, particularly during the most recent decades. Overall, African nations with veterinary schools have seen increasing numbers of women entering higher education, including veterinary studies. Other nations, such as Tunisia, Algeria, Sudan, and the island nation of Madagascar, also have higher levels of participation. Gradually, African female veterinarians have also entered higher earning and leadership positions. For instance, after various African countries had established veterinary associations, female vets became presidents of those associations in Botswana, Ethiopia, and Uganda.

Asian Nations

In Asian nations, the picture is different depending on location. In Japan, both public universities and private veterinary schools provide accredited education.

About 30 students are admitted to each of 11 national or public universities per year, and about 120 to each of 5 private schools. The veterinary student population became half female around 2010, and this trend is expected to continue. In Thailand in 2018, about 65% of veterinary students were women, and other nations such as Sri Lanka and Malaysia also have quite a high representation of women in veterinary medicine. Data from the College of Veterinary Medicine from Seoul National University (South Korea), in Figure 6.6, shows that the feminization process started in the 1990s there. The percentage of women students has fluctuated around 40% until today.

Explanations for the Increase in Women Veterinarians

The most remarkable aspect of the feminization of the veterinary profession is that it happened basically concurrently around the world. Various explanations are given for this phenomenon. Some scholars claim that the higher influx of female students coincided with the second feminist movement in the Western world. However, in interviews of Dutch female veterinarians graduated in the 1970s and 1980s, the majority stated that they did not consider themselves as active feminists. Instead, they concentrated on the development of various fields of veterinary medicine during their career. They did not want to be judged on the fact that they were women, but – just like their male colleagues – on the quality of their veterinary work. Nevertheless, they played an important role in the acceptance of women in Dutch veterinary medicine. Interviews with 161 female vets who had studied in schools in France and Belgium between 1950 and 2010 confirm this picture. Despite some obstacles and misogynist remarks, they kept working and they were positive about the way they had overcome the obstacles.

Another explanation reflects the fact that the veterinary profession in high-income countries has become oriented toward companion animal practice. Women, who are supposed to "love animals," could be more attracted to companion animal practice than male vets. That sector also offers more part-time jobs. Indeed, most women veterinarians work in practices that exclusively treat companion animals (primarily dogs and cats), rather than in the mixed or large-animal practices. However, most men do, too – because there are far more jobs in companion animal practice than in mixed or large-animal practice. In the Western world, most female students report being interested in working with companion animals. However, feminization of the veterinary profession has also occurred in African countries, where companion animal practice is a much smaller sector of the economy. Both women and men work in government positions with food-producing animals.

Workforce issues are also tied to changing economic realities in much of the world. Livestock or general practice, the old image of a veterinarian's work, has declined in nations where populations have urbanized (and acquired pets) and farm practice has become high-tech preventive veterinary management. The small, mixed animal veterinary practice of the past is becoming rarer. It is not clear how these trends affected the increase in women in veterinary medicine. But it is a problem for the veterinary profession that the earnings and employment for necessary veterinary work, such as livestock care and meat inspection, have decreased. Moreover, fewer male students are attracted to veterinary medicine because they can make more money and work under better conditions in other professions. Compared with human medicine, or working as scientists in industry, veterinarians earn far less money per hour worked but still pay similar costs for their education. For a student, the cost-benefit analysis does not look favorable for veterinary medicine. (In the United States, veterinary students now expect that they must acquire large debts to pay for university and veterinary school.) Research shows that men are far more motivated to achieve a high salary than are women, who tend to choose according to personal preference. This factor may explain some of the feminization of veterinary medicine over the past forty years: men have left veterinary medicine as earnings in other professions have outpaced it.

Another explanation for veterinary feminization is demographic. More and more female students entered universities from the 1960s onward. In many countries, this trend followed from legislation that guaranteed access to education for women. In the United States, the federal government forced veterinary schools to allow women to enroll, using legislation in the 1970s. Female enrollment immediately increased. In Europe, girls have also achieved better grades throughout secondary education than boys, which made it more likely that universities would recruit more women with the top grades. Finally, although this is much more difficult to study, social and cultural values seemed to liberalize throughout the 1960s and 1970s. Progressive policies, and workforce needs, meant that the percentage of women increased over all professions. Veterinary medicine was merely following this larger trend.

As with most major social changes, many factors probably contributed to the feminization of veterinary medicine in the late twentieth century. The convergence of economics, demographics, social and cultural changes, the modernized livestock industry, and the growth of commercialized pet keeping all encouraged the influx of women into veterinary medicine. Was the profession ready for such a dramatic transformation?

Concerns and Criticisms of the Changing Veterinary Profession

The feminization of veterinary medicine was initially seen as a problem by many male veterinarians. Veterinary schools only reluctantly accepted female students. For instance, when the Veterinary College of Helsinki opened its doors in 1946, there were 16 female and 21 male applicants. However, the professors decided that women could not be successful in the veterinary profession and allowed 13 male and only 2 female students to enter. Despite this setback, feminization increased on average from 8% in the period 1946–1958 to 26% in 1959–1965 and 44% in the years 1966–1973.

Ample examples and anecdotes exist about the hostile attitude of some male professors. Many did not consider women intelligent enough to study science, and not physically strong enough to become a good vet. Female students were sometimes openly discriminated against or harassed. Well known is the story of professors who persisted in opening their lectures with "good morning gentlemen," despite the fact that there were more and more women in the lecture halls. Women were accused of only wanting to work with dogs and cats, but those who expressed interest in livestock were told they could not do so because it was a "man's job." A 1976 report by the U.S. Department of Health, Education, and Welfare found that veterinary school alumni and agricultural interests pressured school administrators to limit women's enrollment, assuming that women would not work once they married and would therefore deprive qualified men of the opportunity to become veterinarians. The concern that women would deprive men of education and employment survives to this day, in surveys that point out how many women are "not actively practicing," presumably to manage a household and raise children. Until the recent advent of corporate veterinary practice, few part-time jobs existed for veterinarians.

For many male practitioners, the masculine, rough culture of veterinary medicine persistently excluded women, no matter how skilled or knowledgeable they were. Women studied and worked in a climate filled with sexual jokes and comments, a distrust of anyone who "loved animals" or was sentimental, and livestock owners who openly refused to allow women to treat their animals. The idea of women veterinarians not only threatened the professional aspirations of veterinarians but also violated masculine livestock culture. This is an important reason why, in the 1970s and 1980s, women encountered entrenched discrimination within the veterinary colleges, the veterinary profession, and among traditional animal owners, particularly farmers. By the 1990s, with larger numbers of women veterinarians in the workforce, farmers had to learn to accept the presence of female vets in their barns and meadows. In most countries and cultures, skilled female vets have gradually won the confidence of farmers, who then have slowly lost their prejudice against having their animals treated by female vets (a continuing process).

In the 1980s and 1990s, veterinary professional leaders also watched the growing feminization of their profession with some concern. They believed that the biggest problem was the veterinarian's salary. Almost everywhere, women earned (and still earn) less than men. There was a persistent idea that women would "work for less," and therefore more women meant lower earnings for all vets. It would be a vicious cycle: as the salaries and earnings decreased, men would leave the profession and veterinary medicine would become a "pink-collar," lower-status profession. Many surveys were done to assess the impact of women on the profession, and almost all their conclusions found that veterinarians' earnings tracked the general economy and the value of animals, not the numbers of women. In the United States, for example, veterinary earnings had already begun to decrease before numbers of women increased in the profession. Although data did not support professional leaders' fears, this anxiety has persisted in the face of increasing costs for veterinary education and stagnant profits for practicing vets. Economics, as well as social status, has always been a concern for the profession's leaders, and undoubtedly this will continue in the future.

Shattering the Glass Ceiling?

The "glass ceiling" refers to how high women might rise in the profession. Will they assume the leadership roles? Will they become top earners? The integration of women into all areas of the veterinary profession has been a gradual process. Except for in the former Soviet bloc countries, European veterinary public health, and particularly meat inspection, proved to be rather conservative in its acceptance of female veterinarians. Despite more women in the profession, the representation of female veterinarians among policy-making officials, leading veterinary authorities, and academic staff is still relatively low. In 2010, women occupied 78% of faculty positions in U.S. veterinary schools, but women were still underrepresented in leadership (department heads and chairs and deans). Apparently, it remained difficult for women to break through the "glass ceiling" in veterinary medicine.

In Europe and the United States today, male veterinarians still dominate the top earning positions (partners, owners, or directors of practices), compared to their female colleagues. Women are working more often as associates or assistants in practices owned by others. Statistics demonstrate not only that female veterinarians are less likely to be elected or appointed to leadership roles, but also that their average earnings are lower than their male counterparts. In the Western world, women earn about 20% less than men in comparable positions. This is the case elsewhere, although the earning gap is not always quite so large. For instance, in Mozambique women earn 10% lower salaries and those in Thailand have 11% lower earnings. From this point of view, veterinary medicine could still be considered as "a man's job," or at least a profession that disproportionately rewards men. Despite the fact that the profession is now female dominated, veterinary medicine has remained gendered masculine in some ways.

Over the past forty years, both men and women veterinarians have responded to the shift toward caring for companion or pet animals. The still growing numbers of companion animals in cities will continue to provide much work for urban vets. Pet keeping is certainly not new, but its impact on the veterinary profession was particularly dramatic in the last decades of the twentieth century. In the next chapter, we examine how the veterinary profession responded to the challenges of changing human–animal relations, the demand for expertise in companion animal medicine, and the other challenges and opportunities of the twenty-first century.

Conclusions

From this survey of the period 1900–1960, we can conclude that:

1. As wealth increases, people consume more meat, milk, yoghurt, cheese, eggs, and other animal products. Intensive animal agriculture, "factory farming," developed as a way to produce large numbers of food-producing animals cheaply. Combined with a vast global network of distribution, factory farming has revolutionized the production of foods from animals.
2. This increased food production came with a price, however. Confining large numbers of animals indoors makes them vulnerable to diseases and undesired stress behaviors, causing concerns about animal welfare. Factory farms have also caused large-scale waste disposal problems and contributed to the production of greenhouse gases (climate change).
3. Meat production quadrupled between 1961 and 2018 worldwide. In 1960, Asia nations produced only about 12% of the world's meat; today they produce 42% (with China the leading producer). By weight, pigs and poultry supply most of the world's meat, with beef and buffalo third.
4. Ninety-six percent of mammals living on the earth today are either humans or domesticated animals (only 4% are wild); and 70% of all birds living on the earth are domesticated poultry. Although humans are only 0.1% of life on earth, we are causing the biggest changes in the composition of the earth's animals due to our vast production of livestock.
5. Veterinarians have contributed to this massive increase in food-producing animals by helping to develop intensive livestock husbandry methods. These methods included new reproduction practices, such as artificial insemination, and the use of vaccines and treatments, such as antimicrobials to control disease outbreaks in closely confined animal populations.
6. Veterinarians shifted to herd health and preventive medicine after World War II, partially in response to international efforts from the FAO, OIE, and WHO. Becoming herd health managers meant changing veterinary education, also. Animal husbandry with the subdisciplines of breeding,

genetics, statistics, animal handling, and farm management obtained a more prominent position in the veterinary curricula. New specializations were developed in swine, beef, and dairy practice and preventive medicine.

7. The growing global production networks quickly spread diseases such as classical swine fever, foot and mouth disease (FMD), and many others. Veterinarians worked to control diseases locally, using test and slaughter, culling, and vaccines (if available). The FMD outbreak in the UK illustrated the tensions between preserving markets (especially for export) and preventing disease outbreaks. Animals that had been vaccinated against FMD became seropositive, the same as infected animals; other nations stopped importing British cattle and products; and FMD exploded into an international diplomatic and economic problem in 2001.

8. Bovine spongiform encephalopathy (BSE) illustrated how veterinary problems stimulated important scientific discoveries. Veterinary pathologists identified BSE in British cattle in 1986 and related it to scrapie and other diseases. Physicians linked BSE to sick humans who had consumed beef from infected cattle. The cause of BSE was something entirely new: rather than a living microorganism, the causative agent was misfolded proteins known as prions that jumped between species.

9. The animal industries (and veterinarians) were targets of social and cultural criticism that increased from the 1970s on. Some critics focused on poor animal welfare conditions in factory farms and slaughterhouses; others worried about food safety and diseases spread to humans. The overuse of antimicrobials (for growth promotion and disease control) was linked to increasing pathogen resistance, making some of these drugs useless in human medicine.

10. Another challenge for veterinarians has been the control of parasitic and vector-borne diseases, such as scabies, hydatid disease (*Echinococcus*), screwworms, and trypanosomiasis. The most successful campaigns against these problems have been internationally led and included education, local farmers' cooperation, surveillance, and treatment and traceback of any infected animals.

11. Veterinarians are at the vanguard of food safety, using both traditional techniques and new technologies (risk assessment, etc.). Systems such as Integrated Quality Control (IQC) seek to coordinate these efforts in the whole production chain of food of animal origin.

12. Responding to client demand, new paradigms in veterinary practice have included traditional Chinese and Ayurvedic treatments; ethnoveterinary medicine based on botanical knowledge of Indigenous people around the world; competing Western medical systems such as homeopathy and osteopathy; and everything else that was not taught in a traditional

Western veterinary curriculum. Today, some veterinary schools offer courses in "Integrative Veterinary Medicine" (IVM), which combines conventional medicine with complementary and alternative veterinary medicine (CAVM).

13. Traditionally opposed to educating and admitting women to the profession, the veterinary profession included few women (with some exceptions, such as the Soviet Union). In the late 1970s, veterinary medicine began feminizing in several places around the world. The uneven pace of this shift, from men to women as veterinarians, reflected the cultural attitudes and social realities of each region or nation. By 2000, women were the majority of veterinary students and veterinarians in many places. This complex change can be traced to several factors, including legal changes, the women's movement, changes in veterinary practice, and economics. The shift to women veterinarians was controversial with older generations of male veterinarians. Today, women are still underrepresented in veterinary leadership. The profession does not include much racial and ethnic diversity; veterinary medicine remains one of the Western world's most ethnically homogenous professions.

Question/Activity: What kind of animal food production methods and veterinary food inspection system developed in your country or region of the world? Which major animal disease challenges and veterinary responses were connected to the food chain in your nation? What major changes in veterinary practice took place in your country during the last decades of the twentieth century, particularly regarding feminization and ethnic and racial diversity?

7   Veterinary Medicine and Animal Health, 2000–2020

Introduction

This final chapter considers recent veterinary history, focusing on companion animal practice; technological developments, especially the digital revolution; One Health; and finally, the challenges facing veterinary medicine today. As a result of growing prosperity from the 1960s onward in some areas, more and more veterinary practitioners obtained their income from pet animal owners. This sector of veterinary medicine, together with wildlife and zoo veterinary medicine, has received much positive public attention which resulted in a higher image and status for veterinarians. In response to a changing need for veterinary services, further differentiation and specialization within education institutes and veterinary practice have also developed in the twenty-first century. The growth of companion animal medicine was also an expression of changing human–animal relationships and the changing position of animals in society in large parts of the world.

Other striking developments that changed society and veterinary medicine in significant ways were technological innovations. These include molecular biology, biochemical techniques (genome, DNA typing), and pharmaceutical and medical technology enabling new diagnostic tools (CT scans) and new generations of drugs and (chemo)therapies (monoclonal antibodies). As part of the digital revolution, personal computers, email, and the Internet were introduced in the 1980s and 1990s. This has created an increasingly interlinked online community. This also brought about a huge and constant flow of digital scientific information, with applications in research, diagnostics, online databases, and websites, as well as global electronic communication and knowledge exchange.

The beginning of the twenty-first century also witnessed an increasing awareness among veterinarians of the importance of the environment, including climate change and the sustainability of livestock production. Emergent and reemergent infectious human diseases, about 70 percent of which are transmitted between animals and humans, have stimulated the growth of interdisciplinary research and disease control strategies involving veterinarians. In 2011, a major triumph for the veterinary profession and animal health officials was the eradication of rinderpest, the cattle killer that had caused so much suffering, famine, and death for centuries. The veterinary profession combined its celebration of rinderpest eradication with the anniversary of the proclamation establishing the first modern veterinary school in 1761.

We end our journey through the history of veterinary medicine in the year 2020. This *annus climactericus* (a turning point year) witnessed an overriding zoonotic pandemic, COVID-19, which disrupted the functioning of societies worldwide. This pandemic has highlighted the significance of the One Health triad: the inseparable connections between humans, animals, and the environment. These are only some of the important challenges and events that the veterinary profession and other animal healers have faced in recent decades. Within the limited space of this book, it is impossible to describe all these changes and topics in detail over time, and we urge veterinary historians around the world to analyze these changes in their own regions and nations. For veterinarians and veterinary students, these larger themes and how they influence your local area are important in shaping your career and the whole veterinary profession.

The Importance of Companion Animal Medicine and Animal Welfare

Valuing Animals for Companionship

Companion animals, especially dogs, have been associated with humans for millennia. We do not have much information about the nature of the relationship between people and these animals, which probably included using the animals for religious purposes, for food, as workers, and for companionship. The rise of commercialized pet keeping is relatively recent, developing since the mid-twentieth century in most regions. It depends on owners valuing their animals for sentimental reasons, and it is often associated with high income and increases in leisure time. Even this is not new; the urban middle and upper classes in many nations accepted animals in the home as domestic companions, and sought health care for them, at least since the eighteenth century. What has changed is the increase in numbers of animals kept for companionship, the rise of widely available goods and services for pets, and the veterinary profession's attention to these animals. These trends are among several indications that human–animal relationships have become important social and cultural concerns in recent decades.

This change has been reflected in the field of history and historical texts. Since historian William McNeill argued in 1976 that animals and microbes have changed human history on a large scale, more interdisciplinary research was initiated on the topics of human–animal relations and animals as important actors in history. Knowledge about animals, society, and veterinary medicine has increased considerably due to new academic fields such as animal studies, gender studies, and environmental and global history. These animal-centered approaches have enriched and extended veterinary history, as well as historical studies in general. Historians have become increasingly interested in topics about animals, in the relationships between humans and animals, and the role and status of animals in modern society. In recent decades, veterinary history has been building upon this scholarship in human–animal relationships.

Affection for animals took on economic value through sociological and cultural changes. Remarkably, sentimental reasons were often given a higher value, even without any economic benefits from these animals as sources for transport, food, or other products. In wealthy nations, households incorporated the companionship and affection – implicit in pet keeping – into two major social structures, namely, mass popular and consumer culture. For centuries, keeping animals just for fun was an isolated luxury hobby only for nobility and the rich. In the second half of the twentieth century, affection for and keeping of companion animals became a widespread consumer activity in higher-income areas. In addition, social and demographic change in society, particularly the individualization, loneliness, and the proportional increase in elderly people (in the Western world, at least), stimulated the increase in numbers of pets. Increasingly, more and more owners considered their companion animals as family members. For instance, sociological research in England revealed that many people preferred talking to their cat or dog rather than to their family members. Prints of the dog's or cat's paws appear on obituaries as signs that the pets of the lost family member are also in mourning, assuming that the pet has human-like feelings.

This process of attributing human characteristics and behavior to animals in households is called "anthropomorphism. " Seeing their companion animals as human-like or as family members, many people tended to treat (and spoil) pets in the same way. This concept explains why some pet owners view their animals as members of the family. Owners may express their love for their pets by spending money on goods and services for them. Pets were provided with attention, empathy, and pet-related products and services such as luxury pet food, (fashion) gadgets, toys and clothes, hair dressing, nail clipping, animal insurance, and veterinary care. Along with veterinary practices, shops, asylums, kennels, trimming salons, babysitting, walking services, elderly homes, hotels, cremation centers, and cemeteries for pets shared in the booming pet business. In the late 1990s, Americans spent more than $5 billion on pet food and $7 billion on veterinary care every year on dogs alone. In the Netherlands, for instance, the economic significance of the pet-keeping sector has become larger than that of the poultry sector. Among the world's wealthier people, certain pet breeds, particularly purebred animals, became fashionable, thereby forcing up prices for the animals themselves. Purebred breeders contributed to this demand because owners were willing to pay more and more money for buying such expensive (purebred) animals as well as for their health care and well-being. (In fact, pedigree animals are more likely to become ill, particularly due to inherited weaknesses.) This vast economy of goods and services revolved around owners' consideration of their pets as "priceless" family members entitled to full lives (Fig. 7.1).

Not only horses, but also cows, pigs, sheep, goats, llamas, and donkeys have been turned into companion animals. Hobby-farmers often have a few live-stock pets, but in some areas, the hobby farmers outnumbered the large-scale farmers (producing for the markets). This caused problems during eradication campaigns of foot and mouth disease, swine influenza, and other diseases among livestock being produced for the market. Owners considered their animals family members, not market production animals. These owners refused to have their livestock pets vaccinated, controlled, or killed to stop transmission of the diseases. Next to the rise of dogs, horses, and mules as companion animals, their function as war animals continued, although at much lower numbers than in World War II. Horses and mules remained important for pack transport in difficult mountain terrain (Afghanistan, for example). However, it seems that dogs have become the main military animal: dogs were deployed in the conflicts in Korea, Vietnam, Northern Ireland, Iraq, and Afghanistan. They were used for guard duties and as tracker dogs for enemy soldiers, and to locate caches of arms and explosives, including mines. In addition, dogs were very effective in detecting narcotics, have worked as service dogs, and have been important companions to treat people with post-traumatic stress disorder. Most people living in earlier time periods would probably be amazed at the sensibility toward animals today: about the ways we talk about and treat our pets as companions or as children; how we spend money on them and view them as objects of beauty, status, or pleasure; and how concerned many societies are about animal welfare.

They would also be amazed at the sheer numbers of animals kept as companions. The dramatic increase in pet animal populations in wealthy nations is as spectacular as the increase in livestock numbers. It is estimated that worldwide over 470 million dogs and 370 million cats were kept as pets in 2018. This number continues to increase dramatically: European countries had a population of 157 million pets in 2015; within 5 years, they had almost doubled that number (290 million by 2020). In France, the number of cats and dogs grew from 7.5 to 18.5 million in the period 1967–2008. In China, pet keeping has increased at a high rate since the partial privatization of the Chinese economy in 1989. From almost none in the late 1980s, 20% of Chinese households now include pet animals. Between 1988 and 2019, the percentage of U.S. households with one or more pets rose from 56% to 67%.

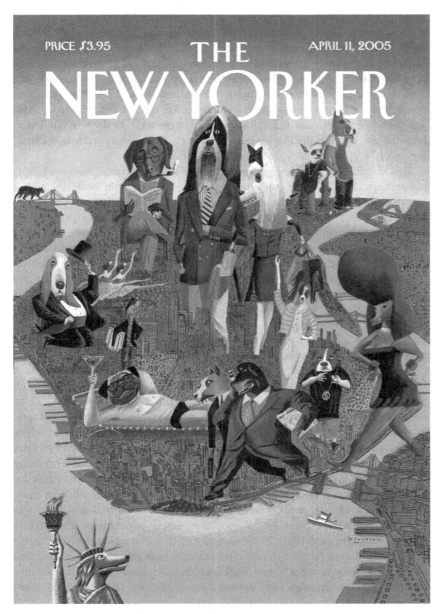

Figure 7.1 Position of pets in postmodern society. Mark Ulriksen, "City Dogs," *The New Yorker*, April 11, 2005.

The United States counted 25 million dogs in 1961; in 2017, this figure was 77 million, next to nearly 58 million cats. Japan counted an estimated 12 million dogs and 10 million cats by 2015. In 2019, a small country like the Netherlands counted 27 million companion animals (compared to a human population of 17 million). About 8 million pond fish, 8 million aquarium fish, 3 million cats, 2.4 million songbirds, 1.7 million dogs, 1.5 million chicken, geese, and ducks, 1.5 million pigeons, 0.6 million rabbits, 0.5 million rodents, 0.3 million reptiles, and 0.3 million horses were kept in 48% of all Dutch households. The top three species, with one or more animals per household, are cats (23%), dogs (18%), and ornamental fish (7%).

This distribution of species reflects changes over time in companion animal populations. For example, the number of cats has risen in societies with a larger percentage of households in which all the adults are out of the house, working, during the day. Cats can easily stay alone for longer periods; the same is true of reptiles, rodents, fish, birds, and exotic animals, and their numbers have been steadily increasing. During the COVID-19 pandemic of 2020–2021, early reports and surveys have shown that pet ownership increased, with owners working from home and seeking companionship and comfort from their pets during stressful times. "Pandemic puppies" and kittens were brought into many homes without pets; also about 20 percent of pet-owning households added a second or third pet during 2020. Almost three-quarters of these owners took their pets to a veterinarian during 2020, reflecting increased attention to their pets' health and well-being.

Numbers of horses, kept as backyard pets or for riding or sports, have increased in recent decades as well. After World War II, horse numbers fell globally. Horses in the armies became redundant after the war and due to mechanization in transport and agriculture. Due to postwar food shortages, many horses were slaughtered and consumed in the war-torn regions, such as the European mainland and Southeast Asia. In the United States, many farmers sold their horses to pet food companies, helping pet food to become a booming business as a result of the growing market for pets. Specialized niches for horses, such as racing, remained important in some countries, while in more rural and low-income areas, horses continued to perform traditional tasks in transport and agriculture. Overall, however, horse populations dramatically decreased until around 1970. In the second half of the twentieth century, horses themselves slowly became companion animals in higher-income areas. This unforeseen factor brought horses back into the landscape of many regions for the first time in decades (and ensured the continuity of equine veterinary medicine).

Elite equestrian recreation and sports date from antiquity but became popular and widespread in high-income countries in the Middle East, Europe, North America, and other regions. Flat and harness racing worldwide, rodeo and related activities in North America, and dressage, jumping, vaulting, and endurance competitions in Europe and the United States flourished as never before. Equestrian sports gained headline status in the world Olympic Games, with lucrative television contracts and millions of fans. The FEI World Equestrian Games were held for the first time in Stockholm in 1990. These elite activities have, in turn, stimulated the participation of amateur equestrians. In many high-income countries, equestrian recreation and sports rank among the top five in terms of people actively practicing it. A small country like the Netherlands has about 1,000 riding schools whose clients are mainly female teenagers. In this country, equestrian sports are second to soccer only; in France, equestrian activities rank third after soccer and tennis. Equestrian sports are gaining in popularity around the world overall.

With horses now considered companions and sport animals, we have traced a full circle from the horse-oriented economies of the early modern period, through the eighteenth and nineteenth centuries, to the dramatic decline in horse numbers due to mechanization in the twentieth century and the restoration of horse populations in some areas today. Of course, in many parts of the world, horses (and other equids) have always remained important, particularly in rural areas, for transport and work. Regardless of the species, those animals that have been designated by various human societies and cultures as companions or pets have drawn special attention. Not only have they have become key drivers of consumerism, but owners' concerns about their welfare have been ethically elevated almost to the level of human welfare. An excellent example of this is the politicization of animal welfare, especially in particular nations and regions.

The Politicization of Animal Welfare at the End of the Twentieth Century

Animal protectionists put forward the centuries-old questions about what animals feel or think. Do they have life expectations? Is it possible to measure discomfort, suffering, and pain? Answers to these questions are crucial in our thinking about animals because these factors help determine how we should treat animals. The more similarities between humans and animals that people notice, the more they are inclined to treat animals like humans. By contrast, greater emphasis on human–animal differences support the more businesslike approach, in which animals are merely economic property. Consuming foods of animal origin, hunting, trading animals, and seeing livestock as mere production units are examples. In previous chapters, we have discussed how animal protectionists united in movements to achieve their goals. Until the 1960s, it was mainly upper-class activists who campaigned against cruelty to animals and tried to improve animal welfare in general.

In the last decades of the twentieth century, animal welfare activism changed in two ways: the broadening of membership to all layers of society and the politicization of animal welfare issues in several European countries. Due to larger and more influential animal protection pressure groups, animal rights and welfare became political issues. Many political parties in Europe included animal welfare issues in their programs. In Germany the *Tierschutzpartei* [Animal Protection Party] was established in 1993, but in 2006 the Dutch *Partij voor de Dieren* [Party for the Animals] became the first political animal protection party worldwide to obtain seats in a parliament. Since then, this political party together with similar (green) domestic and foreign parties promoted an animal- and environmental-friendly policy and succeeded in obtaining animal welfare legislation on national and international levels. This included a ban on animal fights (cocks, dogs, bulls), tail and ear docking and other procedures such as declawing of cats, further regulation of animal husbandry (transport, size of cages, number of animals kept in a certain area), slaughtering methods, and breeding.

Even the economically oriented livestock industry came under scrutiny for the welfare of animals produced for food. Well known is the research by U.S. animal scientist Temple Grandin (b. 1947). She is an expert on animal behavior, particularly livestock being slaughtered. She measured behavior and stress exposure during transport, handling, and restraint and in different ways of killing (pre-stunning, kosher, halal), thereby providing a deeper insight into the extent to which animals experience suffering or pain. She determined how long animals remained conscious after various ways of killing and stated that slaughter animals are not aware of the oncoming killing. New technologies and equipment were developed, as well as slaughterhouses designed to be more animal friendly. Due to Grandin's work, the humane treatment of livestock for slaughter has increased considerably. Finally, the societal debate on animal welfare also triggered changes in veterinary practices. For centuries, veterinarians focused on healing animals, often ignoring suffering and pain in their patients. The past decades witnessed a shift to analgesia during treatments for both livestock and especially for companion animals. This new interest in alleviating animal pain reflected the public's concern about animal welfare (a success for animal protectionists).

Animal protectionists also renewed their battle against the use of animals in biomedical research and education. Changing ideas about animal welfare contributed to a significant reduction of laboratory animals in the late twentieth and early twenty-first centuries. For example, 6 million animals were used in laboratories in Britain and 1.3 million in the Netherlands in 1980. Under the pressure of anti-vivisection activists and politicians in various European countries, the European Union enacted a directive in 1986 (updated in 2010), ordering each member state to incorporate legislation to regulate the use and welfare of laboratory animals. Since then, European countries have reduced their usage of laboratory animals by more than 50 percent by applying the "3-R" principles: replacement, reduction, and refining. Live animals were replaced wherever possible with *in vitro* or other methods; the numbers of animals were reduced per experiment or test; and experiments were refined to be more efficient. These principles have been incorporated into legislation worldwide and have stimulated research in alternatives for animal use (human stem cells, molecular biology and genetics, bioinformatics, modeling, and other methods).

Similar to the 3-Rs approach used in reducing laboratory animal use, basic and uniform principles were sought on which animal welfare in general could be defined, and hence regulation and legislation could be built. However, neutral assumptions supported by all parties involved are hard to find, since so many different – and often emotional – ideas about animal welfare exist. Compromises between different stakeholders are hard to find, since growing affection and sentiment for more animal species has conflicted with the traditional businesslike approach in farm animals. Within political debates on animal welfare, some books and authors have proved to be very influential. An important new impetus was the book *Animal Machines*, published in 1964 by English writer and animal welfare activist Ruth Harrison (1920–2000). Her description of abuse and the poor quality of farm animal life had a profound impact on public opinion in Britain. It prompted a government enquiry, resulting in a 1965 report by a committee presided by Irish zoologist Roger Brambell (1901–1970). By analogy with the United Nations Universal Declaration of Human Rights of 1948, the Brambell Committee published basic needs for animals: freedom from hunger or thirst, discomfort, fear, distress, pain, injury, or disease, and the freedom to express (most) normal behavior by providing sufficient space, proper facilities, and company of the animal's own kind. These minimal standards for animals' lives were designed to be implemented in all settings, from farms to laboratories.

Similarly influential for the further development of animal rights and veterinary ethics were studies by philosophers in the 1970s–1990s. The Australian Peter Singer published *Animal Liberation: A New Ethics for Our Treatment of Animals* (New York, 1975), and American philosopher Tom Regan followed with *The Case for Animal Rights* (Berkeley, 1983). Animal "rights" differed from animal welfare, these authors argued, because animals were no longer defined as "things" but as sentient beings who possessed "intrinsic value." This philosophical movement extended to veterinary medicine. For example, American philosopher Bernard Rollin published *An Introduction to Veterinary Medical Ethics: Theory and Cases* in 1999. Rollin argued for new attitudes in the profession toward animals: veterinarians would need to be guardians of what was best for the animal, even if it cost the owner money.

Based on these studies, some new standards of animal welfare were defined and used in developing regulation and legislation. Also, several traditional uses and roles for animals have been questioned and regulated. In some countries, this has led to a strong limitation in keeping, trading, or exhibiting exotic animals as well as a ban on wild animals in circuses, carnivals, and exhibitions. Currently under debate is whether certain animal species should be kept in zoos, children's farms, and natural parks. Some cities (such as San Francisco in the United States) have even passed legislation stating that animals, as individuals with intrinsic rights, cannot be "owned" but instead have human "guardians."

Within debates on politics and legislation concerning animal welfare (and health) it became very clear that emotions and strong convictions often dominated the discourse. This complicated policy, law, and regulation because scholars from various disciplines argued that scientific facts, not emotion, should be the basis for decision making. Veterinarians joined research that was aimed at obtaining scientific facts and evidence that was desperately needed to gain deeper insight into how animals feel and behave. For scientists, measuring is knowing. Therefore, ethologists and neurobiological scientists are researching cognition and consciousness in animals. They occupy themselves with major question such as, How do animal brains work? What are the differences between brains of certain species (humans, other mammals, birds, fish, reptiles, amphibians, insects)? What does this mean for their perception of positive factors such as comfort, well-being, and pleasure on the one hand or discomfort, fear, stress, and pain on the other hand? Based on results, these scientists have tried to determine (objective) parameters for the welfare of kept animals. Basic needs such as food, water, mobility, and shelter from hostile animals and elements of nature are obvious. More problematic is the prerequisite that kept animals should be able to show their natural behavior, within the limits of their ability to adapt. Dogs for instance, originate from wild canids that roamed freely. If roaming is "natural" behavior for domesticated dogs, most pets do not have that ability. Should they therefore be banned from our homes? Animals in confinement indeed have less control over their natural behavior. During the past decades, more animal-friendly houses and facilities have been designed and built, allowing for more animal behavior needs to be met and a certain feeling of control which are crucial for welfare.

"Man's Best Friend" or "Danger to Society"?: Inconsistent Attitudes toward Animals

Beliefs and concerns about the welfare and rights of animals are cultural and social ideas. Therefore, they will differ from one place to another, and even from one observer to another. In many parts of the world, the notion that animals have rights equivalent to those of people would be incomprehensible. For many people in low-income areas, human survival and well-being are the important issues, not animal welfare or rights. Yet, because people with few resources depend on their animals, they are careful with them. Animal health contributes to human health, and animals may have high value in a family setting for that reason. The animal welfare movement has often been classist and selective: lower-class people have been disproportionately blamed for ignoring animal welfare, while middle- and upper-class pet owners have been blind to their own violations of animal welfare. Finally, it is important to recognize that multiple attitudes toward pet species exist at the same time, sometimes even for the same animals. A dog can be a pet, a war hero, or "man's best friend"; and that dog can also be a nuisance or a danger, a stray, or a laboratory animal without a name.

Critics of the companion animal industry in high-income societies have pointed out many problems and inconsistencies. While accusing farmers of not vaccinating their animals, pet owners themselves often forgot the (annual) vaccinations of their pets against rabies, parvovirus, kennel cough (*Bordetella* or viral infection), canine distemper, and feline leukemia, as well as antiparasitic treatment. Many pet owners prefer purebred and cosmetically altered animals that suffer health problems as a result of genetic anomalies or unnecessary surgeries. Gradually, cosmetic surgeries, such as trimming the ears and docking the tails of dogs or declawing cats, have become more widely considered to be violations of the animal's welfare, physical integrity, and rights. Another major problem has been the breeding of pedigree dogs and cats, resulting in hereditary defects. A well-known example is the French bulldog, bred for a brachycephalic head shape that results in a constant shortage of breath, headache, and bulging eyes due to the small skull. Other skeletal deformities, spinal abnormalities, and patellar luxation are common problems in this breed. French bulldogs' slim hips make it difficult, if not impossible, for these dogs to breed naturally, and they must be artificially inseminated. In this and other breeds, puppies must be born by caesarean section due to abnormally shaped bodies. Despite these abnormalities, the French bulldog is a popular breed in the UK, Australia, and the United States.

Another downside of pet keeping is that owners may lack knowledge about keeping certain animals. Do people know the proper food, housing, and care of regular and exotic animals? Poor nutrition, obesity, vegetable foods lacking necessary proteins for carnivores, insufficient exercise, and confinement are common problems veterinarians see in pet dogs. Do owners know how to train their dogs and to control them? Apparently not, since accidents with dog bites are widespread and sometimes even fatal. This is the case with people who are keeping aggressive dogs as defending or attacking weapons. Pet owners often don't believe that they or their children can become ill from or injured by their beloved pets. However, animal bites are a problem and outbreaks of rabies still occur. Other zoonotic diseases result from intense close contacts between humans and their pets (petting, kissing, licking, sharing food, sleeping together). Parasites can also be transmitted between pets and people, including roundworms in children and toxoplasmosis in pregnant women who have been in contact with pet feces. Veterinarians play a crucial role here in informing future and existing owners of companion animals. Finally, human cruelty toward animals remains a problem, despite the increasing emphasis on love for animals. Research has shown that cruelty to animals is often the preliminary stage of domestic violence; therefore, veterinarians have an important responsibility to recognize injuries in pets resulting from cruelty. In some countries courses for vets are given to recognize such injuries, how to discuss this with involved owners, and the duty to inform responsible authorities.

Unfortunately, pet animals can very quickly change status, from pampered pet to homeless and hungry. Many pets are abandoned once owners are no longer able to pay for food or (veterinary) care, or when they go on holidays, or when their pets get sick, old, start to smell, or cannot be controlled any longer. Fish and reptiles end up in the sewage system. Abandoned cats become strays, surviving by killing songbirds and suffering from illnesses and injuries. If shelters or facilities for abandoned animals are available, these animals may have a second chance to find a home. But shelters for abandoned animals do not exist in many parts of the world. According to the World Health Organization (WHO), there are more than 200 million stray dogs worldwide. These animals have hard lives and die at younger ages, and they can spread diseases. For example, rabies virus persists in the stray dog population worldwide. Rabies in India represents a major public health problem, with 20,000 human deaths every year due to bites from infected dogs.

The contradiction between sentiment and indifference toward animals has also challenged veterinarians because they work on both sides of this changing market for veterinary services. It has caused tensions between different interest groups within veterinary associations. Gradually, veterinarians went along with the shifting attitudes of the general public toward what is considered ethical in our handling of animals. Vets had their own thoughts about it, but eventually realized that they could make good money with treating pets. The veterinary profession responded with further differentiation in education and specialization and accreditation in practice, all aimed at providing high-quality care. Modern medical technologies enabled more complex and expensive treatments of such animals, and many owners were willing to pay for the best treatment for their beloved animals.

"The Profession Goes to the Dogs": Veterinary Services for Companion Animals

A century ago, veterinarians expected few of their patients to have sentimental value; nor would many veterinarians have considered the treatment of such animals to be a primary mandate of their profession. Economic value determined whether an animal would get veterinary care. Veterinary medicine served the commercial interests of livestock owners and the public health, not owners determined to pamper their pets. This was one of the reasons given for excluding women from the profession. In 1897, a British veterinarian acknowledged that women could make good "pet-doctors," but he also indicated his disdain for this type of veterinary practice: "If the practice of veterinary surgery consisted in making a round of visits among lap-dogs, ... and simply diagnosing their diseases ... then, and only then, the profession might be a suitable one for women possessed of any delicacy of feeling."[1] Women did not belong in the stable, barn, or pasture. This long-standing attitude continues today in some sectors of the veterinary profession.

As we have seen, both the increase in women veterinarians and the shift to companion animals in veterinary practice have turned this quote into reality within a century. Companion animals became valuable for sentimental reasons, and their owners sought veterinary care for their animals. This development challenged the traditional focus veterinarians had on animal health because the veterinary profession had to adapt to new ideas about companion animals. Some veterinarians quickly saw the advantage of a new patient population whose owners would be willing to pay well for veterinary services. Gradually, companion animal veterinary practice has grown since the 1960s to be the majority of veterinarians' work in urban areas, high-income populations, and even in some rural areas. Veterinarians turned care for companion animals into a very successful and popular domain of the market for veterinary services within a couple of decades.

Of course, this has not been a universal trend, and veterinary practice varies between different regions and different animal populations. A special category is that of animals valued for a combination of sport, honor, and a kind of close companionship. For example, pigeons are very popular with rural men in Pakistan, who collect and train their birds to fly to targets and return. Pigeon flying competitions are popular, both for honor and economic reward, and the birds are quite valuable. Special *ūstad* (masters) provide health care for pigeons, using a combination of traditional Pakistani and Western biomedical treatments (such as antibiotics). Qualified veterinarians almost never treat these

---

[1] Bell, R. (1897). editorial. *American Veterinary Review* vol. 21, pp. 595–596, quote on p. 596.

valuable birds; instead, *ūstad* are considered the experts in pigeon physiology, nutrition, and diseases. Another popular type of bird in rural Pakistan, the fighting cock, usually receives most of its health care from its owner, the local imam (for prayer), and – when it is very sick – from a veterinarian who administers Western biomedical treatment. For the local veterinarians, it is frustrating because they are often not consulted until the animal is already dying. Nonetheless, these examples demonstrate that veterinarians have varied roles in providing health care for valuable small animals around the world, and that they are often considered supplementary to other animal healers.

In many areas, however, companion animals became big business for the veterinary profession over the past century. The emotional value of pets and their higher status in society influenced this change, but the veterinary profession has also worked hard to encourage the market for pet health and care. This could occur only after veterinary practitioners learned to accept the new paradigm, in which animals were valued for sentimental rather than economic reasons. Within this context, veterinarians also had to change their traditional focus on animal health alone to also include animal welfare, because pet owners demanded it. In higher-income parts of the world, veterinarians began to characterize their profession as the experts in animal welfare as well as animal health during the mid-twentieth century. This strategy served the veterinary profession well because it defined a higher moral purpose for their work and supported the valuation of animals based on sentiment. They based many of their strategies and standards of care on the model of physicians' practices and human hospitals. Veterinary researchers developed vaccinations for companion animals, which veterinary practitioners then integrated into an "annual wellness check-up" for companion animals. Similar to human medicine, pet owners received friendly reminders to visit the veterinarian for their pet's annual vaccinations and health check. By cooperating with other animal industries, such as pharmaceutical and pet food companies, veterinarians' office visits became an important component of expert care of the modern pet.

Veterinarians built clinics and hospitals, incorporating medical technologies formerly available only in human hospitals. Today, such interventions as open heart surgery, replacement of the lens in the eyes of older dogs, and long-term chemotherapy at very high cost are not exceptional. High-level imaging and genetic testing are also available for animals. Although expensive, these treatments can more easily be applied to smaller animals. Along with these technological innovations, veterinarians offer a suitably caring attitude toward companion animals' owners, recognizing the owner's love for their pet. For example, in the past thirty years, veterinary practices began sending condolence cards and letters to owners whose beloved pet had died. Obviously, the huge increase in the number of pet animals provided ample employment for companion animal veterinarians. To meet the medical needs of their dogs, an average household in the United States visited a veterinarian 2.4 times each year (and for cat owners, 1.3 times per year). In 2018, U.S. dog owners spent an average of $410 each year on veterinary care; cat owners spent $182 per year. Increasingly, veterinarians have specialized: for example, feline-only veterinary practices have grown rapidly in numbers since the 1990s and have their own certification.

The shift to companion animals has proceeded at a different pace in different parts of the world, of course. But the trend looks similar: as income and leisure time increase, so does the demand for veterinary services for companion animals. Veterinary practices focusing on companion animals were not common in China until after 1989, with the partial privatization of the Chinese economy. That year, the first private veterinary practice focusing on small animals opened in the country's third-largest city, Guangzhou. By 2015, Guangzhou counted more than 150 private small animal practices. Other Chinese cities are also experiencing this same trend. Today, about 20 percent of all Chinese households own a companion animal. Most of these pets are dogs, although numbers of other animals (cats, birds, and others) are slowly increasing.

In China, the veterinary marketplace is quite varied. In cities, the registered private small animal hospitals (*Yi-yuan*) employ state-qualified veterinarians; there are over 5,000 of these in China. Also in cities, there are small clinics (*Xiao-zhen-suo*, often attached to pet stores) that are largely unlicensed and unregistered. These clinics may employ both licensed veterinarians and "veterinary technicians," which are often veterinarians who have graduated from a three-year curriculum or, after graduation from the five-year curriculum, have not yet passed the national veterinary qualifying examination. In rural areas, the veterinary technicians provide most small animal care. A small, but increasing, sector of this market is corporate veterinary medicine, with one company owning several private practices. The corporate model, imported from the West, serves both Chinese and expatriate clients and their companion animals.

A unique factor in China is the combination of traditional Chinese medicine (TCM) and Western veterinary medicine. In the 2010s, cooperation between Chinese and U.S. veterinary schools and organizations led to international training courses in acupuncture and herbal medicine. This reflected the increasing interest in acupuncture and other components of TCM on the part of U.S. companion animal owners. These treatments have been used on dogs with arthritis and performance horses with injuries or stiffness, for example. An estimated 6,000 American veterinarians have completed the certified veterinary acupuncture courses offered in the United States. Also in the 2010s, close cooperation between some Chinese and U.S. veterinary schools began, with exchanges of students and collaborative educational programs. The major U.S.

formulary, *The Merck Veterinary Manual*, has been translated into Chinese. While international politics and diplomatic relationships will affect these types of cooperative programs, the combining of Chinese and Western veterinary knowledge and practice is likely to continue because companion animal owners in the West and in China are demanding it.

With a long-standing capitalist economy, the situation is somewhat different in Japan. In 2013, the Japanese Veterinary Medical Association reported over 13,000 small animal practitioners, which was 76 percent of all private practitioners in the country. The rise of companion animal practice reflected the increase in ownership of these animals. Japan counted an estimated 12 million dogs and 10 million cats by 2015. As with other capitalist countries, companion animal ownership closely reflects the state of the economy, per capita income, and amount of leisure time. Expecting this trend to continue in the future, Japanese veterinary leaders have called for more continuing education programs on the topic of companion animal medicine and for veterinarians to work with animal humane organizations on animal welfare. Many nations around the world report that a majority of veterinarians today specialize in "small animal" or companion animal practice: South Africa, Brazil, most European nations, the United States, Canada, and many more. Worldwide, the pet care market is growing fastest in Asia and Latin America.

We cannot predict whether the veterinary profession will continue to shift toward focusing on companion animals, but many indicators point in this direction. Privately owned veterinary practices are more likely to treat the animals whose owners will pay for their services. This has been true since the era of the horse as veterinarians' most valuable patients. These veterinarians' work will be most responsive to broader economic shifts, closely following the development of wealth. The other major sectors of veterinary medicine, public, government, military, and industrial employment, respond not only to per capita income but also to international markets and regulation. For all of these market sectors, one of the keys to success is the development and adoption of new technologies.

Technological Developments and Backlash at the Turn of the Twenty-First Century

Technological developments have influenced veterinary medicine for centuries, from the thermometer to the microscope to the radiograph (X-rays). The turn of the twenty-first century witnessed another rapid increase in the adoption of new technologies by veterinarians. Often, veterinary medicine has adapted technologies built for human patients to the needs of individual animal patients. Basic tools that we take for granted today – indwelling catheters, echocardiograms, detailed blood cell and body chemistry tests – were not widely available in veterinary practice until a few decades ago (and are still rare in some parts of the world). The development of nuclear science during World War II enabled new technologies that could trace molecules moving through the body's metabolism and allow clinicians to see inside the body at high resolution – all without penetrating the skin. As we have seen, new pharmaceuticals revolutionized the ability of veterinarians to heal both individual animals and protect entire herds. Biotechnologies have developed at a rapid pace since then, including molecular genetic techniques such as polymerase chain reaction (PCR) that have facilitated new knowledge about conditions such as cancer and new vaccines and therapeutics such as interferons.

By the late 1900s and early 2000s, readily accessible high-speed computing also brought important new tools to veterinary research and practice. Veterinarians now use computerized axial tomography (CT scanning), magnetic resonance imaging (MRI), and other digital tools for diagnosis and treatment of individual patients. Herd management and herd health have also become computerized, solving the problem of how to organize and access information about large numbers of animals. Even in the remotest places, satellite communications, remote sensing, and other technologies enable veterinarians to communicate and send samples to central laboratories. Life without digital tools is hard to imagine these days. The benefits are tremendous: veterinarians can do much more for our animal patients, food safety, and animal husbandry. The advantages for veterinarians are undeniable; but these major changes also have critics. What are the consequences of, and responses to, technological and digital innovations in the veterinary profession and practices of veterinarians and animal healers?

The Digital World: New Opportunities, Old Challenges

Today it is hard to imagine that only a few decades ago everyone was writing on paper with a pencil or pen or using a typewriter. In veterinary hospitals and practices, data about patients and pharmaceutical inventories were kept in paper files and card catalogues. From the 1970s onward, copy and fax machines became more common, while calculations and statistics could be done on electronic calculators. The digital revolution in veterinary practices started in the 1980s, when hospitals and larger practices began acquiring personal computers with programs that facilitated word processing, collecting and storing data, and applying statistics. Originally developed in the 1960s, the digital Internet (a vast network of computers) and electronic mail came into general use during the 1990s, allowing fast exchange of information and data that also changed scientific research. In 1996, 16 million people in the world used the Internet. By 2006, 1.6 billion people used it to buy things, get information, and communicate.

Another major innovation, the mobile phone, was originally installed in vehicles. Although expensive, a mobile phone was very useful for veterinarians traveling to farms and distant villages. The development of cellular networks and standardized equipment meant that mobile phones could be used beyond local areas; by the early 2000s, these networks had connected people around the world. More remote areas used satellite technology for networking. As hand-held cellular phones became smaller and cheaper, their availability and use exploded around the world in the 2000s. By 2010, cellular networks and the Internet were both available on smartphones. The smartphone's user could carry a device that combined phone, computer, and camera in their pocket, enabling face-to-face online communication at any time. The digital world has now become an essential part of people's daily lives.

The digital and technological developments at the turn of the twenty-first century also reached into animal husbandry. These innovations brought blessings but also caused new problems. Biomedical science and technology and the development of GMOs (genetically modified organisms) contributed to even more intensive livestock raising and higher efficiency and productivity. Farmers requested veterinary guidance for preventive medicine and detailed electronic invoicing to improve their herd management. Exchange and accountability were also facilitated by computers when identification and registration of animals became required by veterinary legislation, either in tracing and tracking during campaigns against animal diseases or in the use of veterinary drugs. At first, identification of animals was done with sketches of exterior characteristics or ear tags. Transponders facilitated the identification and storage of specific data of individual animals, and computer programs now monitored large livestock herds. Technologies for processing livestock (slaughter lines, butchering, deboning, meat technologies such as preservation, irradiating, dielectric heating, etc.) became more automated, controlled by computers. Workers had to adjust to faster assembly lines. Food companies used digital media to expand the impact of their message: that their meat, milk, and other animal products were very safe and cheap. Using the Internet, pet food and veterinary drug companies also advertised and sold their products widely. Consumers now had even easier access to information, products, supplements, and drugs for their animals.

Veterinarians had to adapt to the digital world, with its technological opportunities but also its consequences. Like physicians, vets encountered clients whose "Internet education" enabled them to question veterinary authority. Farmers could evade veterinarians altogether by ordering medications on the Internet (a long-standing problem that only increased with Internet access). Veterinary medicine and veterinarians themselves also used the Internet (and, increasingly, social media) to advertise and compete for clients. Veterinary professional ethics had long discouraged advertising as undignified and unfair;

but healers and veterinarians had always found ways to market their services and compete with each other. The Internet enabled them to reach far larger groups of potential clients, however, and made the crowded, contentious veterinary marketplace more visible. Computer-based recordkeeping, for patients and inventory, has become common in even smaller veterinary practices. The veterinary profession has also gained new visibility due to the media. In some countries, television documentaries and series on animals and veterinary medicine became very popular, bringing the profession and its professionals out of the shadows into the spotlight. Most portrayed veterinarians as medical heroes, bringing comfort and health to people and animals.

However, many familiar social problems accelerated during the 2000s with the rise of virtual web-based networks and communities (social media), which changed everyday life considerably. This intensified the general feeling that everyone should be available continuously within a 24-hour economy, increasing workers' stress and fatigue. Digital social networks' lack of regulation, and little education for consumers, led to the spread of deceptive information that caused uncertainty, xenophobia, digital fraud, crime, hacking, and deliberate deception by dissemination of false data. For veterinarians, similar to other medical fields, the output of information dealing with all facets of veterinary medicine grew dramatically. Due to Internet search engines, such as Google and PubMed, an endless stream of publications in an ever-increasing number of digital scientific journals became available, also to the wider public. The pressure on research scientists to publish ("publish or perish" – lose their jobs) in high-impact journals became stressful and did not always improve the quality of the research performed. For researchers, practicing veterinarians, and the public, it has become more difficult than ever to navigate through the overload of information to find what they need.

To be successful, veterinarians need information-processing skills and even more sophisticated communication skills. Convincing a client to ignore misinformation found on the Internet can be very difficult; likewise, clients may have unrealistic expectations. For example, discussions with clients about anthropomorphizing their pets represent a common challenge for companion-animal veterinarians. "Anthropomorphizing" is defined as attributing human characteristics or behavior to animals and treating them as if they were human. In wealthy countries, some companion animals now have the same problems as their owners: obesity, cancer, mental illness, and other chronic lifestyle conditions. At the same time, abandoned animals or those seen as merely an economic resource may not receive appropriate feed, shelter, and medical care. Even if treatments are available, many owners cannot afford to spend a lot of money treating their animals.

Veterinarians occupy a difficult position: they are independent scientific experts and animal advocates, but they are also entrepreneurs often competing for clients. Do they discuss the premise that humans as reasonable beings have a moral duty of care for kept animals (which means that suffering should be avoided)? Do they outline limits? Must everything that is technically possible be done? At what point should an individual animal be euthanized? These daily decisions for practicing veterinarians must be effectively negotiated and communicated with animals' owners. Given the wide availability of information, and the ever-increasing complexity of veterinary medicine and surgery, good communication skills are absolutely essential to today's veterinarian. Recognizing this, veterinary schools are increasingly requiring students to study the so-called soft skills such as communication, deontology, ethics, and decision making.

Traditional Expertise First, Technology Second

One interesting aspect of technologies is the fact that people must decide how and when to use them. As we know, European-style veterinary medicine is a relative newcomer to much of the world. In many areas, both rural and urban animal owners provided their own animal health care first and then decided how to partner with veterinarians (if vet services were available). Owners had a great deal of expertise in preventing and treating animal injuries and diseases. They had developed and circulated expert knowledge during years of raising livestock. This local expertise included ideas about contagion and preventing disease spread; practices to protect animals from environmental problems such as insect vectors of disease; and which problems were likely, given climate conditions. This knowledge influenced veterinarians, both those educated within the country of their birth and those who emigrated.

For example, the disease "redwater" (bovine babesiosis) was unknown to European-trained veterinarians when they arrived in Kenya in the early 1900s. This disease, known as *Alembo* in the local *Dholuo* language, was common in cattle in the Kenyan district of Kisumu on Lake Victoria and also in the Bukusu community in western Kenya. Cattle owners understood that it came from ticks, and that nonlethal infection of young animals raised locally made them immune to the disease. But European cattle brought to these areas died of acute disease, and early veterinarians noted the high fever, weakness, nervous system signs, and dark red urine (thus the name "redwater"). Only after learning about the connection to ticks did European animal owners and veterinarians begin to apply arsenic-based and other insecticides to prevent infection, after 1910.

To fight tick-borne diseases, cattle owners had (and still have) their own regimes of control that included tick removal and destruction, burning pastures and grazing areas, and applying insect repellants. Wycliffe Wanzala, surveying the Bukusu community in 2012, found that the cattle owners applied an integrated method of tick control into which they could insert commercial insecticides when available and affordable. Every morning, family and community members hand-picked ticks off the cattle and destroyed them. Cattle were deliberately herded into areas frequented by tick-eating birds, the *Kamacharia* or oxpeckers (*Buphagus africanus*). At night in enclosures, they burned grasses and branches to create smoke to make the ticks drop off the animals. Pastures and grazing areas were regularly burned to kill the ticks. Local animal healers sold proprietary ethno-botanical products, which owners applied to the animals as tick repellents. Commercial chlorinated hydrocarbon insecticides worked faster and were highly effective in the worst-affected areas. However, these chemicals were expensive; very toxic to people, birds, and mammals; and not always available; and the ticks developed tolerance to them. For these reasons, even after veterinary control and cattle dipping were instituted in the 1960s, cattle owners in western Kenya continued to rely on their own expertise and practices to prevent tick-borne diseases such as redwater and East Coast fever. They simply added periodic dipping to their usual practices.

In rural Tanzania, cattle owners also reported tick-borne diseases (mainly East Coast fever and anaplasmosis) as the major cause of mortality and morbidity in their animals. Here, the problem was more severe: almost half the young cattle died within the first year of life, despite farmers' attempts to control ticks. East Coast fever, caused by a blood-borne parasite, was a good example of the need for targeted technological development: a vaccine, preferably. To immunize animals, veterinarians used the "infection and treatment method," consisting of immunization with extracts from infected ticks followed by a dose of long-acting oxytetracycline. This method caused symptoms but not severe clinical disease while seroconverting about 80 percent of animals, so it was effective. However, the problems with immunization reflected societal factors: the vaccine was not heat stable and refrigerators were rare; it was expensive; and it was packaged in vials with large numbers of doses, which was not practical for the small herds kept by most livestock owners. Technological development of vaccines and immunizations against East Coast fever and other diseases had not been targeted to serve small-scale rural farmers. Most small-scale farmers continued to rely on their own strategies of prevention: tick removal (by hand) and keeping animals away from wildlife and areas known to be infested with ticks. Cattle owners decided how to combine their own treatments with those available from veterinarians.

This pattern continued in other areas. In rapidly urbanizing African nations such as Ethiopia, people brought their livestock with them to the city to ensure that they would have a reliable food supply. In Dar es Salaam, for example, almost 75 percent of residents kept livestock even in densely populated parts of the city. This practice was illegal but tolerated by the local government, so that citizens could feed themselves. In Kenya, half a million people lived in the city of Kisumu and its municipal area, which contained many rural-like open spaces (roadsides, unused lands, and rubbish dumps). A study by veterinarians J.M. Kagira and P.W.N. Kanyari estimated that 60 percent of Kisumu's citizens participated in urban agriculture and kept cattle, chickens, goats, and other livestock. Most of these animals were grazed in open spaces and housed in bomas at night. Kisumu's citizens brought rural knowledge with them and adapted it to urban livestock raising.

In 2007, the major disease problems in Kisumu's urban cattle included lumpy skin disease, worms, diarrhea, respiratory problems, foot and mouth disease, and impaction from ingesting rubbish (plastic bags). The municipal area was served by veterinarians and local animal healers, while farmers provided many treatments themselves. These treatments included traditional ethno-veterinary products and remedies obtained from pharmacies and agro-veterinary shops. Veterinarians relied heavily on vaccine technologies to carry out anti-disease campaigns against foot and mouth disease and rinderpest; anthelmintics to treat parasites; and antibiotics for serious infections. However, the cost of veterinary services was the main limitation to using even basic technologies in places such as Kisumu. The authors of the Kisumu study concluded that the best way to provide veterinary services was through the government-sponsored district veterinary offices. When these governmental veterinary services were privatized, due to the World Bank's financial restructuring programs in the late 1980s, farmers could not afford to pay for vaccinations and other veterinary care. This set of social problems – urbanization, poverty, and government versus privatized veterinary services – limited the ability of veterinarians to employ the necessary technologies.

"We Need These Technologies": Veterinary Responses to Technological Innovations

In wealthy areas around the world, veterinary practice has become dependent on medical technology to a large extent during the past few decades. Patient owners want the same high-tech instruments, equipment, techniques, and drugs used in human medicine to be applied by veterinarians in treating their animals. Noninvasive diagnostic imaging with advanced X-ray, ultrasound, CT scanning, electron and scanning electron microscopy, MRI, and nuclear perfusion scintigraphy have increasingly enabled veterinarians to "see inside" their patients' bodies while avoiding invasive procedures. Special courses and advanced training in radiography and imaging became widespread in veterinary schools' curricula. Beyond imaging, other relatively noninvasive procedures such as endoscopy, laparoscopy, and arthroscopy were made possible by the development of accurate and less expensive instruments, which veterinary students could learn to use during their education. Diagnostic veterinary internal medicine benefited from ever-more sophisticated laboratory tests: biochemistries to analyze organ function; hematology to assess immune function; histopathology; monoclonal antibody testing; and many others. Introduced in the last decades of the twentieth century, new generations of drugs as well as more sophisticated inhalation anesthetics were and have improved diagnostic and therapeutic possibilities. Double-blind, randomized, and (placebo)controlled clinical trials and evidence-based veterinary medicine became the standard for testing efficiency of drugs and therapies.

New materials and techniques have also changed human and animal surgery. For example, in university and specialist veterinary hospitals, improved fracture fixation methods and the development of prosthetic body parts have greatly decreased amputations and improved recovery. During the past decade, the development of patient-specific 3D implants – new knees for dogs, for example – is gaining ground in the veterinary world. In 2018, veterinary surgeons in Canada and the Netherlands succeeded in printing new titanium craniums (skull caps) and implanting them into dogs who had large tumors removed from the skull. An advantage of 3D printing of prostheses is that each part can be perfectly tailored for the individual animal (Fig. 7.2).

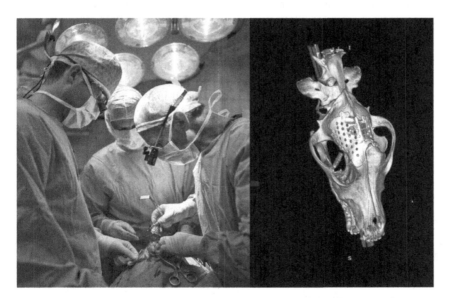

Figure 7.2 Surgery on a dog's skull, Utrecht 2018. After removal of a large tumor, a 3D-printed titanium implant is fixed on the skull. Printed from porous titanium, the edge allows the bone to grow into the implant and integrate it into the skull.
Courtesy: Faculty of Veterinary Medicine, Utrecht University.

Technological innovations have also helped the veterinary profession address public concerns about animal welfare by reducing the number of laboratory animals used by researchers and almost eliminating the use of animals to train veterinary and medical students. Instead of using laboratory animals, tissues, and organs, students now learn practical veterinary skills such as drawing blood, suturing, and 3D anatomy and physiology on models made of plastic, silicon, or plastinated organic tissue (which has the added benefit of being environmentally sustainable). For students planning to work with live-stock production, it is essential to become proficient in the determination of a cow's estrus cycle stage and dating of pregnancies. Until recently, this meant subjecting pregnant practice animals to repeated examinations by dozens of inexperienced students, which caused discomfort and bleeding for the animals. Recently, haptic technology (kinesthetic communication or 3D-touch) has begun to be applied in high-tech robotic artificial cows and horses in a few veterinary schools. This simulator allows students to practice conducting rectal examination in a safe environment before they move on to real animals, resulting in less discomfort for animals and more practice for students. Students learn to confidently locate, palpate, and determine the position, consistency, and shape of reproductive organs. Pressure sensors attached to the silicon organs also allow students to see what they are feeling.

Recent advances in genetic and genomic technologies raise new issues about the ability to manipulate animal production in the future. For example, research on human and animal genomics has increased knowledge about the relation between genome and disease and has resulted in genetic tests to identify a high risk of disease. Another well-known example is cloning animals. In this procedure, a biopsy of tissue DNA is extracted from the animal to be cloned. Scientists then prepare recipient fertilized eggs by remov-ing their DNA and replacing it with the DNA from the animal they wish to clone. This procedure was very complex, and it took years to create viable cloned eggs that could be implanted into surrogate mothers. In 1996, scientists at the Roslin Institute near Edinburgh, Scotland, successfully cloned a sheep they named Dolly. This Finn Dorset sheep, the first clone of an adult mammal, lived until 2003. Just a few years later, a multi-million-dollar project was started in the United States with the goal of cloning a beloved dog named "Missy." Although the "Missyplicity Project" failed, South Korean scientists succeeded in cloning a dog they named "Snuppy" in 2005. Two years later, they achieved a clone of "Missy." Named "Mira," this dog was the world's first clone of a family pet.

What began as an interesting laboratory project for genomic scientists now has the capability to produce identical animals for anyone wealthy enough to pay for the service. In February 2000 a company was founded in response to the growing demand of customers who wanted to clone their beloved companion animals. Since then, gene-banking technology has been used to preserve DNA to clone dogs and cats, a technique which costs between US $25,000 and $50,000 per animal. As with many new technologies, however, cloning will probably become cheaper and easier over time if there is a market for it. Possibly during the lifetime of today's veterinary students, cloning of pets and livestock could become routine. The "ideal" animal may be within our reach, designed by and for human desires. To some observers, these procedures present ethical problems. To others, genetic manipulations are acceptable because they are only the latest version of animal breeding practices that have become more and more human controlled. For decades, artificial insemination has been used to increase the impact of superior bulls, rams, and boars on livestock herds. Frozen sperm of superior animals is used worldwide in artificial insemination. In the 2000s, DNA patterns of young male animals are now routinely compared with markers from a reference group of high performing animals to select good breeding animals. The latest breeding methods include embryo-transplant and *in vitro* fertilizations in livestock.

Veterinarians' adoption of new technologies has depended on several factors: the type, size, and location of the veterinary clinic; the patient populations; the relative wealth of the animal owners; and the education of the veterinarian. Research has shown that veterinary practices employ newer technologies when they are viewed as effective for a common veterinary problem and cost-effective, and when the veterinarian feels comfortable using them. Medical supply companies spend huge amounts of money advertising, running educational seminars and workshops, and demonstrating the uses of new veterinary technologies (including pharmaceuticals). While these newer technologies are protected by patent, they are expensive and mainly used by veterinarians working with wealthier clients. However, once generic versions are available, newer pharmaceuticals are often used in remote areas of the world, if they are not too expensive and if they do not require frozen storage. Veterinarians in remote areas caring for livestock find that their clients are often willing to adopt vaccines and treatments from Western veterinary medicine and integrate them with more local, traditional treatments. Portable scanners and X-ray machines and in-field blood sampling are quite commonly used by veterinarians even in remote areas.

However, technological advancements have also caused concerns and some issues for the veterinary profession. In wealthy countries, many people are worried about the welfare of the animals living in factory farms, despite the best veterinary care. Consumers have questioned the safety of their food, produced in high-output slaughterhouses. Critics have sometimes accused modern veterinary medicine of ignoring the ethical problems of high-intensity animal agriculture and food production. In the area of companion animal practice, some animal owners have criticized veterinarians for suggesting very expensive diagnostic techniques and treatments. These clients are suspicious that veterinarians are simply trying to make more money or satisfy their scientific curiosity, at the owner's expense. Finally, veterinary care was not equally available to all people, and studies showed that veterinarians commonly chose to work in the wealthiest areas. This meant that only wealthy people and their animals were entitled to benefit from the almost limitless possibilities of the digital information explosion and its associated technologies. For the veterinary profession, this mismatch between the distribution of veterinarians and the needs of societies was a workforce problem. But it was also a larger social problem – public investment in veterinary education has often been insufficient. Many areas of the world remain underserved and many animal owners cannot afford to pay for veterinary care. This uneven social investment has limited the use of many of the latest technologies, no matter how effective they are.

Success in meeting veterinary goals comes with the right combination of technology and social investment, and an excellent example is successful disease control campaigns. By 2010, veterinarians eagerly anticipated one of the profession's greatest triumphs: the eradication of rinderpest, the "cattle killer" that had devastated livestock and wild animal populations for centuries.

The End of the "Cattle Killer" and Celebrating World Veterinary Year

Today, only two diseases have been eradicated from the earth: smallpox and rinderpest. Rinderpest eradication gained traction in the 1960s when the Food and Agriculture Organization (FAO) and Office International des Épizooties (OIE) helped coordinate national and regional programs. At the same time, veterinary pathologist Walter Plowright and colleagues, working in Muguga (Kenya), developed a new tissue culture vaccine against the rinderpest virus. After years of work, Plowright had a vaccine that was safe and cheap, and produced lifelong immunity in animals susceptible to rinderpest (however, this vaccine required refrigeration – a significant disadvantage in the field). In East Asia, the vaccine developed by Junji Nakamura and colleagues during World War II had been used to create disease-free belts and regions. Using this vaccine and strict campaigns of stamping-out and surveillance, rinderpest was eradicated in China and Taiwan by about 1960. In Japan, Kazuya Yamanouchi and colleagues developed a new vaccine in 1976. They noted the close genetic relationships between the rinderpest, measles, and canine distemper viruses – thus potentially linking the evolution of viral infections in humans, dogs, cattle, and sheep. Rinderpest remained a problem in the Middle East, India, and eastern Africa, but the tools necessary for a global eradication campaign – technologies and expertise – were now available. How would these tools be used?

Successful eradication campaigns are rare because they require not just technologies and expertise, but also governments' commitments, international cooperation, a lot of money, and good luck. The "good luck" refers to the nature of the virus itself: how rapidly it mutated, whether its various subtypes would evade vaccine-induced immunity, and so on. Rinderpest virus did not mutate rapidly, and the important strains belonged to the same serotype, so that was lucky. But there were other challenges: rinderpest traveled the world with armies and with the global economy of animals and animal products; and because it infected wildlife, rinderpest could hide from veterinary surveillance. Both these challenges made this disease difficult to eradicate, and earlier campaigns to control it had not succeeded in preventing further outbreaks. An African resurgence of rinderpest in cattle in the 1970s, probably originating in wild giraffes and kudus, touched off another pan-African epizootic. From South Asia, armies carried the disease to the Middle East and Southeast Asia. In the 1980s, the FAO and OIE again began lobbying governments and international agencies to fund international rinderpest eradication campaigns.

Emboldened by the success of the WHO's smallpox eradication campaign, the OIE, FAO, and international veterinary leaders developed the "Rinderpest Pathway" to eradicate the disease from the earth. This "pathway" did not always make sense to livestock owners: used to depending on vaccination, they were reluctant to stop vaccinating as a test to see whether the virus was truly gone from the area. As with foot and mouth disease, available serological testing could not differentiate between an animal that had survived a natural infection and one that had been vaccinated. Both carried antibodies to the virus. If an unvaccinated region remained free of rinderpest cases for three years, it was declared free of the disease; after two more rinderpest-free years, the region had eradicated the infection. That five-year wait was excruciating for small-scale farmers, who feared losing their unvaccinated livestock. Veterinarians worked hard to educate and encourage farmers, but their reaction shows how rinderpest had different effects on small-scale subsistence livestock raisers than it did on the big producers selling to the intensive global economy. Subsistence farmers had more to lose (their family's livelihood), while large producers in wealthy countries had mostly disease-free herds and could expect compensation. In this way, the type of production was an important predictor of whether national governments and international organizations were willing to fund global eradication.

In the summer of 2011, the OIE and FAO officially announced that infections of the dreaded cattle killer, rinderpest, had been eradicated from the earth's animals. Throughout its long history with humans and their animals, rinderpest virus caused almost unimaginable misery, starvation, destitution, death, and the dissolution of whole societies. By some measures, this disease drove the establishment of modern veterinary schools, services, and regimes in many parts of the world. It was a major reason for founding the OIE. After almost a century of effort, rinderpest eradication was a major triumph for veterinary medicine. The timing was almost perfect: 2012 would be the 250th anniversary of the first European veterinary school at Lyon in France opening its doors. Since the Royal Decree establishing the school dated to 1761, vets around the world decided to celebrate both the Lyon École's anniversary and the declaration that rinderpest was eradicated in 2011, during a celebratory "World Veterinary Year." At the World Veterinary Congress, held in Cape Town, South Africa, OIE Director General Bernard Vallat called the activities of the veterinary profession "a global public good" and reminded the audience that veterinarians were not only doctors for animals but were also essential to human welfare and public health. Veterinarians aided animal protein production, worked in food safety and prevention of human diseases, and therefore helped alleviate poverty around the world. Veterinary medicine has had many successes and accomplishments in its 250-plus years. Clearly, the profession had broadened its mandate: from mainly caring for armies' horses during the 1700s, veterinarians in the 2000s treated companion animals, contributed to global food security, and worked to control zoonoses. Vallat saw the veterinary profession as a strong partner in ongoing international efforts to deploy scientific developments (such as vaccines) for the betterment of both animals and humans around the world.

The rinderpest campaigns proved that it was feasible to eradicate an animal disease *if* all the necessary factors were in place: international and national cooperation, with fairly stable political and military regimes; funding; the availability of veterinary and other trained personnel; and persistence and patience. However, as expected, wiping out the rinderpest in wild animals was the final challenge. Particularly in regions of Africa, scientists needed to understand the broader ecology of rinderpest in wild ungulates (antelopes, buffaloes, wildebeest, giraffes, and wild pigs). Only then could they be sure that smoldering infections would not flare up to cause epizootics in domesticated animals and threaten the survival of Africa's wildlife heritage. We next turn to the major challenges facing the veterinary profession and its partners, now and in the future.

The 2010s: Veterinary Medicine, Now and the Future

The first decades of the twenty-first century witnessed the emergence and re-emergence of global outbreaks of infectious diseases that were closely related to environmental disruptions and changes. It became clear that ecological and epidemiological methods were needed to understand disease that could not only be explained by the reductionist approach of germ theories. These emerging and reemerging diseases were a reminder that most human infectious diseases are zoonoses (shared by humans and animals) and are influenced by environmental conditions. The field of disease ecology, overshadowed during the second half of the twentieth century by reductionist molecular biology and microbiology, further developed to provide answers to the disease challenges imposed on animals, humans, and veterinary medicine by environmental change. In this final section, we discuss how the complex and dynamic interactions between groups of animals, humans, plants, ecosystems, and microorganisms influenced ideas and actions regarding the control of animal and human diseases during the 2010s. For the veterinary profession, the usual concerns about economics and workforce were joined by fears of zoonotic disease outbreaks and epidemics. In response, the veterinary profession has been a major driver of a recent approach that builds on disease ecology and comparative medicine – One Health. This approach broadened during the early 2000s in response to growing alarm about climate change, ecosystem destruction, and the human impact on the planet.

Sustainable Animal Production in a Globalizing World

As agricultural historian Paul Brassley has described, the global economy intensified when producers from the Americas, Australia, and New Zealand entered the European markets. At first this was international trade with movement of commodities, but in the course of the twentieth century this global economy also included the transfer of labor and technology, foreign investment, and advertising/branding. This was true for rich countries, where big high-tech international companies sold branded goods in an essentially global food chain (subject to national and international politics) for a market of consumers that spent about 20 percent of their disposable income on their food. However, this global economy did not reflect the food system in many parts of the world. Small producers, using traditional production methods, supplied food for the local market for less wealthy consumers, who spent about 70 percent of their income on food. Much of this local meat and milk production did not rely much on formally trained veterinarians, and its impacts on the labor supply and environment usually remained local.

However, the *global* economy for animal-derived foods required huge amounts of basic resources (animal feed, water, land) and international veterinary cooperation to create systems of food inspection for safety and quality control. When the quality and safety of these goods was compromised by food scandals or food poisoning, it immediately became a very sensitive political matter. As we have seen, this was not a new problem for veterinarians, but it certainly became more complex during the past half-century. From the 1960s onward, the "Green Revolution" yielded a spectacular increase in crop production in many countries achieved by the use of new chemical fertilizers, synthetic herbicides, pesticides, and high-yield crop varieties. In China, India, and Mexico, international scientific collaborations changed the cultivation patterns of wheat, rice, and other crops. Livestock raising changed, also, with a shift to bigger populations of animals, often raised in high densities (intensive animal production). With more supply came more consumer demand for meat, milk, and other animal-origins foods. More areas of the world were becoming incorporated into the global economy as the new millennium began in 2000. The benefits for the global food production were obvious, even if this increased production caused the decline of traditional agriculture.

The global economy, and its cycle of growing demand for animal foods and increasing populations of animals, meant that huge quantities of land, water, and animal feed were required. "Factory farms" (raising animals in high densities) in the Global North have been notorious for poor animal welfare; producing huge amounts of manure and greenhouse gas emissions (methane, CO_2); and overuse of water, land degradation, and erosion of biodiversity. In Figure 7.3, the amount of plant-based animal feed necessary to produce foods of animal origin in one year (2016) is shown. The problems with these livestock feeding practices also led directly to other environmental impacts

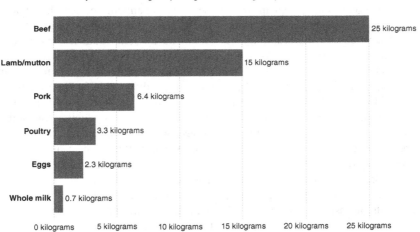

Feed required to produce one kilogram of meat or dairy product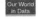
This is measured as dry matter feed in kilograms per kilogram of edible weight output.

Beef — 25 kilograms
Lamb/mutton — 15 kilograms
Pork — 6.4 kilograms
Poultry — 3.3 kilograms
Eggs — 2.3 kilograms
Whole milk — 0.7 kilograms

0 kilograms   5 kilograms   10 kilograms   15 kilograms   20 kilograms   25 kilograms

Figure 7.3 Globalization of animal feed. Required amount of feed to produce 1 kg of meat, eggs, or dairy products, measured as dry matter feed in kg per kg of edible weight output.
Source: Hannah Ritchie and Max Roser, "Meat and Dairy Production," Our World in Data, 2016/2019, https://ourworldindata.org/meat-production.

such as deforestation in Brazil and Thailand, and nutrient deficits throughout the Global South. In recent years, many groups of people have expressed concern about environmental damage, the reduction of agricultural biodiversity, and the loss of more sustainable farming practices. Many have called for a "new green revolution" based on less pollution, ecosystem disruption and global sustainability. Environmental health became a very important political issue in the first decades of the twenty-first century, as shown by the 2015 Paris Climate Accords, a legally binding international treaty on climate change.

Concerned scientists, critical consumers, and environmentalists have urged governments to change the global food economy and livestock industries and turn to more sustainable food production practices. For example, small-scale organic farming has increased in recent years, and some consumers prefer organic products over the mass-produced products of factory farming. They assume that this food is healthier and that the animals in organic farming systems experience a higher level of welfare (the animals are more comfortable). Free-roaming animals, outdoors with more space, are more able to behave naturally and do not have the stress of confinement. They are also not fed antibiotics, growth-promoting hormones, and other artificial substances that may pass into the meat and milk. On the other hand, research shows that some animals raised organically are sick more often than those in confined systems in which antibiotics, de-wormers, and other medications are heavily used. Free-ranging chickens, pigs, and goats have more infections because they are in contact with possible carriers of pathogens in their environments. Small-scale organic production is also more expensive for the consumer. Largely for this reason, the organic food market has remained small, at about 2 to 6 percent of mainstream factory farming. Of course, many people around the world do not eat animal products, either by choice or due to the cost. However, the global animal products economy has continued to grow in recent years, and it still depends mainly on factory farming practices.

For veterinarians, public concern about factory farming and the call to return to earlier farming practices represented a challenge. Since the end of World War II, the veterinary profession had increasingly shaped itself to the needs of animals raised in high densities. Keeping animals alive and well in the global economy required eliminating the infections and parasites that could kill them quickly when living in high-density populations. Using large amounts of antimicrobials, anthelmintics, and other chemicals was the basis of veterinary herd health. This became increasingly controversial, however. From the 1960s onward, global antibiotic use in livestock caused growing concerns about risks of drug residues and antimicrobial resistance. Methicillin-resistant *Staphylococcus aureus* (MRSA) posed a problem in hospitals. The veterinary profession was blamed by the medical authorities for causing antimicrobial resistance due to the widespread use of antibiotics in treating animals. In return, veterinarians claimed that research showed that veterinary use was responsible for about 20 percent of such resistance, while the rest was due to widespread use of antibiotics and unhygienic circumstances in hospitals. Either way, the pathogens responsible for many long-standing infectious diseases had developed some degree of resistance to traditional antibiotics, urging new ways of treatment.

Animals raised in lower-density, outdoor, "natural" surroundings no longer required the same type of high-tech preventive care veterinarians provided for factory farms. Animals raised outdoors were exposed to (and became infected with) parasites and microbial infections that previous generations of veterinarians had battled. The concerns about drug residues led to regulations forbidding or restricting the use of antimicrobials and other chemicals in animals raised for human consumption. Therefore, veterinarians working with small-scale, organic farming had to learn new ways – or re-learn old ways – of keeping animals healthy without relying on feed additives and "magic bullet" chemotherapeutics. They were not trained to provide herd health care for natural production and had to improvise in practice. Veterinary schools' curricula only began to change in the mid-2010s, with a few schools in the United States and Europe beginning to offer some instruction in "alternative" modalities of treatment and prevention. One survey of midwestern U.S. veterinarians found that, although organic livestock raisers were a very small proportion of their clients, about half said they would be interested in knowing more about how to serve these clients. Over half of all veterinarians surveyed admitted that they had little knowledge about treatment options for organic animal production; but they believed that better veterinary knowledge would help the farmers and increase their profits.

Veterinarians seek training and knowledge to meet the needs of their clients and to respond to regulations and laws governing animal production. Of course, these conditions differ from place to place. Much of the world's food, purchased directly from the farmer or at local open markets, is not raised under veterinary care or sold under veterinary inspection. Especially if such food is kept without proper preservation, cooling, inspection, or supervision, food safety may be compromised. Chemotherapeutics may also be unregulated, leading to improper use of antibiotics and other chemicals freely available to farmers. Regulating the distribution and sale of veterinary pharmaceuticals has been a long-standing problem for the profession. The veterinary profession now, as in the past, will adapt and help shape the ways livestock are raised for food in the future.

Environmental health is another growth area for veterinary medicine. This approach, closely allied with veterinary public health, calls for a broader education and working with environmental scientists. This field grew from concerns about environmental residues of chemicals, for example, with insecticides used to kill vectors of diseases in humans and animals. A good example is the chemical DDT, which began mass production as an insecticide around 1940 and was used to kill disease-carrying lice affecting World War II troops and civilian refugees. By the 1960s, DDT was being used as a very effective agent against the mosquito responsible for spreading malaria. Malaria incidence and deaths decreased dramatically in many parts of the world. However, scientists noticed as early as the 1950s that mosquitos developed resistance to DDT. As more mosquitos survived being sprayed with DDT, operators applied higher and higher doses. Unfortunately, excessive amounts of DDT were applied to huge tracts of land in the Americas, Africa, and Asia without an understanding of its environmental effects. DDT, with a half-life of about 20 years in the environment, accumulated in the bodies of humans, fish, birds, and mammals and caused problems. For example, it killed birds acutely exposed to it and led to the near-extinction of several bird species by interfering with calcium uptake and egg laying. The environmental movement, triggered by the publication of U.S. biologist Rachel Carson's book *Silent Spring* (1962), opposed the broad use of DDT. In the 1970s, nations began developing regulations targeting DDT and other pesticides, and research on nonchemical management of insects and pests greatly increased. Today, national and international regulation has led to a decreased use of pesticides and new ways of controlling pests and diseases.

Another problem increasingly attributed to the unregulated growth of livestock raising is the destruction of huge parts of the natural environment and an alarming decline of wild populations of mammals, fish, birds, reptiles, and amphibians. According to the World Wildlife Fund's Living Planet Report 2020 (livingplanet.panda.org), wild animal populations have declined an average of 68 percent between 1970 and 2016 around the world. This decline is an important marker for the overall health of ecosystems. The exponential growth of human consumption, population, global trade, and urbanization since the 1960s has had a negative impact on biodiversity. Recent research has definitively linked biodiversity loss and other ecosystem disruptions to an increasing rate of disease spillover from wild animals to human populations. Spillover leads to increasing rates and severity of epidemic or pandemic zoonotic diseases, such as COVID-19. The WHO, FAO, and World Veterinary Association (WVA) have developed warning systems, procedures, and guidelines to tackle disease threats in terms of dynamic interactions at the human–animal–ecosystems interface. Whether watching for local outbreaks of zoonotic diseases, inspecting food, or working in governmental veterinary public health, all veterinarians are important parts of disease prevention systems today. This broad understanding of veterinary responsibilities is guided in the 2010s and 2020s by the One Health framework.

Reinvention of the One Health Approach

One Health is not new. As we have described, natural philosophers and biomedical scientists have stressed the importance of comparative medicine from antiquity onward to obtain a deeper insight into diseases in both humans and animals. Today's One Health framework emerged from zoology, comparative anatomy, and comparative medicine. In the mid-1800s, Rudolf Virchow's "One Medicine" promoted the ideas that animal and human bodies worked in similar ways, suffered similar diseases, and could be treated similarly. This approach also led to scientific advances. Experimental animals were proxies for humans in experiments that contributed to cell theories, germ theories, and the understanding of zoonotic diseases. Observed homologies between animal and human bodies, and their pathologies, were the foundation for One Medicine. The most obvious cases were zoonoses, diseases transmitted between animals and humans.

Today, about 70 percent of human infectious diseases (emergent and reemergent) are actively zoonotic or vector borne (Fig. 7.4). Humans living closely with animals have probably observed that diseases could be transmitted between them for thousands of years. Since at least the late 1800s, scientists have elucidated the complex life cycles of the microorganisms and their interactions with insect, animal, and human populations. Zoonotic diseases are caused by a variety of microorganisms: viruses (HIV-AIDS, SARS, MERS, COVID-19, rabies, encephalitis, West Nile virus, etc.); parasites (giardiasis, echinococcus, etc.); bacteria and protozoa (anthrax, plague, tuberculosis, brucellosis, salmonellosis, Lyme disease, etc.); and prions (BSE/new variant Creutzfeldt-Jakob disease). Many are vector borne (mainly spread by insects). An important function of the One Health approach is to establish the origin of the disease, often traceable to other species, and to understand how it is spread (transmission). For example, acquired immunodeficiency syndrome (AIDS) is caused by a virus (HIV) traced back to a simian (monkey) virus present in wild primates in Cameroon. Humans were probably exposed to this virus by hunting and consuming infected monkeys. Influenza viruses (human type A), which have caused periodic pandemics in humans, have been genetically linked to influenza viruses in swine and wild birds. Proximity to these animals is a risk factor.

Over the past century, recognizing the potential wildlife and domesticated animal origins of these and other important diseases has broadened epidemiology to include the ecological and environmental sciences. This approach has been especially important in the Soviet Union (today, the Russian Federation and several other nations) where scientists developed the "natural focus" theory of disease transmission in response to outbreaks of encephalitis, plague, and other diseases. In the West, scientists rediscovered ideas from the 1800s

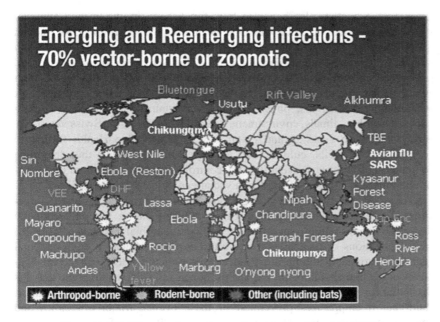

Figure 7.4 World map of emerging and reemerging infections; 70% are vector borne or zoonotic.
Source: https://onehealthinitiative.com/.

One Medicine framework a century after Virchow proposed it. Veterinarians such as Karl Friedrich Meyer (1884–1974), Calvin Schwabe (1927–2006), and James Steele (1913–2013) argued for a return to the One Medicine approach between the 1910s and 1970s. These pioneers' training and experiences convinced them that this approach was valuable. All three were trained in both veterinary medicine and (to some degree) human public health, so they felt comfortable crossing disciplinary boundaries. All had worked internationally and had confronted zoonotic diseases. They understood disease as a larger biological phenomenon, not just from the perspective of human medicine and epidemiology.

They also joined with physicians and microbiologists, such as René Dubos (1901–1982), to advocate for the importance of a healthy environment to human health. As medical historian Roy Porter has pointed out, environmental improvements and better living standards today contribute more to health than curative medicine. From this point of view, it is more worthwhile to invest in public health, environmental hygiene, and nutrition, especially in less wealthy countries lacking basic infrastructure, than in advanced clinical medicine programs. Scientists also began to look for disease origins in wild animals' environments, and in 2008 the One Health Initiative group (USA) added "Environment" to the One Health framework to create the One Health "Triad": Human–Animal–Environment. This broader vision has been embraced and promoted by WHO, FAO, OIE, and WVA. The One Health Concept can be defined as a global framework that unites professionals (including veterinarians, physicians, and environmental scientists) working toward healthy animals, environments, and humans. In 2011, Swiss veterinary professor Jakob Zinsstag and co-authors expanded One Health further to emphasize the social, cultural, and ecological entanglements that determine outcomes of disease prevention and control strategies. These authors concluded that One Health is "health in social-ecological systems (HSES)."[2]

Today, One Health is the strategy most often used to study zoonotic infections and emergent/reemergent diseases. It encompasses not only zoonotic infections, food safety, surveillance, and antimicrobial resistance, but also the applications of comparative and translational medicine to environmental and occupational health hazards, cancer, metabolic disorders, and the implications of the human–animal bond. The proponents of One Health argue that it is essential for prevention of zoonotic disease spillover and potential epidemics, and that it emphasizes prevention of these events. Major epidemics and pandemics caused by influenza viruses in 2009 and SARS-CoV-2 in 2019 have reinforced this claim. The major questions include how surveillance of wild animals (bats, rodents, and other common host species) can predict where spillover is likely to occur; the roles of pets or domesticated livestock in spreading zoonoses; and how to break cycles of zoonotic transmission. Along with encouraging interdisciplinary collaboration, One Health investigations scale up from the molecular level to the ecosystem level. All these advantages make the One Health framework crucial to preventing and responding to a broad range of serious problems at the human–animal–environment interface.

Of course, the One Health framework has its critics. Veterinary leaders have been disappointed that physicians and leaders of the human medical profession have been less keen to cross disciplinary lines and truly collaborate. (This reflects the often-troubled history of physician-veterinarian disciplinary relationships discussed throughout this book.) One Health has been criticized for being too focused on human diseases to the detriment of non-human problems. In addition, research scientists may be reluctant to participate because their reputations are built on specializing narrowly, which is the opposite approach to the broad collaborative One Health approach. Citizens of poorer nations

[2] Zinsstag, J., Schelling, E., Waltner-Toews, D., and Tanner, M. (2011). 'From "One Medicine" to "One Health" and Systematic Approaches to Health and Well-Being'. *Preventative Veterinary Medicine* vol. 101, nos. 3–4, pp. 148–156.

view One Health with skepticism. The One Health framework reflects a particular view of *which* diseases are important and *how* we should respond to them – the view controlled by Western biomedicine. As scholars have pointed out, deploying this framework effectively reproduces a kind of health colonialism: the diseases we focus on are often those that elites in wealthy countries see as a threat. Responses to these diseases may not address the basic problems related to poverty and food and health insecurity present around the world. Once an acute problem (such as a pandemic) dies away, we forget about protecting the environment or improving the basic living conditions of poorer people and their animals. While this historical pattern is common, it is not inevitable. Already environmental scientists are seeking to expand One Health to a new, broader framework: "Planetary Health." Whatever framework is available at the time, it is the duty of all veterinarians to advocate for better health outcomes for the environment, wild and domestic animals, and human populations.

Conclusions

From this survey of the early twenty-first century, we can conclude that:

1. Worldwide, over 470 million dogs and 370 million cats were kept as pets in 2018, along with many other species too numerous to count (fish, birds, small mammals, and reptiles). Horses have increasingly become companions and sport animals. Commercialized pet keeping developed since the mid-twentieth century in most regions. The numbers of pets, the wide availability of goods and services for them, and the veterinary profession's attention to animals kept for companionship have all increased. Worldwide, the pet care market is growing fastest in Asia and Latin America.
2. Since the 1970s, historians have increasingly analyzed animals and human–animal relationships. Anthropomorphism is defined as attributing human characteristics and behavior to animals. This concept explains why some pet owners view their animals as members of the family. Owners may express their love for their pets by spending money on goods and services for them; this has become a vast global industry. Veterinary history has built upon this scholarship to explain developments in veterinary medicine.
3. In the last decades of the twentieth century, animal welfare activism changed in two ways: the broadening of membership to all layers of society, and the politicization of animal welfare issues in several European countries. Due to larger and more influential animal protection pressure groups, animal rights and welfare became political issues.

Changing ideas about animal welfare contributed to a significant reduction of laboratory animals. This also affected veterinary practice, with more attention paid to animal suffering and pain and new developments in analgesia during treatments.

4. Attitudes toward animals have been inconsistent because they are social and cultural ideas. They change from one time period to another, from one place to another, and between different groups of people. Some veterinary procedures, such as declawing cats, became controversial, while owners demanded purebred cats and dogs with high levels of genetic and congenital health problems. Some pet animals are treated very well, while others are not. Diseases and behavior problems, such as rabies, parasites, and canine aggression, cause controversy. Finally, pet animals can be abandoned, leading to suffering, disease, and injury since the pet does not know how to survive. Veterinarians must confront these inconsistent attitudes and realities.

5. Companion animal veterinary practice has grown since the 1960s to become the majority of veterinarians' work in urban areas, high-income populations, and even in some rural areas. In many parts of the world and for certain animals (such as falcons, racing pigeons, and fighting cocks), health care is provided by local healers as well as veterinarians. Traditional healing systems are often combined with Western veterinary medicine.

6. Veterinarians have turned care for companion animals into a very successful and popular domain of the market for veterinary services within a couple of decades. The standard of care was based on the model of physicians' practices and human hospitals. Animal hospitals and clinics adopted new technologies, developed surgical procedures and medical treatments, and offered a caring attitude toward companion animals and their owners. Companion animal practitioners are now the majority of veterinarians in nations such as Japan, South Africa, most European nations, the United States, Canada, Brazil, and many more.

7. Veterinarians have incorporated new technologies, from echocardiograms and detailed body chemistry tests to CT scanning and MRIs and genetic testing. Although expensive, these technologies work well for smaller animals whose owners are willing to pay for them. In food-producing animals, the development of technologies such as GMOs (genetically modified organisms) contributed to even more intensive livestock raising and higher efficiency and productivity.

8. The digital revolution in veterinary practices started in the 1980s, when hospitals and larger practices began acquiring personal computers with programs that facilitated word processing, collecting and storing data, and

applying statistics. The Internet and hand-held mobile phones (and eventually smartphones) have revolutionized veterinary practice (as well as daily life for much of the world). Consumers now have even easier access to information, products, supplements, and drugs for their animals.

9. Life in the digital world has caused some problems for veterinarians: workload, fatigue, and stress have increased; animal owners believe deceptive or false information; digital fraud and crime have increased; and it is almost impossible to keep up with the huge amount of information available. To be successful, veterinarians need information-processing skills and even more sophisticated communication skills.

10. Social problems – urbanization, poverty, and government versus privatized veterinary services – have also limited the ability of veterinarians to employ the available technologies. Sometimes technological developments (including some much-needed vaccines) do not work well under field conditions. Animal owners in many areas have continued to rely on their own expertise and practices to maintain animal health, adding the biomedical technologies when they work well within the local situation. Uneven social investment has limited the use of many of the latest technologies, no matter how effective they are. Public investment in veterinary education has often been insufficient. Many areas of the world remain underserved, and many animal owners cannot afford to pay for veterinary care.

11. Rinderpest was declared eradicated from the earth in 2011, after the OIE, FAO, and international veterinary leaders cooperatively implemented the "Rinderpest Pathway" to eradication for over three decades. This was a major triumph for organized veterinary medicine, which was established in part due to the devastation caused by rinderpest over the past 400 years.

12. In 2011–2012, veterinarians celebrated the "World Veterinary Year," the 250th anniversary of the first European veterinary school at Lyon, France. Veterinary medicine has had many successes and accomplishments in its 250-plus years. Clearly, the profession has broadened its mandate: from mainly caring for armies' horses during the 1700s, veterinarians in the 2000s treated companion animals, contributed to global food security, and worked to control zoonoses.

13. In response to increasingly common outbreaks of zoonotic diseases, the veterinary profession has been a major driver of "One Health," a recent approach that builds on disease ecology and comparative medicine. One Health is generally defined as a worldwide strategy for expanding inter-disciplinary collaborations and communications in all aspects of health care for humans, animals, and the environment. Veterinarians collaborate with physicians, environmental scientists, and other specialists to address

complex disease problems. While important, One Health has been criticized for being too focused on human diseases and for working on diseases that wealthy countries see as a threat – without addressing the basic social needs of poorer countries. This approach broadened during the early 2000s in response to growing alarm about climate change, ecosystem destruction, and the human impact on the planet. Veterinarians are also beginning to work in environmental health, and with organic farming, both of which advocate decreasing the use of chemicals and other agricultural technologies that cause harm to ecosystems, add residues in food, and create resistance to antimicrobials.

Question/Activity: Did the veterinary profession shift from focusing on food animal health to companion animal welfare in your country or region? Did animal welfare become a political or societal issue in your country? Which veterinary services for companion animals have developed in your nation? To what extent did technological innovations as well as sustainable animal production affect veterinary practice in your part of the world? What are the most important characteristics of the One Health approach, and what impact does this have on veterinary medicine, animal health, and human health in your country?

Epilogue
Veterinary Medicine in the Postmodern World

We began this book with the ancient Ayurvedic, Chinese, Indigenous American, and many African peoples' frameworks of understanding animal health and disease. These frameworks included sophisticated theories about the body, environment, and spirit that guided practitioners in their choices of treatments for sick or injured animals. These ways of knowing are still strong today and are often combined with modern veterinary medicine. Both the Hippocratic tradition of holistic medicine (taking into account the whole body of the patient and its environment) and the more reductionist analysis of disease (focused on organs, tissues, cells, and molecules) have continued in veterinary medicine. Biomedicine and veterinary medicine are also the products of the European Enlightenment. They share the Enlightenment's successes and its problems: not only the development of Western science, but also the reliance on capitalist economics and the close ties to imperialism. Throughout its history, veterinary medicine has been influenced by beliefs about the human–animal relationship and major social and political events such as wars. Since 1500, the animals themselves have changed, adapting and evolving to new environments and new circumstances.

Historians cannot predict the future, but the one conclusion we can make is that veterinary medicine and animal healing will continue to be affected and molded by changing sociocultural and environmental conditions. Unforeseen events and trends happen regularly: disease outbreaks, the rise of pet keeping, wars, the feminization of the workforce. Veterinary medicine is constantly shaping, and being shaped by, these broader social and cultural forces. Over time, the changing needs of societies, and the value they have placed on animals, have often determined the tasks undertaken by the veterinary profession. As human–animal relationships have changed, so has veterinary medicine. As scientific knowledge has developed and traveled around the world, veterinary medicine and animal healing have become increasingly complex. Today, the major concerns for veterinary medicine's future depend on one's point of view, including veterinary students and practicing professionals, animal owners, public health officials, political leaders, and people concerned with animal welfare.

The Challenges and Rewards of Working as a Veterinarian

In 1961, more than 161,000 veterinarians were active worldwide. Most of these were in Europe (100,000), followed by the Americas (30,000), Asia (28,000), Africa (1,900), and Australia and New Zealand (1,500). According to the World Veterinary Association, there were over 500,000 veterinarians worldwide in 2018, of which around 300,000 worked in Europe and 115,000 in the United States. The female-to-male ratio was roughly 3:2. It is estimated that about 65% are active as veterinary practitioners, 10% are working in public service, and 5% in industry, while the rest have unknown employment or are unemployed. In some countries with many veterinary colleges (for example, Spain and Italy), unemployment can be high. Due to an influx of younger vets, a shift in age is taking place. Older generations have retired and are being replaced by millennials (people born between 1981 and 1996). In the United States, for example, millennials are now about 39% of active veterinarians.

This newer generation of veterinarians is faced with critical farmers, environmentalists concerned about sustainable animal production and climate change, demanding pet owners, and anxious consumers of animal-origin foods – all with different and sometimes opposite demands. The public image of the profession is linked to consumer culture, international politics, outbreaks of enzootic or zoonotic diseases, and the social value of zoo, wild, farm, laboratory, or companion animals. The veterinary profession, and its members, must be well informed, flexible, and able to change quickly – like our predecessors a century ago, who faced the disappearance of horses, their most important patients. The historical narratives told in this book show that veterinary medicine and its wide range of practitioners regularly had to adjust to the ever-changing and different kinds of human–animal interactions that have existed between and among animal owners, government authorities at different levels, armies, colonies, businesses, consumers, scientists, and animal protectionists. Overall, veterinarians everywhere must contend with meeting animal owners' expectations, feeding the world's people, and controlling animal disease outbreaks without causing harm to societies and ecosystems. These challenges emerge from the inequalities built into the global animal economy and the realities of environmental conditions such as climate change.

Students seeking to become veterinary professionals are well aware of these challenges. They also worry about the lengthy and expensive education, after which they must compete in an often-crowded veterinary marketplace. Some experienced veterinarians report problems with the job: debts from education, more animals to treat in less time, the changing attitude of patient owners (boldness, aggression, delayed payment). These factors, plus economic concerns, more administrative tasks, and the higher number of colleagues to compete with are causing stress and stress-related illnesses, sometimes resulting in burnout among relatively young vets (30 to 40 years old). Unfortunately, the suicide rate among veterinarians has also increased during the past decade. This worrying fact represents a challenge for the veterinary profession, veterinary education, and veterinary associations. In veterinary school, more attention needs to be given to the "soft skills" and "support skills," development and implementation of standardized stress management interventions, such as courses for improving communication, managing stress and caring for one's own mental and physical health, and work–life balance.

Despite these points of tension, veterinary medicine remains a popular career choice for several reasons. Surveys of veterinary students in Western nations almost always show a high level of regard and love for animals. Students joke that they prefer animals to people, at least in terms of caring for them. Another positive factor is the desire to combine the rigorous intellectual aspects of biomedicine with hands-on practical work with animals. Those students who wish to work with livestock enjoy the outdoor life and the farm culture. Finally, students cite their strong desire to improve animal welfare and alleviate suffering, reflecting the cultural emphasis on more humane and sustainable values. As sociologists, philosophers, and political scientists have discussed, critiques of modernism – especially capitalistic modernism, in which profit is the most important consideration – have encouraged a postmodern society that questions powerful institutions such as commercial food producers. Postmodern ideas, offering space for individual autonomy, diversity, and self-expression, have influenced younger veterinarians and cultural ideas on how to keep and treat animals.

Does the Veterinary Workforce Meet the World's Needs?

From the point of view of some government officials and political leaders, the veterinary workforce often does not reflect the nation's needs. In wealthy areas, many veterinarians choose to work in urban companion animal practices, while rural livestock owners often lack access to necessary veterinary care. In less wealthy areas, animal healers and veterinarians will choose among the traditional and biomedical therapeutics, vaccines, and surgical methods available to them rather than expensive, highly specialized technologies that do not meet their needs. Fewer rural veterinarians also lead to less oversight of farmers' husbandry methods, including not meeting animal welfare standards and the use (and misuse) of antibiotics. Because young veterinarians often emerge from school heavily in debt, they cannot afford the lower salaries paid to government employees and meat inspectors, so not enough vets work in these sectors. Yet global food production depends on them: imagine the serious problems society as a whole would encounter if all veterinarians would go on strike at the same time. Food production and supply would stop, while animal owners would be deprived of acute care for their animals. This "workforce mismatch" between veterinarians' career choices and global needs has become more acute since the mid-twentieth century.

Today about 55% of the world population is urbanized; by 2050 this could be 68%. Urbanization has already had consequences for veterinary practice and the profession. In Europe, the United States, Japan, and South Africa, there is already a shortage of vets in rural areas. Not many young vets want to move to the countryside. This is the case despite the popularization of historical veterinary-themed dramas in film and television, including the British James Herriot and Dutch Dr. Vlimmen, both of whom were portrayed as well-regarded professionals in small rural villages. These are nostalgic dramas, however; this type of veterinary practice has almost disappeared. Veterinary medicine is becoming an urban profession again, just as it was over a century ago during the age of working horses. Veterinary professional leaders have begun calling for incentives to encourage young veterinarians to work in food animal practice and food safety. Increased salaries, reduced school fees, or debt forgiveness have all been proposed in return for the young vet choosing to work in an underserved rural area. These economic incentives can also be augmented by attention to work–life balance: group practices, so that vets can share the responsibility for emergency and after-hours work; better availability of diagnostic laboratories and other support services; and transportation, housing, and other benefits.

Despite the triumphs of biomedicine, animal diseases – including zoonoses – have persisted and continued to reemerge. This has highlighted the importance of veterinarians working in disease control, public health, and environmental sustainability. The eradication of rinderpest, "the cattle-killer," was a major achievement for veterinarians; but swine influenza, Newcastle disease, parasitic infections, and many other disease problems continue to kill animals and to impoverish people. In industrialized countries, the drive for efficiency and higher profits as part of modernization has reached a point of reduced benefits in terms of disease control, animal welfare, and environmental health. Unregulated human appetites for exotic foods of animal origin have contributed to the emergence of novel pathogens and outbreaks of zoonotic diseases. Environmental toxins and contamination of fresh food with pathogenic microorganisms have also caused disease in human and animal populations. Veterinarians are an obvious resource pool of professionals to help address these problems, if given the power and resources to do so. When surveyed in 2018, veterinarians from thirty European countries listed the most important resources to meet the changes of the next five years: more specialization; more business training; more training in digital skills; and more legislation supporting the profession.

Despite all these concerns (magnified by the stress of the COVID-19 pandemic), the veterinary histories in this book also speak of the resilience of people and animals, the alleviation of suffering, and the deployment of local expertise and biomedical tools to help achieve these goals. Many people have helped unravel the mysteries of how animals' bodies and disease processes worked: the Ayurvedic and Chinese theories of the body's circulation of vital processes; Ibn al-Nafis' explanation of the pulmonary circulation; Paracelsus' view of digestion as a chemical process; and veterinarian Jean-Baptiste Chauveau's studies of the physiology of the nervous and hepatic systems. Chauveau then used this knowledge to develop techniques such as cardiac catheterization, drug delivery, the separation of red from white blood cells, and vaccines. In southern Africa, the Zulu people struggled against European colonialism while educating White farmers and vets about the importance of the tsetse fly in spreading deadly cattle diseases. African leaders commonly combatted animal diseases by imposing quarantines, while livestock owners burned the bush to eliminate fly and tick vectors. The biomedical discoveries of the late nineteenth and twentieth centuries were built on these early efforts to keep animals alive and well.

Veterinarians contributed greatly to the knowledge necessary for those biomedical discoveries, such as vaccines and medications for both humans and animals. Danish veterinarian Erik Viborg's proof that glanders was contagious came too late to save the father of scientific veterinary medicine in England, Charles Vial de St. Bel, who had died a horrible death due to glanders a few years before. But Viborg's conclusion supported isolating or destroying infected horses to prevent the spread of the infection, which was particularly important in army horses. It also led to an early allergic hypersensitivity test, the mallein test, which helped eliminate glanders from Europe and North America. In the 1890s, Americans Theobald Smith, Fred Kilborne, and Cooper Curtice demonstrated the epidemiology and microbiology of a vector-borne disease, Texas cattle fever; their work led to breakthroughs in malaria control and research on many diseases of animals and humans in the Global South. Veterinarians have played other crucial roles in safeguarding animal and human health: they developed campaigns against bovine tuberculosis and brucellosis; trichinosis and other problems with meat hygiene; and, most dramatically, they were crucial to the eradication of rinderpest (only the second disease in history to be eradicated from the earth). These campaigns, and the lifetimes of work and sacrifices that contributed to them, demonstrated the determination of veterinarians and veterinary researchers to reduce animal suffering and the impact of animal diseases on human well-being.

Veterinary medicine has tremendous opportunities today. Veterinarians and animal healers are key providers of global health care for animals and food security for people. Emerging disease problems (such as COVID-19) have only reinforced the need for a "One Health" or "Planetary Health" approach that brings biomedical scientists together, elevates veterinary public health, and links the well-being of the world's people to that of its animals. Moving forward, veterinarians will contribute to global efforts to address disease, food safety, inequality, disease, and environmental pollution. Animal healers and veterinarians have a long and proud tradition of addressing the societal needs of their time and place, and this will inspire the profession in the future.

Almost twenty years ago, veterinary historian Angela von den Driesch finished her book on the history of veterinary medicine with the remark that the modern veterinarian should act as a mediator between the use and care of animals. Within these conflicting demands, a veterinarian must balance the needs of humans with those of animals. But veterinarians can never forget their duty to their animal patients: *in dubio pro animale* (when in doubt, act in favor of the animal). We will end as we began: we have much work to do. Let us all, as informed citizens and dedicated professionals, pledge to use our abilities to make the world a better place for people, animals, and their environments.

Appendix A Spread of Veterinary Education Institutions around the Globe (List of the First Veterinary School Established in Selected Nations, 1762–1960s)

Year	City	Country
1762	Lyon	France
1767	Vienna	Austria
1769	Turin	Italy
1771	Göttingen	Germany
1773	Copenhagen	Denmark
1775	Skara	Sweden
1787	Budapest	Hungary
1791	London	England
1793	Madrid	Spain
1805	Kharkiv	Ukraine
	Bern	Switzerland
1806	Vilnius	Lithuania
1807	St. Petersburg	Russia
1821	Utrecht	Netherlands
1823	Edinburgh	Scotland
1824	Warsaw	Poland
1827	Cairo	Egypt
1830	Lisbon	Portugal
1836	Brussels	Belgium
1842	Istanbul	Turkey
1848	Tartu (Dorpat)	Estonia
1853	Mexico City	Mexico
1855	Boston	USA
1861	Bucharest	Romania
1862	Toronto	Canada
1876	Tokyo	Japan
1881	Lahore	Pakistan
1883	Santa Catalina	Argentina
	Bombay	India
1898	Santiago	Chile
1900	Dublin	Ireland
1902	Lima	Peru
1905	Montevideo	Uruguay
1907	Havana	Cuba

(cont.)

Year	City	Country
1908	Melbourne	Australia
1909	Guangzhou	China
1910	Manila	Philippines
1912	Rio de Janeiro	Brazil
1918	Brno	Czechoslovakia
1919	Riga	Latvia
	Zagreb	Yugoslavia
1920	Pretoria	South Africa
1921	Bogota	Colombia
1923	Sofia	Bulgaria
1931	Manabí	Ecuador
1932	Kabul	Afghanistan
	Tehran	Iran
1935	Oslo	Norway
1938	Khartoum	Sudan
	Maracay	Venezuela
1940	Bangkok	Thailand
	Santa Cruz	Bolivia
1945	Taipei	Taiwan
1946	Helsinki	Finland
1947	Peradeniya	Sri Lanka
	Seoul	Korea
1949	Kabete	Kenya
1950	Addis Ababa	Ethiopia
	Thessaloniki	Greece
1952	Tirana	Albania
1955	Santo Domingo	Dominican Republic
1956	Asuncion	Paraguay
1957	Baghdad	Iraq
1957	Guatemala City	Guatemala
	Riyadh	Saudi Arabia
	Rangoon	Burma
	Tripoli	Libya
1959	Saigon	Vietnam
1960	Nsukka	Nigeria
1961	Mymensingh	Bangladesh
	Managua	Nicaragua

Data are drawn from: Dieter Breuer, *Weltkatalog der Veterinärmedizinischen Lehranstalten*, Doctoral thesis (Hannover: Tierärztliche Hochschule Hannover, 1957), pp. 213–222; Astrid von Cramon-Taubadel, *Weltkatalog der Veterinärmedizinischen Lehranstalten nach dem stand von 1976/77*, Doctoral thesis (Hannover: Tierärztliche Hochschule Hannover, 1977), pp. 318–326; Angela von den Driesch & Joris Peters, *Geschichte der Tiermedizin* (Stuttgart & New York: Schattauer, 2003), p. 137; Reinhard Froehner, *Kulturgeschichte der Tierheilkunde. Ein Handbuch für Tierärzte und Studierende*. Vol. 3, *Geschichte des Veterinärwesens im Ausland* (Konstanz: Terra Verlag, 1968), pp. 419–422, 458, 529–531, 640–642; Emmanuel Leclainche, *Histoire de la médecine vétérinaire* (Toulouse: Office du Livre, 1936), pp. 237–238. Thanks are also due to Miguel Marquez (Mexico), Myung-Sun Chun (South Korea), and Junya Yasuda (Japan).

Appendix B   Table of Learning Objectives

Learning Objective	Chapters
Recognize the different views of cultures and societies about animal species	1, 2
Understand how scientific ideas have been communicated between cultures	2, 3, 4, 6
Know the relative importance of different health problems according to social needs and cultural values	2, 3, 4, 5, 6, 7
Understand the role of sacred beliefs in animal healing	1
Learn various theories of disease causation and how they inform veterinary treatment and policy	1, 4, 5, 6, 7
Understand the roles of technological development in shaping veterinary medicine	5, 6, 7
Learn the role of comparative sciences (anatomy, physiology, & pathology) in the relationship between veterinary medicine and human medicine	1, 4, 7
Understand the role of warfare in shaping veterinary medicine	2, 3, 4, 5

Appendix C   Key to Main Topics for Use in the Veterinary Curriculum

Main Topics	Chapters
Anatomy	1
Materia medica & pharmacology	2, 4, 5
Physiology	2
Parasitology	4, 6
Pathology	2, 4, 5
Professionalization	3, 4, 5, 6, 7
Cross-cultural	1, 2, 3, 6
Comparative medicine	4, 5, 6, 7
Surgery	2, 7
Microbiology, virology, & immunology	4, 5, 6
Food hygiene	4, 5, 6
Ethics and deontology	2, 4, 5, 7

Further Reading

Introduction: Human–Animal Relationships and the Need for Veterinary Medicine

Martin F. Brumme, *Tierheilkunde in Antike und Renaissance. Historiografische Untersuchungen zur Konstituierung und Legitimierung* (Berlin: Free University, 1997)

Jacalyn Duffin, *History of Medicine: A Scandalously Short Introduction*, 2nd ed. (Toronto: University of Toronto Press, 2010)

Robert H. Dunlop and David J. Williams, *Veterinary Medicine: An Illustrated History* (St. Louis, MO: Mosby-Year Book, 1996)

Erica Fudge, 'What Was It Like to Be a Cow?', in Linda Kalof (ed.), *Oxford Handbook of Animal Studies* (Oxford and New York: Oxford University Press, 2014/2017) 258–280

Koert van der Horst, *Great Books on Horsemanship: Bibliotheca Hippologica Johan Dejager* (Leiden: Brill, 2014)

I. Hershkovitz, H.D. Donoghue, D.E. Minnikin, et al., 'Tuberculosis Origin: The Neolithic Scenario', *Tuberculosis* (2015). doi:10.1016/j.tube.2015.02.021

L.P. Louwe Kooijmans, 'Van jager tot boer in Nederland', *Argos* 41 (2009) 8–14

Saurabh Mishra 'Veterinary History Comes of Age', *Social History of Medicine* 27 (2014) (Special online issue).

F.R. Rozzi and A. Froment, 'Earliest Animal Cranial Surgery: From Cow to Man in the Neolithic', *Scientific Reports* 8 (2018) 5536–5540

1. Animal Healing in Sacred Societies, 1500–1700

James N. Adams, 'The Origin and Meaning of Lat. *veterinus, veterinarius*', *Indogermanische Forschungen* 97 (1992) 70–95

Pelagonius and Latin Veterinary Terminology in the Roman Empire (Leiden, New York & Cologne: Brill, 1995)

R. Tamay Basagaç Gül, 'From Folk Veterinary Medicine to Scientific Veterinary Medicine in Turkey', Conference paper, 37th World Association for the History of Veterinary Medicine Congress, Leon, Spain, 23 September 23, 2006. www.researchgate.net/publication/341106497_from_folk_veterinary_medicine_to_scientific_veterinary_medicine_in_turkey

Bruce Boehrer (Ed.), *A Cultural History of Animals in the Renaissance* (Oxford & New York: Berg, 2007)

Peter E.J. Bols, 'How Andreas Vesalius Inspired Early Veterinary Authors', in R. van Hee (ed.), *In the Shadow of Vesalius* (Antwerp & Apeldoorn: Garant Publishers, 2020) 249–265

Virginia DeJohn Anderson, *Creatures of Empire: How Domestic Animals Transformed Early America* (Oxford: Oxford University Press, 2006)

Jared Diamond, *Guns, Germs and Steel: A Short History of Everybody for the Last 13,000 Years* (London: Vintage, 1998)

Ferruh Dinçer, 'An Analytical Approach to the Veterinary Knowledge of the Islamic Period', in F. Dinçer (ed.), *Veterinary Medicine – Historical Approaches* (Ankara: Ankara University Press, 2002) 177–194

'Some Notes on the Treatment of Human and Animal Diseases in the Folklore of Turkey and Balkan Countries', *Deutsche tierärztliche Wochenschrift* 98 (1991) 179–180

Angela von den Driesch and Joris Peters, *Geschichte der Tiermedizin: 5000 Jahre Tierheilkunde,* 2nd ed. (München: Schattauer, 2003)

Peter Frankopan, *The Silk Roads: A New History of the World* (New York: Vintage Books, 2017) 94–96, 182–186, 194–196

Anita Guerrini, *The Courtiers' Anatomists: Animals and Humans in Louis XIV's Paris* (Chicago: University of Chicago Press, 2015)

Experimenting with Humans and Animals: From Galen to Animal Rights (Baltimore: Johns Hopkins University Press, 2003)

Anita Guerrini and Domenico Bertoloni Meli, 'Introduction: Experimenting with Animals in the Early Modern Era', *Journal of the History of Biology* 46 (2013) 167–170

Robert Hoyland, 'Theonmestus of Magnesia, Hunayn ibn Ishaq and the Beginnings of Islamic Veterinary Science,' in Hoyland and P. Kennedy (eds.), *Islamic Reflections, Arabic Musings* (Oxford: Oxford University Press, 2004) 150–169

Pamela Hunter, *Veterinary Medicine: A Guide to Historical Sources* (London: Routledge, 2016)

J.H. Lin and R. Panzer, 'Use of Chinese Herbal Medicine in Veterinary Science: History and Perspectives', *Revue scientifique et technique (International Office of Epizootics)* 13 (1994) 2: 425–432

Anne McCabe, *A Byzantine Encyclopedia of Horse Medicine: The Sources, Compilation and Transmissions of the Hippiatrica* (Oxford: Oxford University Press, 2007)

Robert B. Marks, The Origins of the Modern World: A Global and Environmental Narrative from the Fifteenth to the Twenty-First Century, 3rd ed. (Lanham: Rowman & Littlefield, 2007)

G. Mazars, 'Traditional Veterinary Medicine in India', *Revue scientifique et technique (International Office of Epizootics)* 13 (1994) 2: 443–451

Ruth I. Meserve, 'Chinese Hippology and Hippiatry: Government Bureaucracy and Inner Asian Influence,' *Zeitschrift der Deutschen Morgenländischen Gesellschaft* 148 (1998) 2: 277–314

'The Terminology for the Diseases of Domestic Animals in Traditional Mongolian Veterinary Medicine,' *Acta Orientalia Academiae Scientiarum Hungaricae* 49 (1996) 335–358

Alan Mikhail, 'Unleashing the Beast. Animals, Energy, and the Economy of Labor in Ottoman Egypt', *The American Historical Review* 118 (2013) 317–348

Vivian Nutton, 'Logic, Learning, and Experimental Medicine', *Science*, New Series 295 (February 2002) 801

David Ramey, Kaoru Tomoyoshi, Dan Sherer, and Katja Triplett, *Horses: Their Care and Keeping in Muromachi Japan* (includes reproduction and translation of historical manuscript on horse medicine). Hong Kong, forthcoming, 2022

Wilhelm Rieck, 'Das Veterinär-Instrumentarium im Wandel der Zeiten und seine Förderung durch die Instrumentenfabrik H. Hauptner', in *H. Hauptner Instrumentenfabrik für Veterinärmedizin Jubiläums-Katalog 1932* (Berlin: H. Hauptner Instrumentenfabrik, 1932) 1–64

Dagmar Schäfer and Han Yi, 'Great Plans: Song Dynastic (970–1279) Institutions for Human and Veterinary Healthcare,' in Roel Sterckx, Martina Siebert, and Dagmar Schäfer (eds.), *Animals through Chinese History: Earliest Times to 1911* (Cambridge: Cambridge University Press, 2019) 160–180

Calvin Schwabe, *Cattle, Priests and Progress in Medicine* (Minneapolis: University of Minnesota Press, 1973)

Hosni Alkhateeb Shehada, *Mamluks and Animals: Veterinary Medicine in Medieval Islam* (Leiden: Brill, 2012)

Alan Shotwell, 'The Revival of Vivisection in the Sixteenth Century', *Journal of the History of Biology* 46 (2013) 171–197

J.F. Smithcors, *Evolution of the Veterinary Art: A Narrative Account to 1850* (Kansas City, MO: Veterinary Medicine Publishing Co, 1957)

Jasmine Dum Tragut, 'Medieval Equine Medicine from Armenia' (Intech Open Online First, 2020). doi:10.5772/intechopen.91379

Nükhet Varlık, *Plague and Empire in the Early Modern Mediterranean World: The Ottoman Experience, 1347–1600* (Cambridge: Cambridge University Press, 2015)

2. Animal Healing in Trade and Conquest, 1700–1850s

Abdurahim Aloud, 'Ibn al-Nafis and the Discovery of the Pulmonary Circulation', *The Southwest Respiratory and Critical Care Chronicles* 5 (2017) 71–73

Karl Appuhn, 'Ecologies of Beef: Eighteenth-Century Epizootics and the Environmental History of Early Modern Europe', *Environmental History* 15 (2010) 2: 268–287

Tülay Artan, 'Ahmed I and *Tuhfet'ül-mülûk ve's-Selâtîn*: A Period Manuscript on Horses, Horsemanship and Hunting,' in Suraiya Faroqhi (ed.), *Animals and People in the Ottoman Empire* (Instanbul: Eren, 2010) 315–332.

Albano Beja-Pereira, Phillip R. England, Nuno Ferrand, et al. 'The African Origins of the Domestic Donkey', *Science* 304 (2004) 1781

Jeremy Bentham, 'Introduction' to Ch. XVII, *An Introduction to the Principles of Morals and Legislation* (London: Payne, 1789)

Nsekuye Bizimana, *Traditional Veterinary Practice in Africa* (Eschborn, Germany: Deutsche Gesellschaft für Technische Zusammenarbeit, 1994)

Karen Brown and Daniel Gilfoyle (Eds.), *Healing the Herds: Disease, Livestock Economies, and the Globalization of Veterinary Medicine* (Athens: Ohio University Press, 2010)

William Bynum, *The History of Medicine: A Very Short Introduction* (Oxford: Oxford University Press, 2008)

Miguel Cordero del Campillo, Miguel Á. Márquez, and Benito Madariaga de la Campa, *Albeytería, Mariscalía y Veterinaria (Orígenes y perspectiva literaria)* (León: University of León, 1996)

Alfred W. Crosby Jr., *The Columbian Exchange: Biological and Cultural Consequences of 1492* (Westport: Greenwood Publishing Group, 1972)
Ecological Imperialism: The Biological Expansion of Europe, 900–1900 (Cambridge: Cambridge University Press, 1986)

Louise Hill Curth, *The Care of Brute Beasts: A Social and Cultural Study of Veterinary Medicine in Early Modern England* (Leiden and Boston: Brill, 2010)

Jim Downs, *Maladies of Empire: How Colonialism, Slavery and War Transformed Medicine*. Cambridge, MA: Harvard University Press, 2021.

Jacalyn Duffin, *History of Medicine: A Scandalously Short Introduction*, 2nd ed. (Toronto: University of Toronto Press, 2010)

Saraiya Faroqi, *Animals and People in the Ottoman Empire* (Istanbul: Erren, 2010)

George Fleming, *Animal Plagues: Their History, Nature and Prevention* (London: Chapman and Hall, 1871)
Travels on Horseback in Mantchu Tartary: Being a Summer's Ride beyond the Great Wall of China (London: Hurst and Blackett, 1863) (Cambridge Library Collection – Travel and Exploration in Asia. Cambridge: Cambridge University Press, 2010). doi:10.1017/CBO9780511709531

Henrico N. Franco, 'Animal Experiments in Biomedical Research: A Historical Perspective', *Animals* 3 (2013) 238–273

Wilma Gijsbers and Peter A. Koolmees, 'Food on Foot. Long-Distance Trade in Slaughter Oxen between Denmark and the Netherlands (14th–18th Century)', *Historia Medicinae Veterinariae* 26 (2001) 115–127

Robert E. Harrist Jr., 'The Legacy of Bole: Physiognomy and Horses in Chinese Painting', *Artibus Asie* 57 (1997) 1/2: 135–156

Constant Huygelen, 'The Immunization of Cattle against Rinderpest in Eighteenth-Century Europe', *Medical History* 41 (1997) 182–196

Susan D. Jones, *Death in a Small Package: A Short History of Anthrax* (Baltimore, MD: The Johns Hopkins University Press, 2010)

D. Karasszon, *A Concise History of Veterinary Medicine* (Budapest: Akadémiai Kiadó, 1988)

Amanda Kluveld, *Mensendier. Verbonden sinds de zesde dag. Cultuurgeschiedenis van een wonderlijke relatie* (Amsterdam, De Arbeiderspers: 2009)

Charles C. Mann, *1493: How Europe's Discovery of the Americas Revolutionized Trade, Ecology and Life on Earth* (New York: Granta Books, 2012)

Nicholas Malebranche, *De la recherche de la verité*, in *Œvres de Malebranche*, vol. 2 (Paris: Charpentier (1842 [1674]).

William Hardy McNeill, *Plagues and Peoples* (New York: Anchor, 1976)

Michel de Montaigne, tr. Charles Cotton (1686). 'Apology for Raymond Sebond,' *Essays*, Book 2, Chapter 12, paragraph 63.

Mireille Mousnier (Ed.) *Les animaux maladies en Europe occidentale (VIe–XIXe siècle)* (Toulouse: Presses Universitaires du Mirail, 2003)

Leon Z. Saunders, *Biographical History of Veterinary Pathology* (Lawrence: Allen Press, 1996)

'Virchow's Contributions to Veterinary Medicine: Celebrated Then, Forgotten Now', *Veterinary Pathology* 37 (2000) 199–207

Frederick Smith, *The Early History of Veterinary Literature* (2 vols.) (London: Baillière, Tindall and Cox, 1919, 1933)

R. Somvanshi, 'Veterinary Medicine and Animal Keeping in Ancient India', *Ancient Agri-History* 10 (2006) 2: 133–146

Clive A. Spinage, *Cattle Plague: A History* (New York: Kluwer Academic / Plenum Publishers, 2003)

Keith Thomas, *Man and the Natural World: Changing Attitudes in England, 1500–1800* (London: Allen Lane, 1983)

Sam White, 'A Model Disaster: From the Great Ottoman Panzootic to the Cattle Plagues of Early Modern Europe', in Nükhet Varlık (ed.), *Plague and Contagion in the Islamic Mediterranean* (Kalamazoo and Bradford: ARC Humanities Press, 2017) 91–116

Lise Wilkinson, *Animals and Disease: An Introduction to the History of Comparative Medicine* (Cambridge: Cambridge University Press, 1992)

Abigail Woods, 'Doctors in the Zoo: Connecting Human and Animal Health in British Zoological Gardens, c. 1828–1890', in Abigail Woods, Michael Bresalier, Angela Cassidy, and Rachel Mason-Dentinger (eds.), *Animals and the Shaping of Modern Medicine: One Health and Its Histories* (London: Palgrave Macmillan, 2018) 27–70

3. Formal Education for Animal Healing: From Riding Schools to Veterinary Schools, 1700–1850

J.M. Arburua, 'History of Veterinary Medicine in the United States', *Journal of the American Veterinary Medical Association* 85 (1934) 4: 10–38

Charles Julian Bishko, 'The Peninsular Background of Latin American Cattle Ranching', *The Hispanic American Historical Review* 32 (November 1952) 4: 491–515

Philippe Blom, *Encyclopédie, The Triumph of Reason in an Unreasonable Age* (London: Fourth Estate, 2004)

Peter E.J. Bols, E. Dumas, J. Op de Beeck, and H.M.F. De Porte, 'De Maréchal-vétérinaire in de Grande Armée van Napoleon (1805–1815)', *Vlaams Diergeneeskundig Tijdschrift* 84 (2015) 333–342

Peter E.J. Bols, 'Is Modern-Day Veterinary Medicine a Product of the Age of Enlightenment?', *Sartoniana* 32 (2019) 229–244

Francesca Bray, 'Where Did the Animals Go? Presence and Absence of Livestock in Chinese Agricultural Treatises,' in Roel Sterckx, Martina Siebert, and Dagmar Schäfer (eds.), *Animals through Chinese History: Earliest Times to 1911* (Cambridge: Cambridge University Press, 2019) 118–138

Miguel Codero del Campillo, 'Medical and Veterinary Reports from Colonial Latin America', in Ferruh Dinçer (ed.), *Veterinary Medicine – Historical Approaches* (Ankara: Ankara University Press, 2002) 143–157

'On the History of Veterinary Knowledge in the Old and New Worlds', *Argos* 30 (2004) 457–469

Ernest Cotchen, *The Royal Veterinary College London: A Bicentenary History* (London: Barracuda Books Ltd, 1990) 11–13

P. Cottereau and J. Weber-Godde, *Claude Bourgelat. Un Lyonnais fondateur des deux premières écoles vétérinaires du monde (1712–1779)* (Lyon: La Maison Chirat, 2011)

Astrid von Cramon-Taubadel, *Weltkatalog der Veterinärmedizinischen Lehranstalten nach dem Stand von 1976/77* (Hanover: Tierärztliche Hochschule, 1977)

Margaret Elsinor Derry, *Horses in Society: A Story of Animal Breeding and Marketing, 1800–1920* (Toronto, Buffalo, London: Toronto University Press, 2006)

Robert H. Dunlop, 'Bourgelat's Vision for Veterinary Education and the Remarkable Spread of the Veterinary "Meme"', *Journal of Veterinary Medical Education* 31 (2004) 310–322

Gülşah Eser, 'The Role of the Military School in the Development of Veterinary Medicine in Turkey', in R. Tamay Basagaç Gül (ed.), *Some Essays on Veterinary History* (Ankara: Ankara University Press, 2012) 103–116

Suraiya Faruqhi (Ed.) *Animals and People in the Ottoman Empire* (İstanbul: Eren, 2010)

Marleen Felius, P. Koolmees, B. Theunissen, and J. Lenstra, 'On the Breeds of Cattle – Historic and Current Classifications', *Diversity* 3 (2011) 660–692

John R. Fisher, 'The European Enlightenment, Political Economy and the Origins of the Veterinary Profession in Britain', *Argos* 12 (1995) 45–51

Reinhard Froehner, *Kulturgeschichte der Tierheilkunde: ein Handbuch für Tierärzte und Studierende. Band 2: Geschichte des Veterinärwesens im Ausland* (Konstanz: Terra, 1952)

Caroline C. Hannaway, 'Veterinary Medicine and Rural Health Care in Pre-revolutionary France', *Bulletin of the History of Medicine* 51 (1977) 431–447

Kit Heintzman, 'A Cabinet of the Ordinary: Domesticating Veterinary Education, 1766–1799', *The British Journal for the History of Science* 51 (2018) 239–260

'History of Veterinary Medicine', *Iowa State University Veterinarian* 2 (1939) 1: 6–10

Ronald Hubscher, *Les maîtres des bêtes. Les vétérinaires dans la société française (XVIIIe-XXe siècle)* (Paris: Odile Jacob, 1999)

Dominik Hünniger, 'Policing Epizootics: Legislation and Administration during Outbreaks of Cattle Plague in Eighteenth Century Northern Germany as Continuous Crisis Management,' in Karen Brown and Daniel Gilfoyle (eds.), *Healing the Herds. Disease, Livestock Economies, and the Globalization of Veterinary Medicine* (Athens: Ohio University Press, 2010) 76–91

Benjamin Kaplan, *Divided by Faith: Religious Conflict and the Practice of Toleration in Early Modern Europe* (Cambridge, MA: Harvard University Press, 2010)

Osamu Katsuyama, 'Veterinary Folk Remedies', *Revue scientifique et technique (International Office of Epizootics)* 13 (1994) 2: 453–463

И.С. Колесниченко [I.S. Kolesnichenko], История ветеринарии [Veterinary History], in Russian (Moscow 2010). Ebook, https://1lib.us/book/3082785/1bb9ae?id=3082785&secret=1bb9ae. Accessed April 10, 2021

Peter A. Koolmees, 'The Professionalization of Medical Professions in the Netherlands 1840–1940', in Johann Schäffer (ed.), *Domestication of Animals, Interactions between Veterinary and Medical Sciences* (Giessen: Deutsche Veterinärmedizinische Gesellschaft, 1999) 54–64

Robert Kreiser, '"La cendrillon des sciences": Toward the Professionalization of Veterinary Medicine in Eighteenth- and Nineteenth-Century France', *Proceedings Consortium on Revolutionary Europe 1750–1850* 13 (1984) 180–197

Emmanuel Leclainche, *Histoire de la Médicine Vétérinaire* (Toulouse: Office du Livre, 1936)

Franklin M. Loew, 'Animals and People in Revolutionary France: Scientists, Cavalry, Farmers and Vétérinaires', *Anthrozoös* 4 (1991) 1: 7–13

A. Mathijsen (Ed.) *The Origins of Veterinary Schools in Europe – A Comparative View* (Utrecht: Veterinair Historisch Genootschap, 1997)

L.A. Merillat and D.M. Campbell, *Veterinary Military History of the United States* (Chicago: Veterinary Magazine Corp., 1935)

Alan Mikhail, *The Animal in Ottoman Egypt* (Oxford: Oxford University Press, 2014)

Tatsuya Mitsuda, 'Entangled Histories: German Veterinary Medicine, c. 1770–1900', *Medical History* 61 (2017) 1: 25–47

Jacques Nicolet, 'La Faculté de Médecine vétérinaire de Berne: une vieille histoire', *Schweizer Archiv für Tierheilkunde* 146 (2006) 1: 33–40

Rahsan Özen and Abdullah Özen, 'Veterinary Education in Turkey', *Journal of Veterinary Medical Education* 33 (2006) 2: 187–196

Zeynel Ozlu, 'An Evaluation on Veterinary Medicine in the Ottoman Empire towards the End of the 19th Century', *Belleten (Türk Tarih Kurumu)* 76 (March 2012) 238–247

Roy Porter, *Blood & Guts: A Short History of Medicine* (London: Penguin Books, 2002)

Filip van Roosbroek, 'Caring for Cows in a Time of Rinderpest: Non-Academic Veterinary Practitioners in the County of Flanders, 1769–1785', *Social History of Medicine* 32 (2017) 3: 502–522

Housni Alkhateeb Shehada, 'Arabic Veterinary Medicine and the "Golden Rules" for Veterinarians according to a Sixteenth-Century Treatise', in Suraiya Faraqhi (ed.), *Animals and People in the Ottoman Empire* (Istanbul: Eren, 2010) 315–332

François Vallat, *Les bœufs malades de la peste: La peste bovine en France et en Europe (XVIIIe–XIXe siècle)* (Rennes: Presses Universitaires de Rennes, 2009)

Karol K. Weaver, *Medical Revolutionaries: The Enslaved Healers of 18th-Century St. Domingue* (Urbana, IL: University of Illinois Press, 2006) Chapter 5

Lise Wilkinson, 'Glanders: Medicine and Veterinary Medicine in Common Pursuit of a Contagious Disease', *Medical History* 25 (1981) 363–384

4. Veterinary Institutions and Animal Plagues, 1800–1900

E. Aalbers and Bent Christensen, *Short History of the World Veterinary Association 1863–2005*. WVA website: www.worldvet.org/about.php?sp=history. Accessed April 10, 2021

Erwin Ackerknecht, 'Anti-contagionism between 1821 and 1867', *International Journal of Epidemiology* 38 (2009) 7–21; reprinted from *Bulletin of the History of Medicine* 22 (1948) 562–593

Ioana Cristina Andronie, Dumitru Curcă, and Viorel Andronie, 'General MD Carol Davila Founder of the Human-Veterinary Medical and Pharmacy Education in

Bucharest-Romania', in R. Tamay Basagaç Gül (ed.), *Some Essays on Veterinary History* (Ankara: Ankara University Press, 2012) 51–62

Sare Aricanli, 'Reconsidering the Boundaries: Multicultural and Multilingual Perspectives on the Care and Management of the Emperors' Horses in the Qing,' in Roel Sterckx, Martina Siebert, and Dagmar Schäfer (eds.), *Animals Through Chinese History: Earliest Times to 1911* (Cambridge: Cambridge University Press, 2019) 199–216

Martine Barwegen, 'For Better or Worse? The Impact of the Veterinary Service on the Development of the Agricultural Society in Java (Indonesia) in the Nineteenth Century', in Karen Brown and Daniel Gilfoyle (eds.), *Healing the Herds: Disease, Livestock Economies, and the Globalization of Veterinary Medicine* (Athens: Ohio University Press, 2010) 92–107

William Beinart, 'Vets Viruses and Environmentalism. The Cape in the 1870s and 1880s', *Paideuma, Journal of Research* 43 (1997) 227–252

William Beinart and Saul Dubow, *The Scientific Imagination in South Africa, 1700 to the Present* (Cambridge: Cambridge University Press, 2021)

Natalia Ye. Beregoy, 'The Fight against Cattle Plague in Russia, 1830–1902: A Brief Overview of Methodological Approaches', *Studies in the History of Biology* (St. Petersburg) 4 (2012) 3: 94–100

Jean Blancou, *History of the Surveillance and Control of Transmissible Animal Diseases* (Paris: Office International des Épizooties, 2003)

Elpidio Gonzalo Chamizo Pestana, Jose Manuel et al., 'A Century of Veterinary Education in Cuba (1907–2007)', *Journal of Veterinary Medical Education* 37 (2007) 2: 118–125

Paul F. Cranefield, *Science and Empire: East Coast Fever in Rhodesia and the Transvaal* (Cambridge: Cambridge University Press, 1991)

A. Cunningham and B. Andrews (Eds.) *Western Medicine as Contested Knowledge* (Manchester: Manchester University Press, 1997)

Dumitru Curcă, Ioana Cristina Andronie, and Viorel Andronie, 'From the History of the Romanian Scientific Societies of Veterinary Medicine', *Scientific Papers, Series C: Veterinary Medicine* LVIII (2011) 3: 1124+. http://veterinarymedicinejournal .usamv.ro/pdf/vol.LVIII_3/Art10.pdf. Accessed January 12, 2021

Diana K. Davis, 'Brutes, Beasts and Empire: Veterinary Medicine and Environmental Policy in French North Africa and British India', *Journal of Historical Geography* 34 (2008) 242–267

Janet Davis, *The Gospel of Kindness: Animal Welfare and the Making of Modern America* (Oxford and London: Oxford University Press, 2016)

Ferruh Dinçer, '100 Years of Veterinary Microbiological Institutes in Turkey,' in F. Dinçer (ed.), *Veterinary Medicine – Historical Approaches* (Ankara: Ankara University Press, 2002) 313–325

Daniel F. Doeppers, 'Fighting Rinderpest in the Philippines 1886–1941', in Karen Brown and Daniel Gilfoyle (eds.), *Healing the Herds: Disease, Livestock Economies, and the Globalization of Veterinary Medicine* (Athens: Ohio University Press, 2010) 108–128

Kari T. Elvbakken, 'Veterinarians and Public Health: Food Control in the Professionalization of Veterinarians', *Professions & Professionalism* 7 (2017) 2. http://doi.org/10.7577/pp.1806

John R. Fisher, 'To Kill or Not to Kill: The Eradication of Contagious Bovine Pleuro-Pneumonia in Western Europe', *Medical History* 47 (2003) 314–331

Anne Fowler la Berge, 'The Paris Health Council, 1802–1848', *Bulletin of the History of Medicine* 49 (1975) 339–352

Daniel Gilfoyle, 'Veterinary Research and the African Rinderpest Epizootic: The Cape Colony, 1896–1898', *Journal of Southern African Studies* 29 (March 2003) 1: 133–154

Vincent Goosseart, 'Animals in Nineteenth-Century Eschatological Discourse,' in Roel Sterckx, Martina Siebert, and Dagmar Schäfer (eds.), *Animals through Chinese History: Earliest Times to 1911* (Cambridge: Cambridge University Press, 2019) 181–198

Constant Huygelen, 'The Early Years of Vaccinology: Prophylactic Immunization in the Eighteenth and Nineteenth Centuries', *Sartoriana* 10 (1997) 79–110

Susan D. Jones, *Valuing Animals: Veterinarians and Their Patients in Modern America* (Baltimore, MD: The Johns Hopkins University Press, 2003)

Edward F. Keuchel, 'Chemicals and Meat: The Embalmed Beef Scandal of the Spanish-American War', *Bulletin of the History of Medicine* 48 (1974) 2: 249–264

Peter A. Koolmees, 'The Development of Veterinary Public Health in Western Europe, 1850–1940', *Sartoniana* 12 (1999) 153–179

'Veterinary Inspection and Food Hygiene in the Twentieth Century', in D.F. Smith and J. Phillips (eds.), *Food, Science, Policy and Regulation in the Twentieth Century: International and Comparative Perspectives* (London & New York: Routledge, 2000) 53–68

'Veterinarians, Abattoirs and the Urban Meat Supply in the Netherlands 1860–1940', in Marjatta Hietala and T. Vahtikari (eds.), *The Landscape of Food: The Food Relationship of Town and Country in Modern Times* (Tampere: Finnish Literature Society, 2003) 17–29

'Epizootic Diseases in the Netherlands, 1713–2002: Veterinary Science, Agricultural Policy, and Public Response', in Karen Brown and Daniel Gilfoyle (eds.), *Healing the Herds: Disease, Livestock Economies, and the Globalization of Veterinary Medicine* (Athens: Ohio University Press, 2010) 19–41

Gary Marquardt, 'Water, Wood and Wild Animal Populations: Seeing the Spread of Rinderpest through the Physical Environment in Bechuanaland, 1896', *South African Historical Journal* 53 (2005) 73–98

Clapperton Chakanetsa Mavhunga, *Transient Workspaces: Technologies of Everyday Innovation in Zimbabwe* (Cambridge, MA: The MIT Press, 2014) Chapter 4

Berfin Melikoğlu, 'A Forgotten Album: École Vétérinaire Civil', in R. Tamay Başağaç Gül (ed.), *Some Essays on Veterinary History* (Ankara: Ankara University Press, 2012) 245–255

'Osman Nuri Eralp' in "Bakteriyoloji dersleri" adlı kitabının veteriner hekimliği tarihi açısından değerlendirilmesi'. Ph.D. dissertation (The Graduate School of Health Sciences of Ankara University: Ankara, Turkey 2007)

Saurabh Mishra, *Beastly Encounters of the Raj: Livelihoods, Livestock and Veterinary Health in North India, 1790–1920* (Manchester: Manchester University Press, 2015)

David A.A. Mossel and Karl E. Dijkmann, 'A Centenary of Academic and Less Learned Food Microbiology Pitfalls of the Past and Promises for the Future', *Antonie van Leeuwenhoek* 50 (1984) 641–663

Türel Özkul and R. Tamay Basagaç Gül, 'The Collaboration of Maurice Nicolle and Adil Mustafa: The Discovery of the Rinderpest Agent', *Revue de Médecine Vétérinaire* 159 (2008) 243–246

Richard Perren, 'The Manufacture and Marketing of Veterinary Products from 1859 to 1914', *Veterinary History* 6 (1989) 43–61

Terrie Romano, *Making Medicine Scientific: John Burdon Sanderson and the Culture of Victorian Science* (Baltimore, MD: The Johns Hopkins University Press, 2002) Chapter 3

Samanta Samiparna, 'Cruelty Contested: The British, Bengalis, and Animals in Colonial Bengal, 1850–1920'. Ph.D. dissertation (Tallahassee: Florida State University, 2012)

Laxman D. Satya, *Ecology, Colonialism and Cattle: Central India in the Nineteenth Century* (Oxford: Oxford University Press, 2004)

Calvin W. Schwabe, *Veterinary Medicine and Public Health*, 3rd ed. (Baltimore: Williams & Wilkins, 1984)

Johann Schäffer, 'The Veterinary Historical Museum at the Hannover School of Veterinary Medicine – History, Conception, Duties and Problem', *Deutsche tierärztliche Wochenschrift* 101 (1994) 8: 326–330

James Serpell, *In the Company of Animals: A Study of Human–Animal Relationships* (Cambridge: Cambridge University Press, 1996)

Thaddeus Sunseri, 'The African Rinderpest Panzootic, 1888–1897', in *Oxford Research Encyclopedia of African History* (Oxford: Oxford University Press, 2018)

'The Entangled History of *Sadoka* (Rinderpest) and Veterinary Science in Tanzania and the Wider World, 1891–1901', *Bulletin of the History of Medicine* 89 (2015) 92–121

Joanna Swabe, *Animals, Disease and Human Society: Human–Animal Relations and the Rise of the Veterinary Regime* (London: Routledge, 1999)

Sandra Swart, *Riding High: Horses, Humans and History in South Africa* (Johannesburg: Witwatersrand University Press, 2010)

H. Tadjbakhsh, 'Veterinary Medicine in Iran', in H. Selin (ed.), *Encyclopaedia of the History of Science, Technology, and Medicine in Non-Western Cultures* (Dordrecht: Springer). https://doi.org/10.1007/978-1-4020-4425-0_8913

Philip M. Teigen, 'William Osler and Comparative Medicine', *Canadian Veterinary Journal* 25 1984) 10: 400–405

Peter Verhoef (Ed.) *'Strictly Scientific and Practical Sense': A Century of the Central Veterinary Institute in the Netherlands, 1904–2004* (Rotterdam: Erasmus Publishing, 2005)

Keir Waddington, *The Bovine Scourge: Meat, Tuberculosis and Public Health, 1850–1914* (Woodbridge: Boydell Press, 2006)

A. Wijgergangs and Ivan Katić, *Guide to Veterinary Museums of the World* (Copenhagen and Utrecht 1997), also published as *Historia Medicinae Veterinariae* 21 (1996) 1–4: 1–77

Lise Wilkinson, *Animals and Disease: An Introduction to the History of Comparative Medicine* (Cambridge: Cambridge University Press, 2005)

Michael Worboys, *Spreading Germs: Disease, Theories and Medical Practice in Britain, 1865–1900* (Cambridge: Cambridge University Press, 2000)

5. Veterinary Medicine in War and Peace, 1900–1960

David Anderson, 'Kenya's Cattle Trade and the Economics of Empire, 1918–1948', in Karen Brown and Daniel Gilfoyle (eds.), *Healing the Herds: Disease, Livestock Economies, and the Globalization of Veterinary Medicine* (Athens: Ohio University Press, 2010) 250–268

Peter Atkins and Ian Bowler, *Food in Society: Economy, Culture, Geography* (New York: Oxford University Press, 2001)

Karen Brown, 'Tropical Medicine and Animal Diseases: Onderstepoort and the Development of Veterinary Science in South Africa 1908–1950', *Journal of South African Studies* 31 (2005) 3: 513–529

C.H. Calisher and M.C. Horzinek (Eds.) *100 Years of Virology: The Birth and Growth of a Discipline* (Vienna: Springer, 1999)

William G. Clarence-Smith, 'Diseases of Equids in Southeast Asia, c. 1800 – c. 1945', in Karen Brown and Daniel Gilfoyle (eds.), *Healing the Herds: Disease, Livestock Economies, and the Globalization of Veterinary Medicine* (Athens: Ohio University Press, 2010) 129–145

'Horses, Mules and Other animals as a Factor in Ottoman Military Performance, 1683–1918', Presented at War Horses of the World, conference, SOAS, University of London, May 3–4, 2014. www.soas.ac.uk/history/conferences/war-horses-conference-2014/

'*Trypanosoma evansi* (surra) in camels,' Presented at The Camel Conference, SOAS, University of London, May 23–25, 2011. www.soas.ac.uk/camelconference2011/

Bryan D. Cummins, *Colonel Richardson's Airedales – The Making of the British War Dog School 1900–1918* (Calgary: Detselig Enterprises Ltd, 2003)

Diana K. Davis, 'Prescribing Progress: French Veterinary Medicine in the Service of Empire', *Veterinary Heritage* 29 (2006) 1: 1–7

Janet M. Davis, 'Where Gasoline Can't Go: Equine Patriotism and the American Red Star Animal Relief Campaign during World War I,' Presented at War Horses of the World, conference, SOAS, University of London, May 3–4, 2014. www.soas.ac.uk/history/conferences/war-horses-conference-2014/

Alanna Demers, 'They Kill Horses, Don't They? Peasant Resistance and the Decline of the Horse Population in Soviet Russia'. Thesis (Bowling Green, Ohio: Graduate College of Bowling Green State University, 2016)

R.L. DiNardo and Austin Bay, 'Horse-Drawn Transport in the German Army', *Journal of Contemporary History* 23 (1988) 129–142

Emmanuel Dumas, 'Les vétérinaires morts pour la France pendant la guerre de 1914–1918', *Bulletin de la Société française d'histoire de la médecine et des sciences vétérinaires* 8 (2008) 123–143

Andrew Gardiner, '"The Dangerous Women" of Animal Welfare: How British Veterinary Medicine Went to the Dogs', *Social History of Medicine* 27 (2014) 3: 466–487

Sigfried Giedion, *Mechanization Takes Command: A Contribution to Anonymous History* (New York: Oxford University Press, 1948)

Daniel Gilfoyle, 'Veterinary Immunology as Colonial Science: Method and Quantification in the Investigation of Horse sickness in South Africa,' *Journal of the History of Medicine and Allied Sciences* 61 (2006) 1: 26–65

Ann Norton Greene, *Horses at Work: Harnessing Power in Industrial America* (Cambridge, MA: Harvard University Press, 2008)

Katherine C. Grier, *Pets in America: A History* (Chapel Hill: University of North Carolina Press, 2015)

José Manuel Gutiérrez Garcia, 'Meat as a Vector of Transmission of Bovine Tuberculosis to Humans in Spain: A Historical Perspective', *Veterinary Heritage* 29 (2006) 1: 25–27

E. Guzman and M. Montoya, 'Contributions of Farm Animals to Immunology,' *Frontiers in Veterinary Science* 5 (2018) 307

Floor Haalboom, *Negotiating Zoonoses: Dealings with Infectious Diseases Shared by Humans and Livestock in the Netherlands 1898–2001*. Ph.D. dissertation (Utrecht: Utrecht University, 2017)

Lotte Hughes, 'They Give Me Fever: East Coast Fever and Other Environmental Impacts of the Maasai Moves', in Karen Brown and Daniel Gilfoyle (eds.), *Healing the Herds: Disease, Livestock Economies, and the Globalization of Veterinary Medicine* (Athens: Ohio University Press, 2010) 146–162

Susan D. Jones, 'Scientific Debates and Popular Beliefs: A Historical Study of Bovine Tuberculosis,' *Argos* 27 (2002) 313–318

'A History of Veterinarians and Biological Weapons during the World Wars,' Revista de Colegio des Médicos Veterinarios del Estado Lara *(Venezuela)* 3 (June 2013) 1. http://revistacmvl.jimdo.com/suscripción/volumen-5/world-wars/

'Defining the Threat: American Veterinarians and Bovine Tuberculosis Eradication in the World War II Era', *Veterinary Heritage* 28 (2005) 2: 33–37

Diana Murphy Jordan, 'Hog Cholera: A Historical Review', *Veterinary Heritage* 21 (1998) 1: 1–8

John Keegan, *A History of Warfare* (New York: Vintage Books, 1994)

Emily R. Kilby, 'The Demographics of the U.S. Equine Population', in D.J. Salem and A.N. Rowan (eds.), *The State of the Animals 2007* (Washington, DC: Humane Society Press, 2007) 175–205

Peter A. Koolmees, 'Meat in the Past: A Bird's-Eye View on Meat Consumption, Production and Research in the Western World from Antiquity to 1945', in W. Sybesma, P.A. Koolmees, and D.G. van der Heij (eds.), *Meat Past and Present: Research, Production, Consumption* (Zeist, Netherlands: TNO Nutrition and Food Research Institute, 1994) 5–32

'The Role of Veterinary Medicine in the Development of Factory Farming', in Francien de Jonge and Ruud van den Bos (eds.), *The Human–Animal Relationship: Forever and a Day* (Assen: Royal Van Gorcum, 2005) 249–264

'From Stable to Table: The Development of the Meat Industry in the Netherlands, 1850–1990', in Yves Segers, Jan Bieleman, and Erik Buyst (eds.), *Exploring the Food Chain: Food Production and Food Processing in Western Europe, 1850–1990* (Turnhout: Brepols Publishers, 2009) 117–137

'Veterinary Medicine in The Netherlands, 1940–1945', in Johann Schäffer (ed.), *Veterinärmedizin im Dritten Reich* (Giessen: Deutsche Veterinärmedizinische Gesellschaft, 1998) 262–275

'From the Marshall Plan to Present Day Prosperity: Veterinary Medicine in the Netherlands 1945–2000', *Schweizer Archiv für Tierheilkunde* 144 (2002) 24–31

'Bovine Brucellosis and Post-War Dutch Veterinary Medicine', in Johann Schäffer (ed.), *Geschichte der Gynäkologie und Andrologie der Haustiere* (Giessen: Deutsche Veterinärmedizinische Gesellschaft, 2008) 198–203

Peter Koolmees and Charlotte Hartong, 'Dierenartsen en chemische wapens in Nederland, 1914–1940,' *Argos: Bulletin van het Veterinair Historisch Genootschap* 64 (2021) 131–142

Milton Leitenberg, 'Biological Weapons in the Twentieth Century: A Review and Analysis', *Critical Reviews in Microbiology* 27 (2001) 267–320

Amanda Kay McVety, *The Rinderpest Campaigns: A Virus, Its Vaccines, and Global Development in the Twentieth Century* (Cambridge and London: Cambridge University Press, 2018)

Berfin Melikoglu, R. Tamay Basagaç Gül, and T. Özkul, 'Paul Ambroise Remlinger: A Pasteurien in Turkey and His Studies on Rabies', *Revue Médecine Vétérinaire* 160 (2009) 7: 374–377

Everett B. Miller, *United States Army Veterinary Service in World War II* (Washington, DC: U.S. Government Printing Office, 1961)

Shaun N. Milton, 'Western Veterinary Medicine in Colonial Africa: A Survey, 1902–1963', *Argos* 18 (1998) 313–322

Martin Monestier, *Les animaux-soldats: Histoire militaire des animaux, des origines à nos jours* (Paris: Cherche Midi, 1996)

Stephen A. Morse, 'Historical Perspectives of Microbial Bioterrorism', in B. Anderson, H. Friedman, and M. Bendinelli (eds.), *Microorganisms and Bioterrorism* (New York: Springer, 2006) 15–29

Arthur W. Moss and Elizabeth Kirby, *Animals Were There: A Record of the Work of the R.S.P.C.A. during the War of 1939–1945* (London, New York, Melbourne, Sydney, Cape Town: Hutchinson & Co., 1946)

Rita Pemberton, 'Animal Disease and Veterinary Administration in Trinidad and Tobago, 1879–1962', in Karen Brown and Daniel Gilfoyle (eds.), *Healing the Herds: Disease, Livestock Economies, and the Globalization of Veterinary Medicine* (Athens: Ohio University Press, 2010) 163–179

Robert John Perrins, 'Holding Water in Bamboo Buckets: Agricultural Science, Livestock Breeding, and Veterinary Medicine in Colonial Manchuria', in Karen Brown and Daniel Gilfoyle (eds.), *Healing the Herds: Disease, Livestock Economies, and the Globalization of Veterinary Medicine* (Athens: Ohio University Press, 2010) 195–214

Roger Roffy, A. Tegnell, and F. Elgh, 'Biological Warfare in a Historical Perspective', *Clinical Microbiology and Infection* 8 (2002) 450–454

Leon Z. Saunders, *Veterinary Pathology in Russia, 1860–1930* (Ithaca, NY: Cornell University Press, 1980)

Boria Sax, *Animals in the Third Reich: Pets, Scapegoats and the Holocaust* (New York & London: Continuum, 2000)

Johann Schäffer (Ed.) *Veterinärmedizin im Dritten Reich* (Giessen: Deutsche
Veterinärmedizinische Gesellschaft, 1998)
  *Veterinary Medicine and National Socialism in Europe: Status and
  Perspectives of Research* (Giessen: Deutsche Veterinärmedizinische
  Gesellschaft, 2018)
James Serpell, *In the Company of Animals: A Study of Human–Animal Relationships*
(Cambridge: Cambridge University Press, 1996)
John Singleton, 'Britain's Military Use of Horses 1914–1918', *Past and Present* 139
(1993) 178–203
Ole H.V. Stalheim, *The Winning of Animal Health: 100 Years of Veterinary Medicine*
(Hoboken, NJ: Wiley-Blackwell, 1995)
  Veterinary Conversations with Mid-Twentieth Century Leaders (Hoboken, NJ:
  Wiley-Blackwell, 1997)
James H. Steele, 'A Personal History of Veterinary Public Health', *Veterinary Heritage*
21 (1998) 1: 9–11
Norman Stone, *World War One: A Short History* (New York: Basic Books, 2009)
Sandra Swart, 'Horses in the South African War, c. 1899–1902', *Society and Animals*
18 (2010) 348–366
Joel A. Tarr and Clay McShane, 'The Horse as an Urban Technology', *Journal of
Urban Technology* 15 (2008) 1: 5–17
Philip M. Teigen, 'Nineteenth-Century Veterinary Medicine as an Urban Profession',
Veterinary Heritage 23 (2000) 1–6
  'Counting Urban Horses in the United States', *Argos* 26 (2002) 267–276
F.M.L. Thompson, *Horses in European Economic History: A Preliminary Canter*
(Reading: British Agricultural History Society, 1983)
Ulrike Thoms, 'Travelling Back and Forth. Antibiotics in the Clinic, Stable and Food
Industry in Germany in the1950s and 60s', in Ana Romero, Christoph Gradmann,
and Maria Santemases (eds.), *Circulation of Antibiotics: Journeys of Drug
Standards, 1930–1970* (Madrid and Oslo: European Science Foundation, 2010)
81–121
Naudy Trujillo Mascia, 'Aportes para la Historia de la Historiografía Médico
Veterinaria Venezolana', *Revista Electrónica de Veterinaria* 11 (2010) 3. www
.historiaveterinaria.org/update/aportes-hist-vet-venez-1457101406.pdf
Y. Zhang, L. Colli, and J. S. F. Barker, 'Asian Water Buffalo: Domestication, History
and Genetics', *Animal Genetics* 51 (2020) 2: 177–191. https://doi.org/10.1111/age
.12911

6. Food, Animals, and Veterinary Care in a Changing World, 1960–2000

Katinka K.I.M. de Balogh, 'De rol van de (vrouwelijke) dierenarts in Africa', *Argos* 23
(2000) 132–137
Raziye Tamay Başağaç Gül, Türel Özkul, Aytac Akçay, and Abdullah Özen,
  'Historical Profile of Gender in Turkish Veterinary Education', *Journal of
  Veterinary Medical Education* 35 (2008) 2: 305–309
Roscoe Bell, editorial, *American Veterinary Review* 21 (1897) 595–596

Hanna E.N. Buenot, 'Témoignages de femmes vétérinaires en France de 1950 à nos jours'. Ph.D. dissertation (Alfort: Ecole Nationale Vétérinaire d'Alfort, 2011)

Martin Brumme (Ed.) *Veterinärmedizin im Sozialismus* (Giessen, Deutsche Veterinärmedizinische Gesellschaft, 1995)

Robert Bud, *Penicillin: Triumph and Tragedy* (Oxford: Oxford University Press, 2007)

Angela Cassidy et al., 'Animal Roles and Traces in the History of Medicine, c.1880–1980', *British Journal for the History of Science* (2017) 2: 11–33

Ana Rodríguez Castaño, 'La veterinaria en femenino: pioneras en España y evolución profesional en la Comunidad de Madrid'. Thesis (Madrid: Faculty of Veterinary Medicine, Complutense University, 2015)

Committee to Assess Current and Future Workforce Needs, *Workforce Needs in Veterinary Medicine* (Washington, DC: The National Academies of Sciences Press, 2013)

Angela von den Driesch, 'Ethnoveterinary Medicine – An Aspect of the History of Veterinary Medicine', in F. Dinçer (ed.), *Veterinary Medicine, Historical Approaches* (Ankara: Ankara University Press, 2002) 131–141

Ronnie G. Elmore, 'The Lack of Racial Diversity in Veterinary Medicine', *Journal of the American Veterinary Medical Association* 222 (2003) 24–26

Lisa Emmett et al., 'Feminization and Stress in the Veterinary Profession: A Systematic Diagnostic Approach and Associated Management', *Behavior Sciences* 9 (2019) 11. doi:10.3390/bs9110114

John R. Fisher, 'Cattle Plagues Past and Present: The Mystery of Mad Cow Disease', *Journal of Contemporary History* 33 (1998) 215–228

Leslie Irvine and Jenny R. Vermilya, 'Gender Work in a Feminized Profession. The Case of Veterinary Medicine', *Gender & Society* 24 (2010) 1: 56–82

Japan Veterinary Medical Association, 'Overview of Veterinary Medicine in Japan.' Tokyo: JVMA, 2013. Available at https://news.vin.com/apputil/image/handler .ashx?docid=8609537. Accessed April 15, 2021

Susan D. Jones, 'Gender and Veterinary Medicine: Global Historical Perspectives', *Argos* 23 (2000) 119–123

'Bringing Veterinary History and History of Science Together: Recent Developments in the English-Language Literature', *Argos* 53 (2016) 94–99

Tjeerd Jorna, 'The World Veterinary Association (WVA) and the Role of the Veterinarian on a Global Level', in R. Tamay Başağaç Gül (ed.), *Some Essays on Veterinary History. Proceedings of the XXXIX International Congress of the WAHVM and the III National Symposium of the TAHVME* (Ankara: Ankara University Press, 2012) 3–5

Rebecca Kaplan, 'Cows, Cattle Owners and the USDA: Brucellosis, Populations and Public Health Policy in the United States'. Ph.D. dissertation (University of California–San Francisco, 2013)

Ivan Katić, "Pioneer Female Veterinarians,' *Medical Sciences* 37 (2012) 137–168

Muhammad A. Kavesh, *Animal Enthusiasms: Life Beyond Cage and Leash in Rural Pakistan* (Abingdon, New York: Routledge, 2021)

Sujoy Khanna, Maneka Sanjay Gandhi, Meenakshi Awasthi, *Gaushala*. Ebook available at www.mkgandhi.org/ebks/gaushala.pdf. Accessed April 10, 2021

Claus Kirchhelle, 'Pharming Animals: A Global History of Antibiotics in Food Production (1935–2017),' *Palgrave Commununications* 4 (2018) 96. https://doi .org/10.1057/s41599–018-0152-2

Peter A. Koolmees, 'Feminization and Veterinary Medicine in the Netherlands,' *Argos* 23 (2000) 125–131

Özgül Küçükaslan, Raziye Tamay Başağaç Gül, and Aytaç Ünsal, 'The First Female Academicians in Turkish Veterinary Education,' *Ankara Üniversitesi Veteriner Fakültesi Dergisi* 64 (2017) 255–260

Phyllis Hickney Larsen, *Our History of Women in Veterinary Medicine: Gumption, Grace, Grit, and Good Humor* (Littleton, CO: Association for Women Veterinarians, 1997)

Kaitlyn Mattson, 'Veterinary Colleges Committed to Anti-Racism, Say Black Lives Matter,' *Journal of the American Veterinary Medical Association* 257 (2020) 4: 348–352

Dennis M. McCurnin and Joanna M. Bassert, *Clinical Textbook for Veterinary Technicians*, 6th ed. (St. Louis, Missouri: Elsevier Saunders, 2006)

Т.Н. Минеева [T.N. Mineeva], История ветеринарии [Veterinary History], in *Russian* (Moscow: LAN Publishing, 2005).

Petrissa Rinesch, 'Pioneer Women Veterinarians in European Society', *Journal of the American Veterinary Medical Association* 212 (1998) 182–184

Marianne Sackmann-Rink, 'Vermeintliche und vereitelte Anfänge des Frauenstudiums an der veterinär-medizinischen Fakultät der Universität Zürich', *Schweizer Archiv für Tierheilkunde* 127 (1985) 793–798

Philip M. Teigen, 'Henry Stockton Lewis, Sr. (1858–1922): An Early African American Veterinarian', *Veterinary Heritage* 25 (2002) 1: 5–6

William H. Waddell, *The Black Man in Veterinary Medicine* (Honolulu, HI: published by the author, 1969, 1982)

Wycliffe Wanzala, 'A Survey of the Management of Livestock Ticks and Other Aspects of Animal Ethno Health in Bukusu Community, Western Kenya', *Livestock Research for Rural Development* 24 (2012) article #173. www.lrrd.org/lrrd24/10/wanz24173.htm. Accessed March 22, 2021

Andrea Wiley, 'Growing a Nation: Milk Consumption in India since the Raj,' in Mathilde Cohen and Yoriko Otomo (eds.), *Making Milk: The Past, Present, and Future of Our Primary Food* (London: Bloomsbury Academic, 2017) 41–61

Abigail Woods, *A Manufactured Plague: The History of Foot and Mouth Disease in Britain* (London: Earthscan, 2004)

'Is Prevention Better than Cure? The Rise and Fall of Preventive Veterinary Medicine, c. 1950–1980', *Social History of Medicine* 26 (2013) 1: 113–131

7. Veterinary Medicine and Animal Health, 2000–2020

Laure Bonnaud and Nicolas Fortané, 'Being a Vet: The Veterinary Profession in Social Science Research', *Review of Agricultural, Food and Environmental Studies* (April 2020). doi:10.1007/s41130-020-00103-1

'Booming Growth of Small-Animal Practice in China,' *DVM 360* (February 28, 2014). www.dvm360.com/view/booming-growth-small-animal-practice-china. Accessed April 14, 2021

Alicia Davis and Jo Sharp, 'Rethinking One Health: Emergent Human, Animal and Environmental Assemblages', *Social Science & Medicine* 258 (2020). doi:10.1016/j.socscimed.2020.113093

Margo DeMello, *Animals and Society: An Introduction to Human–Animal Studies* (New York: Columbia University Press, 2012)

Douwe Fokkema and Frans Grijzenhout, *Nederlandse cultuur in Europese context. Rekenschap 1650–2000* (Den Haag, SDU Uitgevers, 2001) 347–351

Jean-Paul Gaudillière and Ulrike Thoms (Eds.) *The Development of Scientific Marketing in the 20th Century* (London: Pickering and Chatto, 2015)

Edward C. Green, 'Etiology in Human and Animal Ethnomedicine', *Agriculture and Human Values* 15 (1998) 127–131

Harold Herzog, 'The Impact of Pets on Human Health and Psychological Well-Being: Fact, Fiction, or Hypothesis?', *Current Directions in Psychological Science* 20 (2011) 236–239

Ronald Inglehart, *Modernization and Postmodernization: Cultural, Economic, and Political Change in 43 Societies* (Princeton: Princeton University Press, 1997)

Susan D. Jones, 'Framing Animal Disease: Housecats with Feline Urological Syndrome, Their Owners, and Their Doctors', *Journal of the History of Medicine and Allied Sciences* 52 (1997) 202–235

Susan D. Jones and Anna A. Amramina, 'Entangled Histories of Plague Ecology in Russia and the USSR', *History and Philosophy of the Life Sciences* 40 (2018) 3: 1–21

J.M. Kagira and P.W.N. Kanyari, 'Questionnaire Survey on Urban and Peri-urban Livestock Farming Practices and Disease Control in Kisumu Municipality, Kenya', *Tydskrif van die Suid-Afrikaanse Veterinêre Vereniging* 81 (2010) 2: 82–86

Joanna de Klerk, Melvyn Quan, and John D. Grewar, 'Socio-economic Impacts of Working Horses in Urban and Peri-urban Areas of the Cape Flats, South Africa', *Journal of the South African Veterinary Association* 91 (2020). https://doi.org/10.4102/jsava.v91i0.2009. Accessed March 22, 2021

Peter Koolmees, 'Changing Perspectives: World Association for the History of Veterinary Medicine, 1969–2019', in Johann Schäffer (ed.), *Future Needs a Past, the Importance of Historical Research for Veterinary Medicine* (Giessen: Deutsche Veterinärmedizinische Gesellschaft, 2020) 27–59

Mara Miele et al., 'Animal Welfare: Establishing a Dialogue between Science and Society', *Animal Welfare* 20 (2011) 103–117

Barbara Natterson-Horowitz and Kathryn Bowers, *Zoobiquity: The Astonishing Connection between Human and Animal Health* (New York: Vintage, 2013)

Tom Regan, *The Case of Animal Rights* (Berkeley and Los Angeles: University of California Press, 1983)

Harriet Ritvo, 'History and Animal Studies', *Society and Animals* 10 (2002) 403–406 'On the Animal Turn', *Daedalus* 136 (2007) 118–122

Peter Roeder and Karl Rich, *The Global Effort to Eradicate Rinderpest*, White Paper (Washington, DC: International Food Policy Research Institute, 2009)

Bernard E. Rollin, *An Introduction to Veterinary Medical Ethics: Theory and Cases* (Ames: Iowa State University Press, 1999)

Hans Rosling, Ola Rosling, and Anna Rosling Rönnlund, *Factfulness: Ten Reasons We're Wrong about the World – And Why Things Are Better than You Think* (New York: Flatiron Books, 2019)

Matthew Salois, 'Fundamental Shifts in Consumer Behavior: What's Next?', *DVM360* (April 2021) 14–15

Arvind Sharma, Catherine Schuetze, and Clive J.C. Phillips, 'The Management of Cow Shelters (Gaushalas) in India, Including the Attitudes of Shelter Managers of Cow Welfare,' *Animals* 10 (2020) 211–243. www.mdpi.com/journal/animals. doi:10.3390/ani10020211

Peter Singer, *Animal Liberation: A New Ethics for Our Treatment of Animals* (New York: HarperCollins, 1975)

Bernard Vallat, 'Speech by the Director General of the World Organization for Animal Health (OIE)', Cape Town, South Africa, October 14, 2011

VetSurvey. Survey of the Veterinary Profession in Europe ([Brussels]: Federation of Veterinarians of Europe, 2019

René van Weeren, 'Horses and Humans: A Special Bond throughout the Ages', *Argos* 56 (2018) 205–211

Michael S. Wilkes, Patricia A. Conrad, and Jenna N. Winer, 'One Health-One Education: Medical and Veterinary Inter-Professional Training', *Journal of Veterinary Medical Education* 46 (2019) 1: 1116–1117

Abigail Woods, Michael Bresalier, Angela Cassidy, and Rachel Mason-Dentinger, *Animals and the Shaping of Modern Medicine: One Health and Its Histories* (London: Palgrave Macmillan, 2018)

K. Yamanouchi, 'Scientific Background to the Global Eradication of Rinderpest', *Veterinary Immunology and Immunopathology* 148 (2012) 1–2: 12–15

Jakob Zinsstag, Esther Schelling, Kaspar Wyss, and Mahamat Bechir Mahamat, 'Potential of Cooperation between Human and Animal Health to Strengthen Health Systems', *Lancet* 366 (2005) 9503: 142–145

Jakob Zinsstag, E. Schelling, D. Waltner-Toews, and M Tanner, 'From "One Medicine" to "One Health" and Systematic Approaches to Health and Well-Being', *Preventative Veterinary Medicine* 101 (2011) 3–4: 148–156

Index

Printed in the United States
by Baker & Taylor Publisher Services